Medical Radiology

Diagnostic Imaging

For further volumes:
http://www.springer.com/series/4354

Gurdeep S. Mann • Joanne C. Blair
Anne S. Garden
Editors

Imaging of Gynecological Disorders in Infants and Children

Foreword by
Albert L. Baert

Springer

Dr. Gurdeep S. Mann MD
Department of Paediatric Radiology
Alder Hey Children's Hospital
Eaton Road
Liverpool
L12 2AP
UK

Dr. Joanne C. Blair MD
Department of Paediatric Endocrinology
Alder Hey Children's Hospital
Eaton Road
Liverpool
L12 2AP
UK

Prof. Anne S. Garden MD
Department of Paediatric Gynaecology
Alder Hey Children's Hospital
Eaton Road
Liverpool
L12 2AP
UK

and

Lancaster Medical School
Lancaster University
Lancaster
LA1 4YB
UK

ISSN 0942-5373
ISBN 978-3-662-50200-6
ISBN 978-3-540-85602-3 (eBook)
DOI 10.1007/978-3-540-85602-3
Springer Heidelberg New York Dordrecht London

Printed on acid-free paper

Springer is part of Springer Science+Business Media (www.springer.com)

Foreword

During the past decades the field of pediatric gynecology developed rapidly due to the new insights evolving from basic and translation research in this rather small but less well known medical field.

This volume of the Medical Radiology series is focused on the highly important imaging features, which are essential for a better understanding, diagnosis and treatment of gynecological disorders in infants and children. It fills a small but very specific gap in publications on modern medical imaging.

The editors have been very successful in bringing together the considerable expertise of well acknowledged specialists from various disciplines such as pediatric radiology, gynecology, surgery and endocrinology, The result is a comprehensive review of our actual knowledge of gynecological imaging in infancy, childhood and adolescence. On the basis of the embryological development, normal childhood appearances as well as pubertal changes of the female genital tract are described in detail. This morphological introduction is followed by different chapters based on dominant symptoms. This innovative general structure of the book greatly benefits the the process of differential diagnosis for the reader and it makes the work an excellent tool for daily clinical practice. Numerous superb illustrations complete the text.

This volume will undoubtedly become the reference work for every medical doctor, who wants to update her/his knowledge and skills in the area of gynecological disorders in infants and children. It is especially warmly recommended to pediatricians and radiologists.

Prof. Albert L. Baert

Preface

This innovative textbook of diagnostic imaging in paediatric gynaecology is, to our knowledge, the first textbook to address this important and rapidly developing field of paediatric practice. Successful delivery of a paediatric gynaecology service requires close multi-disciplinary collaboration between expert paediatric gynaecologists, paediatric surgeons and urologists, endocrinologists and radiologists. This field of expertise is reflected in the authorship of this text.

Interpretation of clinical information and imaging requires a robust understanding of the physiology of the female reproductive tract. It has therefore been our intention to describe the imaging of the female reproductive tract in the context of normal development from fetal life, through infancy, childhood and adolescence to the development of full adult maturity. We hope we have achieved this by committing two chapters to detailed descriptions of normal development: the first describing the embryology of the female reproductive tract and the second describing normal postnatal development, with a detailed description of the endocrinology that regulates these developmental changes. From these descriptions of normal anatomical development and maturation we have moved on to describe congenital, structural abnormalities, including disorders of sexual development and abnormalities in the timing of puberty. Gynaecological neoplasia is addressed in a separate chapter and we include two chapters exploring the assessment of pelvic pain and disorders of menstruation. Finally, disorders of the breast are covered in our closing chapter.

This textbook is intended primarily for paediatric radiologists, however it should be of interest to all those who care for girls with developmental or acquired gynaecological pathology, including radiologists, gynaecologists, urologists, endocrinologists, neonatologists and paediatricians.

We are most grateful to our colleagues for their sharing their expertise in the development of this textbook. We hope it will become a reference and working resource for all those who work in this fascinating field of medicine.

Liverpool

Gurdeep S. Mann
Joanne C. Blair
Anne S. Garden

Contents

Diagnostic Imaging Techniques 1
Gurdeep S. Mann and Umber Agarwal

Embryology of the Female Reproductive Tract 21
Andrew Healey

Disorders of Sex Development 31
Justin H. Davies, Pat S. Malone, and Jo Fairhurst

Gynaecological Disorders in the Neonate and Young Child 51
Gurdeep S. Mann and Angela T. Byrne

Structural Abnormalities of the Female Reproductive Tract 65
Paul Humphries

Normal Growth and Puberty 81
Caren J. Landes and Joanne C. Blair

Delayed and Precocious Puberty 115
Laurence J. Abernethy, Joanne C. Blair, Julie B. Smith,
and Mohammed A. Didi

Menstrual Disorders and Vaginal Discharge 145
Urmi Das and Gurdeep S. Mann

Gynaecological Causes of Pelvic Pain 173
Gurdeep S. Mann, Angela T. Byrne, and Anne S. Garden

Gynaecological Neoplasia 209
Kieran McHugh, Kirsteen McDonald, and Edwin Jesudason

Breast Disorders 225
Gurdeep S. Mann, Asha Shivaram, and Andrew Healey

Index 247

Contributors

Laurence Abernethy Department of Radiology, Alder Hey Children's Hospital NHS Foundation Trust, Liverpool, L12 2AP, UK, e-mail: laurence.abernethy@alderhey.nhs.uk

Umber Agarwal Department of Fetal and Maternal Medicine, Liverpool Women's Hospital NHS Foundation Trust, Liverpool, L8 7SS, UK, e-mail: Umber.Agarwal@lwh.nhs.uk

Joanne C. Blair Department of Endocrinology, Alder Hey Children's Hospital NHS Foundation Trust, Eaton Road, Liverpool, L12 2AP, UK, e-mail: jo.blair@alderhey.nhs.uk

Angela Byrne Department of Radiology, British Columbia Children's Hospital, University of British Columbia, Vancouver, BC, V6H 3V5, Canada

Urmi Das Department of Endocrinology, Alder Hey Children's Hospital NHS Foundation Trust, Eaton Road, Liverpool, L12 2AP, UK, e-mail: urmi.das@alderhey.nhs.uk

Justin Davies Department of Paediatric Endocrinology, Child Health Directorate, Southampton University Hospital Trust, Southampton, SO16 6YD, UK, e-mail: justin.davies@suht.swest.nhs.uk

Mohammed Didi Department of Endocrinology, Alder Hey Children's Hospital NHS Foundation Trust, Liverpool, L12 2AP, UK, e-mail: mohammed.didi@alderhey.nhs.uk

Jo Fairhurst Department of Radiology, Southampton University Hospital Trust, Southampton, SO16 6YD, UK, e-mail: jo.fairhurst@suht.swest.nhs.uk

Anne S. Garden Department of Gynaecology, Alder Hey Children's Hospital NHS Foundation Trust, Liverpool, L12 2AP, UK, e-mail: a.garden@lancaster.ac.uk

Andrew Healey Department of Radiology, Alder Hey Children's Hospital NHS Foundation Trust, Liverpool, L12 2AP, UK, e-mail: andrew.healey@alderhey.nhs.uk

Paul Humphries Imaging Department, University College Hospital, London, NW1 2BU, UK, e-mail: paul.humphries@uclh.nhs.uk

Edwin Jesudasan Department of Surgery, Alder Hey Children's Hospital NHS Foundation Trust, Liverpool, L12 2AP, UK, e-mail: Edwin.jesudason2@alderhey.nhs.uk

Caren Landes Department of Radiology, Alder Hey Children's Hospital NHS Foundation Trust, Liverpool, L12 2AP, UK, e-mail: caren.landes@alderhey.nhs.uk

Kirsteen McDonald Radiology Department, Great Ormond Street Hospital for Children NHS Trust, London, WC1N 3JH, UK, e-mail: kmcdonald@doctors.org.uk

Pat Malone Department of Urology, Southampton University Hospital Trust, Southampton, SO16 6YD, UK, e-mail: pat.malone@suht.swest.nhs.uk

Gurdeep S. Mann Department of Radiology, Alder Hey Children's Hospital NHS Foundation Trust, Liverpool, L12 2AP, UK, e-mail: gurdeep.mann@alderhey.nhs.uk

Kieran McHugh Radiology Department, Great Ormond Street Hospital for Children NHS Trust, London, WC1N 3JH, UK, e-mail: MCHUGK@gosh.nhs.uk

Asha Shivaram Department of Radiology, Royal Liverpool and Broadgreen University Hospitals NHS Trust, Liverpool, L7 8XP, UK, e-mail: asha.shivaram@rlbuht.nhs.uk

Julie Smith Department of Radiology, Alder Hey Children's Hospital NHS Foundation Trust, Liverpool, L12 2AP, UK, e-mail: julie.smith@alderhey.nhs.uk

Diagnostic Imaging Techniques

Gurdeep S. Mann and Umber Agarwal

Contents

1 **Introduction** 2

2 **Special Considerations and the Imaging Environment, Sedation and Anaesthesia** 3
2.1 Special Considerations 3
2.2 Sedation and Anaesthesia 3

3 **Ultrasound and Doppler** 3
3.1 Indications 4
3.2 Transabdominal US Imaging 4
3.3 Doppler US 6
3.4 Transperineal US 6
3.5 Transvaginal US 7
3.6 Transrectal US 7

4 **Magnetic Resonance Imaging** 8
4.1 Indications 8
4.2 Field Strength 8
4.3 Patient Preparation 8
4.4 Patient Position 8
4.5 Free-Breathing and Breath-Hold Imaging 8
4.6 Spasmolytic Agents 8
4.7 Coils 8
4.8 Scanning Planes 9
4.9 Pulse Sequences 10

5 **Contrast Studies** 11
5.1 Genitography 11
5.2 Vaginography 13
5.3 Cystography 13

6 **Computed Tomography** 13
6.1 Indications 13
6.2 CT Parameters 13
6.3 Intravenous Contrast Medium 13
6.4 Bowel Contrast 14
6.5 Post-processing 15

7 **Radiography** 15
7.1 Bony and Spinal Abnormalities 15
7.2 Soft Tissue Calcifications 15
7.3 Radio-Opaque Foreign Bodies 16

8 **Drainage, Biopsy and Angiography** 16
8.1 Drainage and Aspiration Procedures 16
8.2 Biopsies 17
8.3 Angiography 17

9 **Antenatal Imaging** 17

References 18

G. S. Mann (✉)
Department of Paediatric Radiology, Alder Hey Children's Hospital NHS Foundation Trust, Liverpool, UK
e-mail: gurdmann@yahoo.co.uk

G. S. Mann
Department of Radiology, Liverpool Women's Hospital NHS Foundation Trust, Liverpool, UK

U. Agarwal
Maternal-Fetal Medicine, Department of Obstetrics and Gynaecology, Liverpool Women's Hospital NHS Foundation Trust, Liverpool, UK

Abstract

Imaging of the paediatric gynaecological tract encompasses patients with vastly different physiology ranging from the neonate under maternal hormonal influence to the post-pubertal young adolescent. Ultrasound is the mainstay of imaging of the genitourinary tract. In specific clinical circumstances, cross-sectional imaging may be necessary. Magnetic resonance imaging (MRI) with its intrinsic high soft tissue contrast and multiplanar capability is preferred but will usually necessitate some of form of sedation in the younger child. Computed tomography (CT) is preferably avoided because of ionising radiation exposure. Contrast

G. Mann et al. (eds.), *Imaging of Gynecological Disorders in Infants and Children*, Medical Radiology. Diagnostic Imaging, DOI: 10.1007/174_2010_80,

examinations are specialised imaging procedures for specific conditions. This chapter considers the various imaging modalities available for the investigation of gynaecological disorders in children.

Abbreviations

TVS	Transvaginal ultrasound
TAS	Transabdominal ultrasound
TSE	Turbo spin-echo
FISP	Fast imaging with steady-state precession
3D	Three dimensional
US	Ultrasound
MDCT	Multi-detector computed tomography
CT	Computed tomography
MRI	Magnetic resonance imaging
HSG	Hysterosalpingogram
NG	Nasogastric
AP	Anteroposterior
MRA	Magnetic resonance angiography
LOCM	Low-osmolar contrast medium
TFE	Turbo field-echo
TSE	Turbo spin-echo
BFFE	Balanced fast field echo
2D	Two dimensional
THRIVE	T1 high-resolution isotropic volume excitation
SPAIR	Spectral adiabatic inversion recovery
FOV	Field of view
NSA	Number of signal averages
TR	Repetition time
HASTE	Half fourier acquisition with turbo spin-echo
SSH	Single shot
GRE	Gradient echo
SNR	Signal-to-noise ratio
MHz	Megahertz
mAs	Milliampere second
kVp	Kilovolt peak
EUA	Examination under anaesthesia
MRU	Magnetic resonance urography
TPS	Transperineal sonography
FLASH	Fast low angle single shot
SENSE	Sensitivity encoding
iPAT	Integrated parallel acquisition techniques
ALARA	As low as reasonably achievable

1 Introduction

Imaging of the paediatric gynaecological tract encompasses patients with vastly different physiology ranging from the neonate under maternal hormonal influence to the post-pubertal young adolescent. In the younger child, small size, high-respiratory rate, variable co-operation and a paucity of intra-abdominal fat can present distinct challenges for cross-sectional imaging.

The guiding principle of paediatric radiology is safe delivery of diagnostic imaging. Diagnostic studies involving ionising radiation should wherever possible be used sparingly (Willis and Slovis 2004; Strauss 2007) with age or weight-specific optimised parameters. Each clinical request received for imaging should be justifiable. The radiology team is tasked with ensuring that the imaging study requested can adequately and safely answer the clinical question posed in a timely fashion. Each imaging request should be carefully weighed up against the available alternate imaging modalities and non-imaging-based clinical management.

Ultrasound (US) is the established initial imaging modality of choice in the investigation of suspected paediatric gynaecological disease. Sonography is often all that is required for follow-up. In specific clinical circumstances, cross-sectional imaging may be necessary. Magnetic resonance imaging (MRI) with its intrinsic high soft tissue contrast and multiplanar capability is preferred but will usually necessitate some of form of sedation in the younger child. Computed tomography (CT) is preferably avoided because of ionising radiation exposure. Contrast examinations are specialised imaging procedures for specific conditions. This chapter considers the various imaging techniques available for the investigation of paediatric gynaecology patients.

2 Special Considerations and the Imaging Environment, Sedation and Anaesthesia

2.1 Special Considerations

Most imaging tests in children are performed with a parent or guardian present. Adolescents may elect to decline parental input, often necessitating an alternative chaperone to be present. Any intimate examination of a child should be performed with appropriate forewarning and in the presence of a reliable chaperone. Verbal consent should be obtained and where necessary written consent. This is to avoid confusion as to the purpose and nature of the study. Examinations should be performed with tact, respecting the modesty of the child and preferably in an age appropriate environment.

2.2 Sedation and Anaesthesia

Few imaging examinations of the genital tract require sedation or anaesthesia. Anaesthesia is usually a prerequisite in paediatric interventional practice but there is also a subset of patients undergoing cross-sectional imaging, typically the very young or non-cooperative child, in whom some form of sedation will be required. Most modern multidetector CT (MDCT) scanner acquisition times preclude the need for routine sedation (Pappas et al. 2000) and so the greatest requirement is in MR scanning.

Natural sleep is ideal, avoiding the attendant costs and medical risk of sedation or anaesthesia. Many cross-sectional imaging studies can be safely and reliably performed in young infants following a feed. The ambient temperature of the room is adjusted to suit the baby who is then fed and swaddled. Adequate ear protection or a quiet environment is required to induce natural sleep; this is also referred to as a so-called 'feed and wrap' study. Older children up to the age of 6–8 years old may struggle to co-operate with the requirements of an MRI scan without sedation. Alternatives to sedation include the use of behavioural therapy, simulation (Rosenberg et al. 1997), mock scanners (de Amorim e Silva et al. 2006) and MRI-compatible audio/video systems (Harned and Strain 2001). Play therapy specialists are a particularly valuable resource to help acclimatise the child to the scanning environment and to practise the technique of reproducible breath-holding (Pressdee et al. 1997). Free breathing scans are obtained in natural sleep and with non-ventilated sedation.

Table 1 Practice guidelines for pre-procedural fasting in healthy children

Clear liquids up to 2 h (any age)
Semisolid liquids including breast milk and formula up to 4 h (<6 months)
Semisolid liquids and solids up to 6 h (6–36 months)
Semisolid liquids and solids up to 8 h (3 years and above)
Children with delayed gastric emptying should be discussed with the anaesthesiologist
After (Anesthesiology 1999)

Sedation represents a broad continuum. A variety of sedative agents are available as premedication for imaging studies (Frush et al. 1996). It is recommended that any proposed sedation drug regime is agreed with the local department of anaesthesiology. Strict standards must be observed in the care of the sedated patient. Appropriate equipment and manpower should available to continuously monitor and safely recover the child according to widely available published guidance (Coté et al. 2006; American College of Radiology 2005; Scottish Intercollegiate Guidelines Network 2004). In our institution, all sedation and anaesthesia for paediatric imaging studies is safely conducted under the direct of supervision of an anaesthesiologist. An important safety aspect of sedating children is appropriate pre-procedural fasting to reduce the risk of pulmonary aspiration. The recommended fasting times in our institution are outlined in Table 1.

3 Ultrasound and Doppler

Ultrasound is usually the initial imaging investigation to evaluate the child with suspected genitourinary disease. Wide availability, relatively low cost, portability, lack of ionising radiation, superb temporal and spatial resolution, and excellent anatomic soft tissue contrast make this an attractive first line imaging modality. US is operator dependant but in skilled hands is a highly reproducible technique and

Table 2 The main indications for pelvic ultrasound in girls

Assessment of pelvic maturity in disorders of precocious or delayed puberty
Disorders of sexual differentiation (including ultrasound of the adrenal glands)
Menstrual disorders
Pelvic pain or suspected pelvic mass (appendicitis, ovarian torsion, pelvic inflammatory disease, ectopic pregnancy)
Follow-up of antenatally detected abnormalities
Congenital abnormalities (Müllerian—uterovaginal anomalies)
Neonatal pathology (ovarian cyst, imperforate hymen)
Evaluation following abnormal pelvic examination
Pelvic discharge and bleeding
Gynaecological malignancy
Pelvic vascular malformation
Suspected foreign body
Clinical work-up of eating disorders
Targeting imaging guided therapy

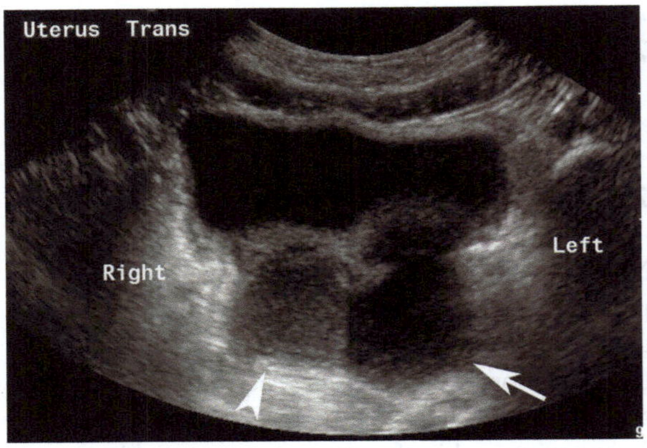

Fig. 1 Transverse wide field of view US scan of the pelvis in a 12 year old with uterus didelphys and duplicated vaginas. The right duplex vagina is obstructed by a distal transverse septum and contains bright internal echoes from debris and blood (*arrowhead*). The left duplex vagina contains anechoic fluid (*arrow*)

frequently the only imaging test required for initial assessment and long-term follow-up.

When a child attends for their first pelvic US, the examination should ideally also include both adrenal glands and kidneys. The adrenal glands should be assessed in those presenting with disorders of sexual differentiation and abnormalities of pubertal development. Congenital obstructive Müllerian anomalies are associated with renal and gastrointestinal tract malformations.

3.1 Indications

The principle indications for pelvic US in girls are summarised in Table 2.

3.2 Transabdominal US Imaging

3.2.1 Patient Preparation

A full urinary bladder is required for transabdominal ultrasound (TAS) of the pelvis. Optimal distension is necessary to sufficiently displace gas filled pelvic bowel loops. The ovaries and uterus are best visualised through the bladder which serves as an acoustic window. The urinary bladder should be assessed at the beginning of an examination. Full evaluation of the pelvis is made once the bladder is sufficiently distended. An under filled bladder should prompt a delay in the examination and where necessary the patient should drink more clear fluids, or an intravenous drip should be sited in those nil by mouth. Reassessment should be performed every 20–30 min thereafter. Over distension of the bladder can be problematic which makes for an uncomfortable scan and can distort normal pelvic anatomy. Post-micturition views can be helpful.

Patient co-operation is critical for high-quality imaging. A variety of techniques can be employed to produce a diagnostic quality study in even the most uncooperative child. Gentle graded compression of the probe should be applied. Image penetration, gain and focal depth should be optimised. Generous use of the cine loop function and large sector width scanning (Fig. 1) provides a useful general overview. For specific areas of interest, the zoom function (Fig. 2) or higher frame rate narrow sector width images can then be obtained (Fig. 3).

3.2.2 Probe Selection

The neonatal pelvis is well suited to TAS owing to a lack of body fat. Small footprint curvilinear, high-frequency (6–9 MHz) probes are ideal for examining the neonatal abdomen and pelvis. High-resolution images are obtained using dedicated paediatric settings. Owing to maternal hormonal influence, the uterus and ovaries are more readily visualised in the

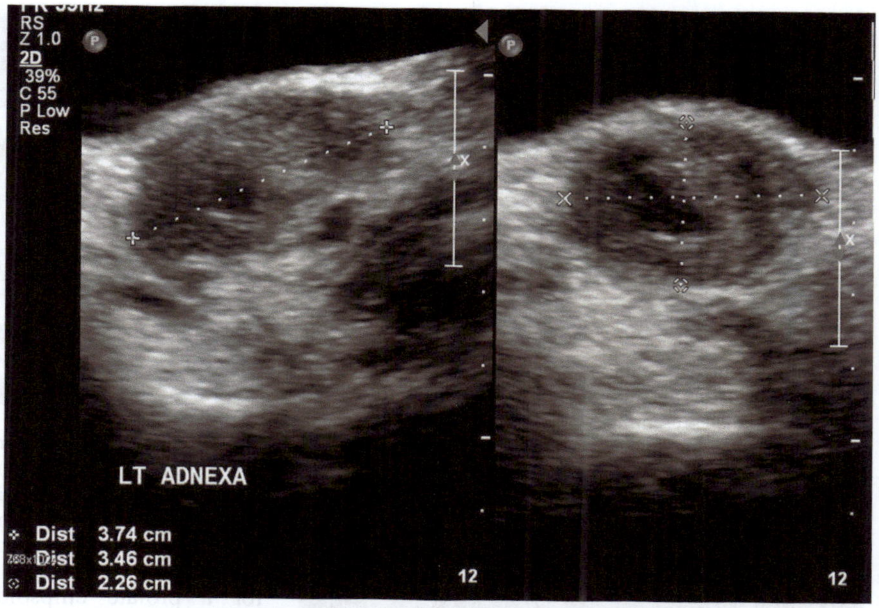

Fig. 2 Dual screen zoomed images of the left ovary (between callipers). The volume calculation here was rejected as two of the three measurements were not obtained along the long axis of the ovary

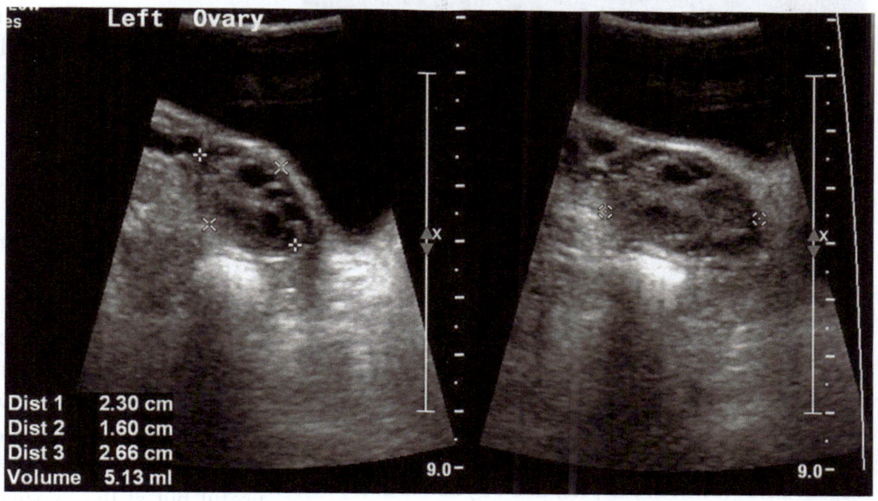

Fig. 3 Dual screen narrow sector perpendicular views about the long and short axis of the left ovary (between callipers). Volume calculated using two measurements about the ovarian long axis and the remaining measure from the mid short axis view

early neonatal period. Neonates should be examined in a warm room, preferably shortly after a feed. The urinary bladder is liable to fill and empty quickly and a further feed may be required to assess the pelvis.

Small children may be scanned using a broadband (4–9 MHz) curvilinear probe. Older children are scanned using adult probes and settings, typically with a 3–5 MHz curvilinear probe. Abnormalities detected on real-time imaging should also be assessed with a linear high-resolution probe (Fig. 4).

3.2.3 Scanning Planes

Transverse and longitudinal scanning through the urinary bladder is normally sufficient to demonstrate the vagina, cervix and uterus. The endometrium, seen as a bright internal stripe within the uterine cavity should be assessed for its echogenicity, outline and thickness (Fig. 5).

The ovaries are identified by scanning transversely through a full urinary bladder typically at the level of the uterine fundus. Oblique parasagittal planes are also obtained, the ovaries typically lie between the iliac vessels and the urinary bladder. Panoramic imaging should be used to demonstrate pathology which cannot adequately be demonstrated in a single field of view (Fig. 6).

3.2.4 Measurements

Endometrial thickness is measured at the maximal depth of the body away from the cervix. Uterine length is measured along the uterine longitudinal axis (Fig. 5). Anteroposterior (AP) measurements are

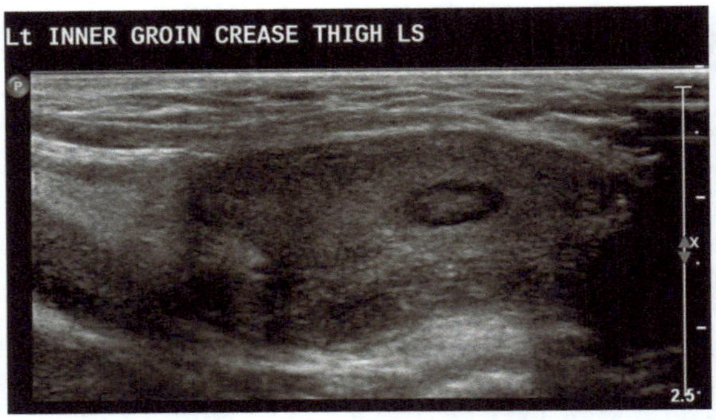

Fig. 4 Linear high resolution: Transverse linear high resolution US scan of the left groin in an adolescent with external female genitalia presenting with primary amenorrhoea. A palpable discrete inguinal gonad was noted at US. Although serum tumour markers were not elevated this was excised and shown to be a testicular hamartoma in this patient with complete androgen insensitivity

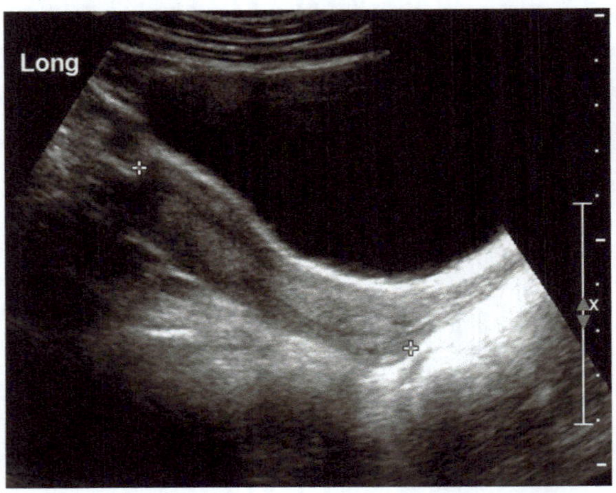

Fig. 5 Longitudinal US scan of the normal post-pubertal 'pear shaped' uterus (between callipers) in a 14-year-old girl

taken at the cervix and uterine fundus. Comparison should be made with age-related normative data for uterine length, transverse dimensions and volume (Orsini et al. 1984; Haber and Mayer 1994). The maturing uterus changes shape with time, and hence, uterine volume estimations are the least reliable measure. Fundal–cervical ratio is expressed as the ratio between fundal and cervical AP diameters. Fundal AP diameter multiplied by uterine length is used to determine uterine cross-sectional area.

The ovaries are measured in three axes (Fig. 3). The premenarcheal ovaries are ovoid in shape. Ovarian volume measurement is calculated using the formula

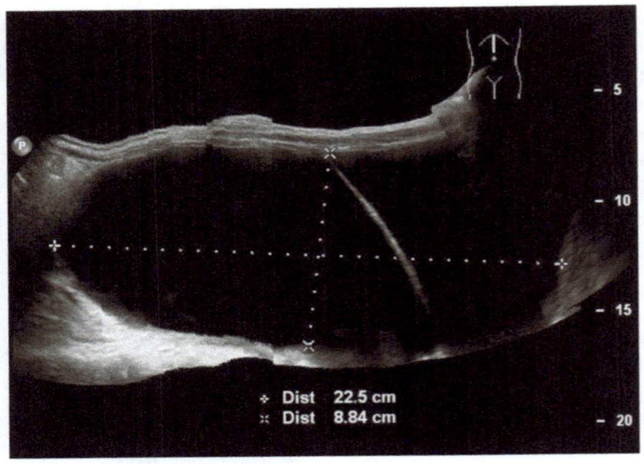

Fig. 6 Longitudinal panoramic ultrasound of a massive ovarian cyst (between callipers) comprising of only a few thin walled septae and anechoic fluid. This was excised and confirmed to be a mature–nonmalignant cystic teratoma

for a prolate ellipsoid body (volume = 0.523 × length × width × thickness). The stromal texture, diameter of the largest follicle, number and distribution of the follicles should also be recorded.

3.3 Doppler US

When pathology is demonstrated on real time greyscale imaging, Doppler interrogation should also be performed (Fig. 7). Optimised steerable pulsed and continuous wave Doppler, colour Doppler and colour power Doppler are useful to characterise lesional flow and to differentiate between solid and cystic tissue. The size of the colour Doppler box should be adapted to cover the pathology. A large colour box is initially useful but at the expense of the maximal achievable pulse repetition and frame rates. Sequential analysis of a lesion with a small colour box enables accurate detection of pulsatile flow and higher velocities shifts.

3.4 Transperineal US

Transperineal sonography (TPS) is useful in demonstrating the perineal soft tissues, urethra, distal gynaecological tract (vagina and cervix), anterior rectum and distal cloacae. The examination is performed using both sector and linear array broadband probes. Scanning is performed supine. A modified lithotomy position is required for the older child. The

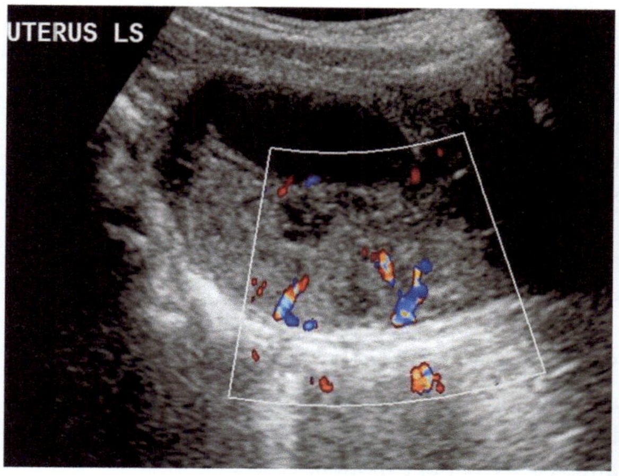

Fig. 7 Longitudinal colour Doppler US in a 2-year-old girl presenting with bloody vaginal discharge showing a heterogeneous solid mass lesion distending and obstructing the vagina. Colour flow is depicted in the solid component of this vaginal rhabdomyosarcoma

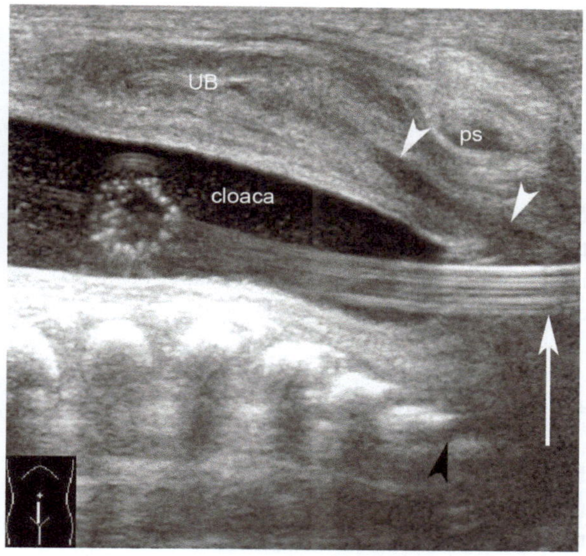

Fig. 8 Longitudinal perineal US in a female with a Foley catheter (arrow) decompressing a complex posterior cloacal malformation. UB indicates the collapsed urinary bladder; pubic symphysis (ps), urethra (white arrowhead). The sacrum is deficient (black arrowhead)

technique is most facile in the newborn and in the first few weeks of life. Scanning planes include the sagittal perineal view aligning the pubic synchondrosis and urethra (Fig. 8), and oblique parasagittal view to show the urethral insertion into vagina. Transverse sector scanning is limited by the narrow near field of view (Teele and Share 1997).

The indications for TPS are varied but include the investigation of incontinence, specifically looking for ectopic ureteral insertion; urethral diverticulum, urethral strictures, anorectal malformations, fistulae, urogenital sinus, cloacae, ambiguous genitalia, pelvic masses and suspected vaginal foreign bodies. TPS in conjunction with TAS provides valuable anatomic information in the pre-operative planning of vaginal agenesis (Scanlan et al. 1990) and has the advantage of avoiding endovaginal or endorectal scanning.

3.5 Transvaginal US

Transvaginal sonography (TVS) also referred to as endocavity US, employs a high-frequency probe placed in a sterile probe cover introduced into the vagina. Clearly, this technique has very limited application in paediatric practice and is not widely advocated or available in many paediatric centres. Where available this facility should be limited to the sexually active patient. Two case series comparing TVS to TAS in adolescents have shown TVS to be well tolerated (Bulas et al. 1992; Bellah and Rosenburg 1991). The main advantages over TAS are improved near field resolution with superior soft tissue resolution of the pelvic viscera and adnexa. TVS is adjunctive to the transabdominal examination.

Transvaginal sonography is useful in individuals who are unable to maintain a full urinary bladder or where bowel gas artefact, body habitus, distorted tissue planes from a surgical incision or inflammation hinder TAS. In practice, if TAS is unhelpful then MRI should be considered. TVS is indicated in the haemodynamically stable sexually active adolescent whom is pregnancy test positive but in whom an intrauterine pregnancy is not revealed by TAS. TVS is better able differentiate between a viable intrauterine pregnancy and an extrauterine gestation sac of an ectopic pregnancy Gynaecological pain.

3.6 Transrectal US

Like transvaginal US very few paediatric imaging centres offer transrectal sonography. Limited cases series have shown the utility of this technique for accurate pre-operative evaluation in children and adolescents with vaginal canalisation disorders (Fedele et al. 1999).

4 Magnetic Resonance Imaging

Magnetic resonance imaging has high-spatial resolution, superb soft tissue contrast and imparts no ionising radiation and is therefore superior to CT in evaluating female pelvic pathology.

4.1 Indications

Magnetic resonance imaging is the cross-sectional modality of choice for the investigation of pelvic masses, congenital uterine anomalies and local staging of gynaecological malignancy. MR is particularly useful in characterising adnexal masses which are indeterminate by US. MR should be considered in the evaluation of unexplained pain of pelvic origin where conventional imaging is unremarkable.

4.2 Field Strength

High-quality imaging is routinely achievable with commercially available 1.5 Tesla field strength MR-scanners. Body imaging at higher field strengths can result in more noticeable image heterogeneity such as shading artefact due to dielectric effects. Motion artefact is more noticeable at higher field strength. Respiratory gating and routine use of anti-peristaltic agents should be considered.

4.3 Patient Preparation

Although no specific preparation for pelvic MRI is required, all patients attending for MRI must complete a standard pre-procedural questionnaire to ensure that they are safe to scan. Common contraindications include children with implanted medical devices such as permanent pacemakers, implantable cardiac defibrillators and neural stimulators. A more comprehensive list outlining detailed advice concerning specific medical devices is provided by standard reference manuals (Shellock 2009).

All patients are asked to change into an MR compatible gown and to place all personal items in a secure locker prior to entering the scanner. Ferromagnetic body jewellery should not be worn. The urinary bladder should not be overly full at the time of scanning as this may contribute to patient discomfort.

4.4 Patient Position

Scanning should be performed in the most comfortable position. The supine position with an under knee bolster or prone positions are least likely to be affected by patient motion.

4.5 Free-Breathing and Breath-Hold Imaging

Prior to coil placement, it is useful to explain the practicalities of gentle respiration for free-breathing scans and to practise the technique of reproducible breath-holding to minimise motion artefact. Clear instructions for each sequence acquisition are necessary.

4.6 Spasmolytic Agents

Small bowel peristalsis can be effectively reduced by a 6 h pre-examination fast. Intravenous administration of antispasmodic agents such as hyoscine-*N*-butylbromide or glucagon should be considered at the commencement of all abdomino-pelvic MRI examinations unless contraindicated.

4.7 Coils

Most commercially available MR scanners offer multi-element pelvic, torso-phased array coils which afford higher signal-to-noise ratio (SNR) compared to standard body coils. A multi-element cardiac coil may also be used. Torso coils enable imaging of the whole abdomen and pelvis. Parallel imaging techniques (SENSE, iPAT) are feasible with phased array coils and enable acquisition of thinner slices with isotropic datasets reducing volume averaging; or, enabling faster scans mitigating motion artefact but at the expense of SNR.

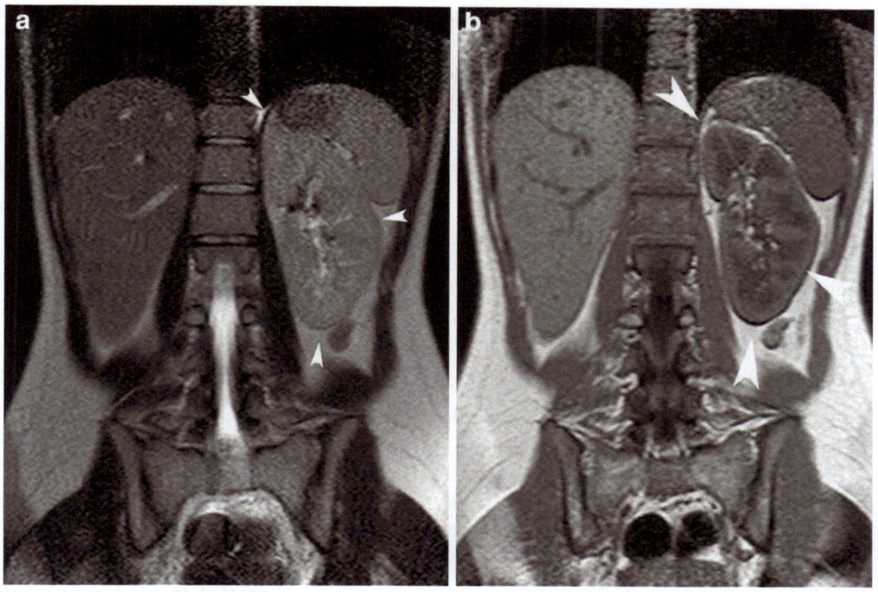

Fig. 9 Coronal large field of view MR images of the upper abdomen in a 14-year-old female with uterus didelphys and duplicated vaginas. **a** T2-weighted single shot SPAIR and **b** T1-weighted TFE MR images showing right renal agenesis and appropriate compensatory hypertrophy of the left kidney (*arrowheads*)

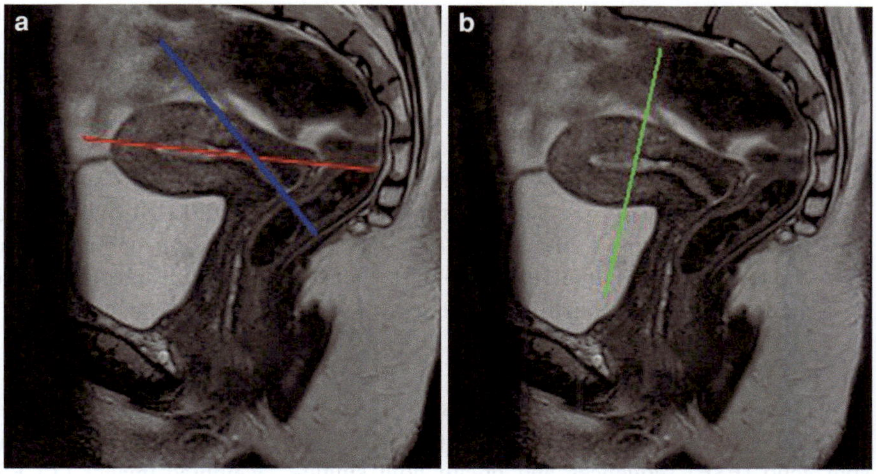

Fig. 10 Sagittal T2 TSE image of the pelvis obtained for planning **a** paracoronal images along the longitudinal axis of the uterine fundus and body (*red line*) and cervix (*blue line*) and **b** paraxial images perpendicular to the uterine long-axis (*green line*)

4.8 Scanning Planes

Imaging orientation is dependent upon the clinical request and target organ(s) of interest. Localiser (scout) images are initially acquired followed by images obtained in at least two perpendicular planes.

The examination should begin with a coronal wide field of view stack of the abdomen and pelvis (Fig. 9). This provides a useful overview of the kidneys, ureters, adrenal glands, liver and pelvic viscera.

In order to assess uterine pathology including congenital Müllerian anomalies Sagittal T2-weighted images of the pelvis are obtained to demonstrate uterine lie. In order to obtain true coronal images of the uterine fundus an oblique sagittal plane is necessary angled parallel to the uterine longitudinal axis also referred to as paracoronal images (Fig. 10a). Images axial to the uterine fundus are obtained perpendicular to the uterine long axis (Fig. 10b uterus lie).

Imaging of the pelvic floor and ischiorectal fossae are obtained in the true axial, coronal and paracoronal planes. True sagittal images are also helpful in demonstrating suspected rectovaginal and vesicovaginal fistulae. With masses of pelvic origin true axial images are obtained to cover the pathology. With pelvic adenopathy the field of view should extend from the

Table 3 Sequence parameters for abdominopelvic body imaging (1.5-Tesla, Philips Achieva; Philips Medical Systems, Best, the Netherlands)

Sequence	FOV (mm)	Thickness/gap (mm)	Matrix	TR (ms)	TE (ms)	Flip angle (degrees)	NSA
Sagittal TSE	200	4.0/1.0	256 × 256	90	3,500	90	3
Axial T2 TSE	200	4.0–5.0/1.0	256 × 256	90	3,500	90	3
Coronal T2 TSE	200	5.0/1.0	256 × 256	90	3,500	90	3
T1 2D TFE	300	7.0	256 × 256	4.6	10	20	1
Axial T1 TSE	250	4.0/0.4	256 × 256	14	340	90	3
Coronal T1 3D THRIVE	400	2.0 over-contiguous	320 × 320	2.4 shortest	4	10	1
Axial T2 SPAIR	200	4.0/1.0	256 × 256	70	2,980	70	1
Cor BFFE	400	4.0/0.4	256 × 256	1.8	3.7	60	2

Alder Hey Children's NHS Foundation Trust, Liverpool. (*NSA* number of signal averages)

region of the pelvic floor to the infrarenal abdominal aorta.

4.9 Pulse Sequences

Pelvic MR imaging has been revolutionised by the advent of turbo spin echo sequences coupled with techniques to suppress motion-related artefact enabling relatively short acquisition times without a significant SNR penalty. A typical protocol pelvic MR protocol comprises of unenhanced T2- and T1-weighted images (summarised Table 3) with T1 post-contrast images obtained if indicated.

4.9.1 T2-Weighted Imaging

T2-weighted sequences are the mainstay of pelvic imaging. Non-breath-hold turbo spin (TSE) or fast spin echo (FSE) sequences and breath hold single-shot TSE (SSH-TSE, HASTE) images of the pelvis can be obtained in 2–3 min and 12–20 s, respectively. Single shot imaging performs poorly compared to TSE imaging when tissues with similar T2 relaxation times are being assessed. TSE imaging offers the best pelvic soft tissue contrast resolution. T2 fat suppression imaging is required in only specific circumstances. Fat signal may be saturated using spectral fat saturation (spectral adiabatic inversion recovery, SPAIR) or nulled using T2 short-time inversion recovery imaging. Steady-state free precession balanced fast field–field echo (BFFE, true FISP) can be used to assess fast motion such a cine imaging of bowel peristalsis in areas of pelvic inflammation.

4.9.2 T1-Weighted Imaging

Axial T1 spin echo (T1 SE) images of the pelvis are useful in evaluating adenopathy and the pelvic muscles but may take between 5 and 7 min to acquire. Nonbreath-hold heavily T1-weighted axial turbo spin (T1 TSE) images of the pelvis can be obtained in around 2–3 min depending on the area of coverage, number of slices and slice thickness. In order to differentiate between fat and haemorrhage T1-weighted imaging with spectral fat suppression is necessary. Axial T1 SE fat-saturated images are used to differentiate an endometrioma from fat. Bright met-haemoglobin signal in an endometrioma will not suppress on this sequence. Axial T1-gradient echo dual echo images (T1-GRE in and out-of phase) can be used to null intralesional fat in an ovarian dermoid cyst. In practical terms, many children will not comply with a lengthy scan. Two- Dimensional Spoiled GE T1-weighted images (T1-FFE, FLASH) can be obtained to cover the pelvis in 15–25 s. The resulting slight reduction in image contrast over conventional T1 SE and TSE imaging in children is a penalty often worth paying in terms of sequence acquisition time.

Conventional planar T1 SE contrast enhanced images can be obtained following IV gadolinium based agents. Pre- and post-contrast fat suppressed 3D ultrafast spoiled gradient echo imaging (THRIVE, VIBE) have the advantage of rapid acquisition time and ability to reconstruct data in any plane.

4.9.3 Diffusion-Weighted Imaging

The role of diffusion-weighted imaging for evaluating solid paediatric tumours is an evolving but promising field. Accurate detection of malignant paediatric neoplasms has been described using non-breath hold single-shot echo planar imaging sequence with *b*-values of 0, 500, and 1,000 mm/s^2. The apparent diffusion coefficient maps depict restricted diffusion which show good correlation with T1-weighted post-contrast images (Alibek et al. 2009).

4.9.4 Magnetic Resonance Urography

Magnetic resonance urography (MRU) images can be obtained to evaluate obstructive uropathy secondary to pelvic disease. Static-fluid and diuretic-enhanced MRU employ heavily T2-weighted images of the urinary tract to generate static, sequential and cine MRU images. Excretory MRU may be obtained during the excretory phase of enhancement following intravenous administration of gadolinium-based contrast agents (Leyendecker et al. 2008).

4.9.5 Contrast

Intravenous gadolinium (Gd) contrast agents principally act by significantly shortening T1 relaxation times and are best appreciated on heavily T1-weighted sequences. The standard contrast medium dose for body soft tissue imaging is 0.1 and 0.2 mmol Gd/kg for MR angiography (MRA). Contrast medium is injected manually, but larger volumes in older children should be automatically delivered using a pump injector, particularly for dynamic contrast enhancement. A saline flush should always follow. Contraindications to IV gadolinium include previous adverse reaction and renal impairment. The latter is associated with the relatively recently recognised idiosyncratic phenomenon of nephrogenic systemic fibrosis (Karcaaltincaba et al. 2009).

4.9.6 MR Angiography

Phase contrast MRA techniques are often adequate to assess the patency of large pelvic vessels without the need for IV Gd-based contrast agents. Contrast enhanced MRA is frequently employed to obviate the need for diagnostic digital subtraction angiography.

5 Contrast Studies

Digital fluoroscopy contrast examinations of the gynecological tract provide high-spatial resolution imaging of the internal genitalia. Fluoroscopic examinations should be performed with appropriate paediatric low-dose settings and collimation (Strauss 2007). The ambient room temperature is maintained to an appropriate level for neonates and infants. Specific techniques and indications for contrast studies are described below.

5.1 Genitography

A genitogram, also referred to as a contrast sinogram is the examination of choice to delineate the appearances of the urogenital sinus and its morphological connections. Its principle indication is in evaluating children with suspected disorders of sex development (see Disorders of Sex Development) .

5.1.1 Indications

The aims of genitography are to:

1. establish the presence of a vagina;
2. demonstrate the relationship of the urethra to the vagina and voluntary sphincter;
3. differentiate between a male or female type urethra;
4. establish the presence or absence of a cervical impression at the vaginal vault (Aaronson and Cremin 1984).

Genitography can also demonstrate the uterine cavity, fallopian tubes and vasa but in most cases these structures are more than adequately depicted by US and MRI.

When performing a genitogram, it is of critical importance to tailor the examination and ensure that all perineal orifices are evaluated (Wright et al. 1995). Genitography is best performed with both the radiologist and clinician in attendance. The advantages of a multidisciplinary approach are to ensure that there is consensus as to the aims of the study and to avoid later confusion in the analysis of the imaging findings. The overall objective of the study is to accurately define anatomical landmarks critical to pre-operative planning.

5.1.2 Technique

A variety of techniques have described to perform genitography (Tristan et al. 1956; Shopfner 1964; Cremin 1974). The flush technique involves deploying a blunt-ended syringe or nipple against the pudendal orifice to occlude the perineal opening (Shopfner 1964). The catheter-based technique involves

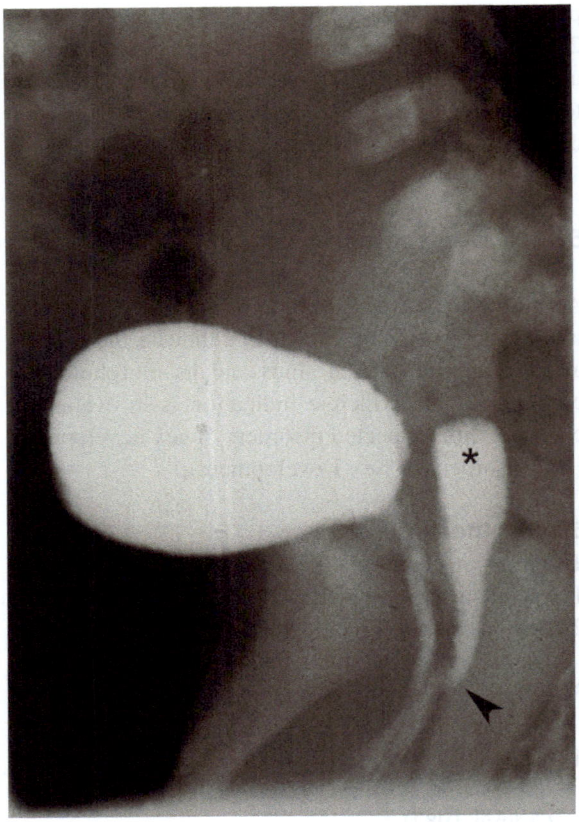

Fig. 11 Genitogram in a child with gonadal dysgenesis demonstrating an elongated urethra, urogenital sinus (*arrow head*) and vagina (*) with no cervical impression. Two catheters have employed the first terminates high in the proximal urethra and the second more distal catheter used to delineate the urogenital sinus

placement of a one or more catheters into the perineal orifices (Cremin 1974). The flush technique is usually sufficient for a common perineal orifice. The use of two or more catheters may be necessary to define complex malformation anatomy (Fig. 11). The study can be combined with a contrast enema if required.

A genitogram must be performed in a sterile fashion using an aseptic technique. The perineum is cleaned under powerful lighting. This enables initial careful inspection to look for fused labia, hypospadias, continuous dribbling and the location and number of the perineal openings which require evaluation. Fused labia can be problematic and if they cannot be separated by gentle manipulation then a topical oestrogen-based cream can be applied locally for several days and the examination rescheduled (Omar 2000).

Water soluble contrast medium is used in our institution. Water soluble contrast medium is not retained for a long period of time but is prone to leak around and bypass the catheter. Only a small amount of contrast medium is typically required. Slow hand injection using 20 ml volume syringes is preferred as it affords much lower injection pressures. The perineum can be outlined by using a barium paste (Grattan-Smith et al. 1966).

The perineal opening may require initial gentle probing with 5F feeding tube catheter. The examination is performed in the left lateral position, with the legs kept firmly together to prevent catheter migration. This catheter is placed a short distance (1–2 cm) into the perineal orifice and only a small amount of contrast (2–4 ml) injected to preserve the morphology of the urogenital sinus. This will usually outline the urethra and the urinary bladder. If the catheter enters the vagina, this enables early demonstration of its relationship to the urethra and status of the cervix, uterus and fallopian tubes. If the catheter enters the urinary bladder then it should not be withdrawn as a standard voiding cystourethrogram may be performed and contrast will eventually outline the urethra during micturition or by backflow. The catheter in the bladder could be withdrawn carefully and contrast injected slowly to try and demonstrate a vagina, but instead this catheter can be left in place and a further catheter can be introduced dorsal to the initial catheter. The catheter balloon is introduced into to the posterior urethra and a further 2–4 ml of contrast medium injected. This will usually show a vaginal orifice if present.

Genitography may occasionally miss a patent vaginal orifice revealed only by careful vaginoscopy. This should prompt the surgeon to perform preoperative selective vaginography.

In infants with congenital adrenal hyperplasia, a limited study is often sufficient. Demonstration of the level at which the vagina opens into the urogenital sinus and the relationship to the external sphincter is all that is required. These observations have important surgical implications in the planning of vaginoplasty (Aaronson 2001).

5.1.3 Catheter Risks

Catheter-related trauma may induce transient bleeding or irritation. The most important risk is to avoid the introduction of infection by observing a meticulous aseptic technique. Antibiotic prophylaxis is not routinely indicated for contrast examinations.

5.1.4 Contraindications

Contrast examinations should not be performed in children with active infection of the gynaecological or urinary tract.

5.1.5 Sedation and Anaesthesia

No sedation is required in infants although catheterisation in older children may occasionally be problematic in terms of patient acceptability. Sedation or anaesthesia in these cases may be unavoidable but should be timed to coincide with any planned examination under anaesthesia (EUA) if possible.

5.2 Vaginography

Vaginography is performed in a similar manner to genitography. Fluoroscopy is performed with the patient in the lateral or lateral oblique positions to evaluate the vagina and its connections.

The main indications for a contrast vaginogram include:

1. evaluation of vaginal size and morphology as a precursor to vaginoplasty;
2. assessment of ambiguous genitalia and common urogenital sinus;
3. evaluation of suspected vaginal fistulae;
4. identification of a 'low' vaginal ectopic ureter (Son et al. 2009).

Vaginography can also be used to evaluate vaginal foreign bodies. Clinical history, physical examination and direct visualisation will usually suffice. An US or MRI for nonferrous foreign bodies (Kihara et al. 2001) may be helpful in the young to confirm a foreign body prior to embarking upon EUA. Vaginography can be performed as part of EUA (Wu et al. 1995).

5.3 Cystography

Cystography alone is rarely indicated in paediatric gynaecological imaging practice although is an integral component of the genitogram examination as described above. Cystography is useful in cases of congenital or acquired vesico-vaginal fistula and in the evaluation of post-operative bladder trauma (Bandhu et al. 2006).

6 Computed Tomography

Computed tomography is widely available and images can be obtained rapidly. Despite this CT has a very limited role in the evaluation of the paediatric gynaecological tract. In most respects, US is best placed to provide initial assessment of the pelvis. Both US and MRI offer superior soft tissue contrast resolution compared to CT and avoid exposure to ionising radiation. Beam-hardening artefact from the bony pelvis can also limit the usefulness of CT.

6.1 Indications

Computed tomography is reserved as a problem solving tool for the acutely unwell but haemodynamically stable patient. Contrast enhanced CT has a useful adjunctive role to US in the assessment of post-operative complications and evaluation of tubo-ovarian abscess complicating pelvic inflammatory disease. CT may guide interventional therapy in cases not amenable to US-guided therapy. CT has a role in staging gynaecological malignancy to look for distant metastases particularly chest disease.

6.2 CT Parameters

The imaging parameters we use with a 16 slice Philips MDCT scanner are summarised in Table 4. kVp and mAs are dependent upon patient weight and should be adapted to each patient according to the specific indication. A detailed discussion of these parameters is beyond the scope of this book. A comprehensive description of the subject is outlined by FRUSH (2005).

6.3 Intravenous Contrast Medium

Most scans of the abdomen and pelvis should be obtained following administration of intravenous contrast medium, typically in the portal venous phase. Pre-contrast scans and multiphase scans are rarely

Table 4 Summary of abdominal and pelvic MDCT (16 slice)

Indication: tumour staging, pelvic abscess		
Coverage: hemidiaphragms to pubic symphysis		
FOV: to cover target axial surface area		
Respiratory phase: suspended end inspiration		
Scanner settings: tube current (mA) based on child's weight		
Weight (kg)	mA	kVp
<10	40	80
11–25	60	80
26–50	80	80
51–70	100–120	100
>70	120–140	120
Rotation time 0.5–1.0 s; collimation 3 mm; pitch 0.75–1.5 (vary according to patient size); reconstruction slice 3 mm		
Contrast:		
IV contrast: 2 ml/kg LOCM 300–350 iodine/ml up to a maximum of either 4 ml/kg or 150 ml (Bhalla and Siegel 2002)		
Hand injection		Mechanical power injector
Flow rate: Tight bolus injection		*Flow rate:* (maximal permissible according to needle size)
		22 gauge—1.5–2 ml/s
		20 gauge—2.0–3.0 ml/s
		18 gauge—3.0 ml/s
Scan delay: 40–60 s from start of injection		*Scan delay:* 40–60 s from start of injection
Oral contrast: optional (see below)		
	Volume of oral contrast (ml)	
Age	45 min prior to study	15 min prior to study
Up to 1 month	60–90	30–45
1–12 months	120–240	60–120
1–5 years	240–480	120–240
6–12 years	480–720	240–320
13 years and above	720–1,080	360–540
Rectal contrast: optional		

indicated in paediatric gynaecologic imaging. Intravenous low-osmolar contrast medium (LOCM—300–350 iodine/ml) is given at a rate of 2 ml/kg up to a maximum of 150 ml. Contrast medium is contra-indicated in renal failure and previous contrast allergy.

Contrast timing in children is dependent on body weight, heart rate, specific cardiovascular physiology and is relative to the completion of the contrast material. A delay of 25 s following complete administration of contrast in children is generally optimal for portal venous phase imaging of the abdomen and pelvis. Bolus tracking and test bolus injection of intravenous contrast can be used to improve scan timing particularly if dynamic imaging is required.

6.4 Bowel Contrast

Oral contrast medium is optional and may be used to opacify pelvic small bowel loops and the large bowel. Oral contrast should be avoided if an urgent scan is required in the context of trauma, contra-indications include active diarrhoea and vomiting, the immuno-compromised child, bowel obstruction or active bowel inflammation (Donnelly 1997). The advantages of oral contrast medium with respect to lesion conspicuity are best seen in thin children who lack intra-abdominal fat. In practical terms, not all children drink the prerequisite amount of oral contrast according to schedule and administration via an NG tube is an alternative. Dilute flavoured water soluble contrast medium (2–3%) can be used according to the suggested schedule in Table 4. Oral contrast should be avoided in sedated children. If contrast opacification of the rectum is desirable but oral contrast does not reach the rectum, then air or water soluble contrast medium can be administered via a rectal catheter.

6.5 Post-processing

Axial contrast enhanced CT with multiplanar-reformatted images (Fig. 12), 3D volume rendered and MIP reconstructions are useful in defining tumour extent and infiltration, vascular supply, vessel encasement, nodal size and to look for liver metastases. Liver metastases and nodal disease are also well depicted by dedicated MRI but CT has a clear advantage when staging for lung metastases. Contrast enhanced CT is also performed in the evaluation of pelvic abscesses prior to image-guided drainage. Delayed imaging in the renal excretory phase is helpful in cases of acquired renal tract obstruction due to a pelvic mass; a repeat-delayed planning scan is a useful low-dose surrogate intravenous pyelogram.

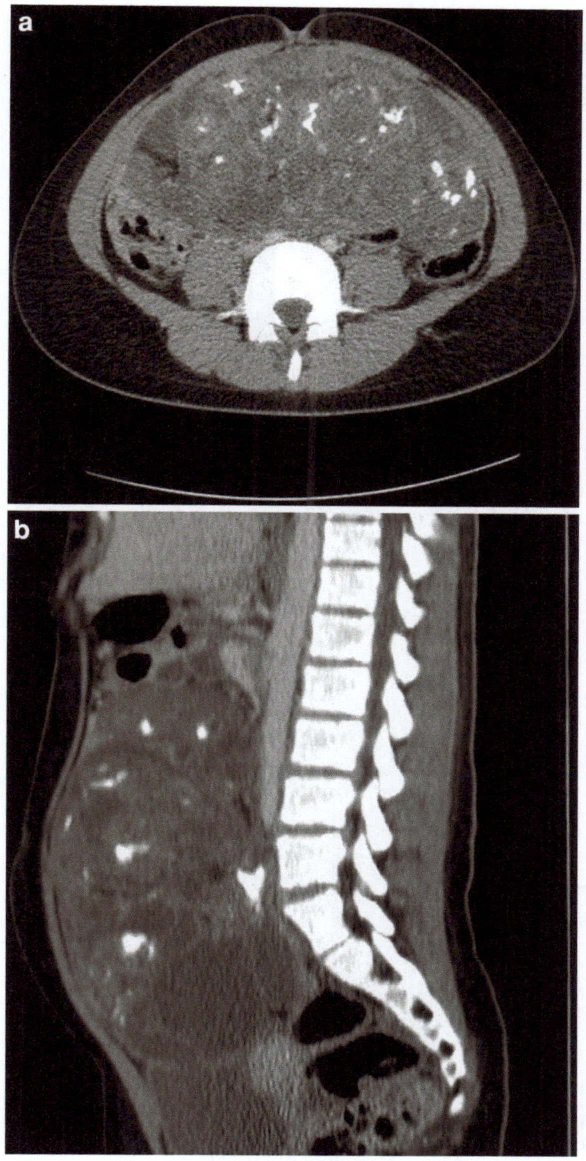

Fig. 12 Contrast enhanced CT scan **a** axial and **b** sagittal reformatted images of a solid part calcified mature ovarian germ cell tumour

7 Radiography

Radiographs are of limited value in assessing the gynaecological tract. The principle role of an abdominal X-ray is in the evaluation of the bowel gas pattern to assess for obstruction and to detect intraperitoneal free air. A full length supine AP view of the abdomen and pelvis can be used to document osseous abnormalities, opaque foreign bodies and abnormal soft tissue calcifications.

7.1 Bony and Spinal Abnormalities

Dedicated views of the spine and pelvis are indicated when evaluating girls with cloacal malformation with caudal regression (Fig 13) or symphyseal diastasis associated with cloacal exstrophy (Fig 14). US and MRI are necessary to fully document intraspinal anatomy.

7.2 Soft Tissue Calcifications

Calcified meconium in urinary tract and colon may be detected in infants with imperforate anus with a fistula

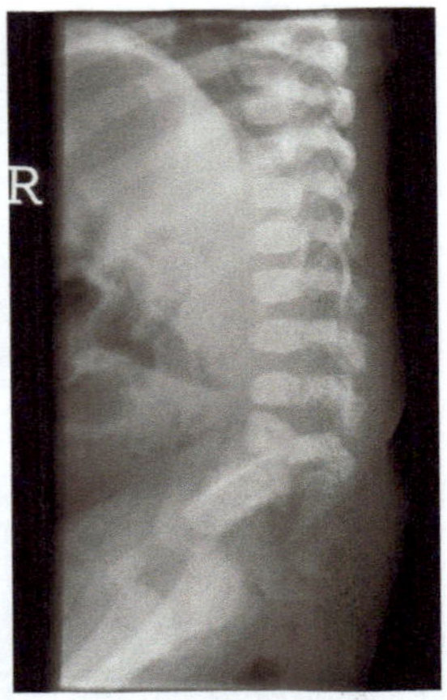

Fig. 13 Lateral X-ray showing termination of the vertebrae at L4 in a girl with caudal regression associated with a cloacal malformation

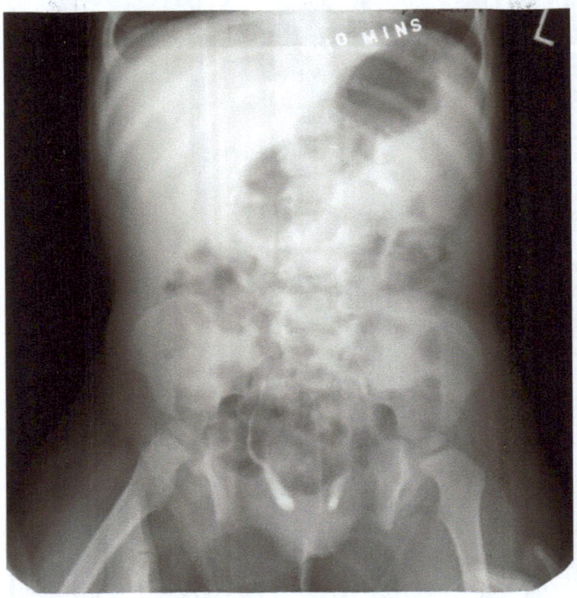

Fig. 14 Renal excretory phase frontal view from an intravenous pyelogram series in a neonate with cloacal–exstrophy complex showing widening of the pubic symphysis

(Selke and Cowley 1978) and cloacal malformations (Chaubal et al. 2003). This finding has also been described in imperforate hymen (Nidecker and Humphry 1978). A tooth from a dermoid can be demonstrated on a radiograph but US and cross-sectional imaging are more appropriate imaging modalities.

7.3 Radio-Opaque Foreign Bodies

Depending on the clinical presentation, US, direct visualisation under anaesthesia and cross-sectional imaging may be required to evaluate for a gynecological tract foreign body but radiographs are a useful starting point when a radio-opaque foreign body is suspected.

8 Drainage, Biopsy and Angiography

Interventional procedures performed in relation to the paediatric gynaecological tract are relatively uncommon. At our institution, such procedures are performed by sub-specialist paediatric interventional radiologists in a dedicated hybrid imaging suite equipped with US, a biplane digital fluoroscopy and angiography unit situated in a paediatric general surgical theatre room. The principles of ALARA should apply in the interventional suite. Where possible image-guided therapy is delivered under US guidance, and radiation is used is sparingly (Connolly et al. 2006).

8.1 Drainage and Aspiration Procedures

Drainage procedures form the most common clinical request for image-guided therapy. Pelvic abscess drainage following acute appendicitis or pelvic inflammatory disease (Fig. 15) are typical indications. Occasionally a large ovarian cyst may require aspiration.

Drainage can be performed using a variety of modalities including US, US combined with fluoroscopy, fluoroscopy alone or rarely under CT fluoroscopic guidance. Most procedures are performed transabdominally under US which enables real-time evaluation without radiation exposure. Bowel gas artefact and overlying bowel loops may make the transabdominal approach impractical. In these cases, the transrectal (Pereira et al. 1996; Chung et al. 1996), transperineal or transvaginal approach can be more efficacious. Deep pelvic abscesses may necessitate transgluteal drainage under CT guidance (Gervais et al. 2000). Drainage can be achieved with the trochar technique, but the Seldinger technique generally allows more precise catheter placement.

Following drainage clinical follow-up should be undertaken jointly by the supervising clinical team and the interventional radiologist. Careful attention should be paid to the results of any biochemical and microbiological tests performed on the drainage aspirates. Catheter drainage rates may tail off

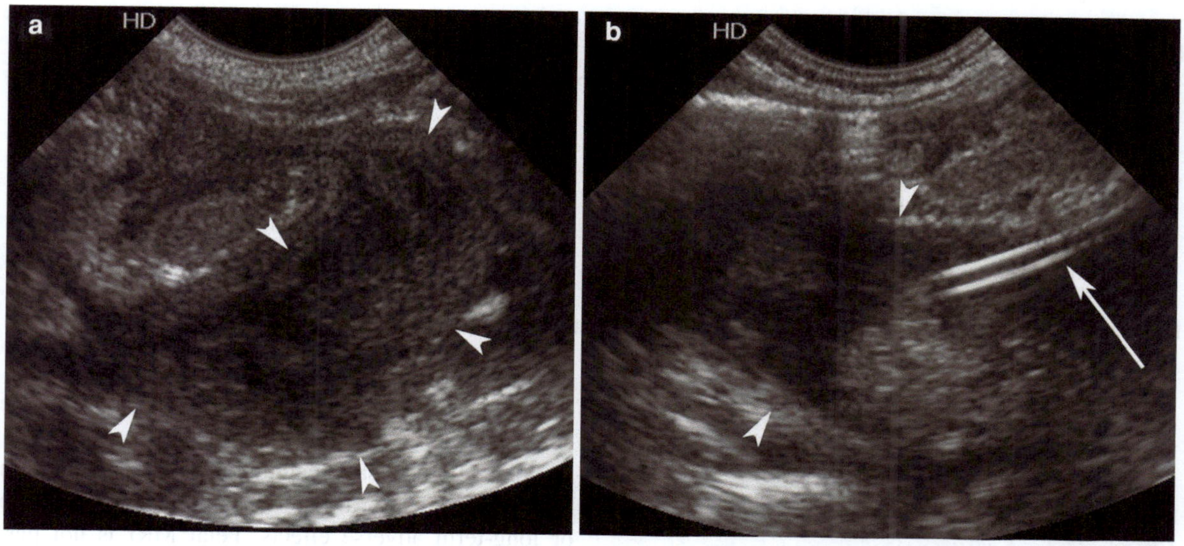

Fig. 15 Ultrasound guided drainage of a right iliac fossa pelvic abscess. **a** Pre-drainage, abscess (between *arrowheads*). **b** Post-drainage with locking percutaneous pigtail catheter (*arrow*) introduced under US guidance

indicating successful drainage, impaired catheter patency, catheter migration or incomplete drainage of a multi-septated abscess. Additional catheter placement should be considered against catheter repositioning and the use of per catheter thrombolytic treatments. Follow-up imaging is dependant upon initial imaging findings and the clinical course of the child.

8.2 Biopsies

Very few biopsies of the gynaecological tract are performed by an interventional radiologist at our institution. In most cases, these are undertaken as a surgical procedure in the context of suspected gynaecological malignancy or as gonadal biopsies in children with disorders of sex development. Of utmost practical importance is that any samples obtained are correctly handled and submitted in a timely fashion to the histopathologist, cytologist and geneticist.

8.3 Angiography

Doppler US, noncontrast MRA and gadolinium enhanced MRA have largely supplanted diagnostic angiography. Digital subtraction angiography should be reserved for therapeutic interventions such as in the planning and treatment of pelvic vascular malformations and chemo-embolisation of tumours.

9 Antenatal Imaging

Most pregnant women undergo a detailed fetal sonographic examination referred to as an anatomy scan. This is preferably scheduled around 18 and 22 weeks gestation when organogenesis is largely complete. The maternal examination is performed transabdominally with a full urinary bladder using a curvilinear broadband probe (3.5–7 MHz). Transvaginal US is used in mothers where fetal position, liquor volume or maternal body habitus hinder adequate transabdominal views.

The role of antenatal imaging is to:

Detect abnormalities and aid in confirmation of diagnosis;

Identify associated anomalies;

Enable constructive parental counselling including prenatal karyotyping and long-term prognosis;

Formulate postnatal management.

Constant improvements in US technology mean that high-quality antenatal imaging of the fetal genitourinary tract and adrenal glands is routinely feasible. Antenatally detectable conditions include

Table 5 Sequence parameters for fetal body imaging (1.5-Tesla, Philips Achieva; Philips Medical Systems, Best, the Netherlands)

Sequence	FOV (mm)	Thickness/gap (mm)	Matrix	TR (ms)	TE (ms)	Flip angle (°)	Number of slices	NSA
T2 SSH-TSE	320–200	4.0–6.0/0.0	256/256	Shortest	140	90	18	1
High-resolution T2 SSH-TSE	345–295	4.0/0.53	320/512	Shortest	250	90	16	1
T1 2D GRE	300	5.0–8.0/0.5	256/256	Shortest	4.6	15	12–14	5

Fetal MRI, Alder Hey Children's Hospital NHS Foundation Trust, Liverpool. (*NSA* number of signal averages)

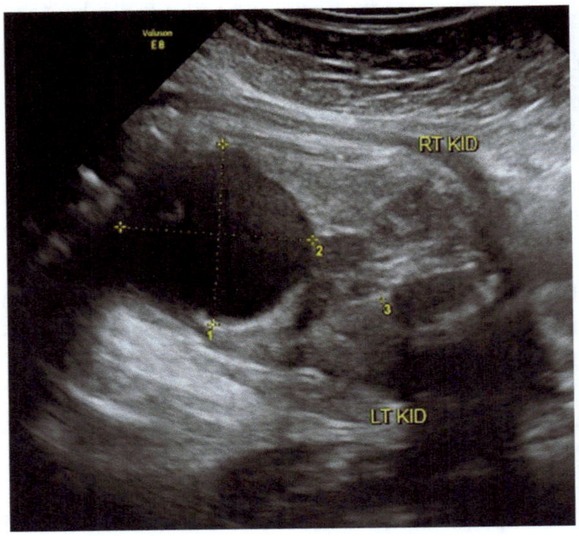

Fig. 16 Fetal ultrasound: Transverse section through fetal pelvis (female) at 36 weeks gestation showing an anechoic ovarian cyst (between callipers)

ambiguous external genitalia (Pajkrt et al. 2008), congenital adrenal hyperplasia (Chambrier et al. 2002), cloacal malformations (Warne et al. 2002; HSU) hydrocolpos (Winderl and Silverman 1995; Dhombres et al. 2007) and ovarian cysts (Fig. 16) (Bryant and Laufer 2004).

The role of fetal body MRI is limited and is adjunctive to US. Fetal MRI should be reserved for problem solving where sonographic views are inadequate or there is doubt concerning the underlying diagnosis. Fetal MRI may be used in fetuses at risk of a specific antenatally detected condition such as a familial disorder. MRI will often confirm prenatal US findings but often provide additional information helpful in planning delivery and postnatal care. In some cases, however, the final diagnosis cannot be confirmed until after delivery.

Fetal MRI is a safe technique. To date no study in humans has demonstrated any significant short-term or long-term adverse effects. Fetal MRI is not performed in the first trimester owing to incomplete organogenesis and very poor fetal SNR. Prior to scanning, the mother is asked to fast to prevent fetal motion. An empty urinary bladder helps to reduce maternal discomfort and movement in the scanner. Scanning is performed in the most comfortable position, typically supine or the left lateral decubitus position, the latter to avoid inferior vena cava compression. Maternal sedation is rarely required. Although no adverse effect has been demonstrated to the fetus following intravenous gadolinium administration it is relatively contraindicated and not necessary.

Following localiser images relative to the mother, fetal body MRI is performed with single shot T2-weighted and T1 2D gradient echo sequences, acquired in orthogonal planes relative to the fetus. Suggested sequence parameters are outlined in Table 5.

References

Aaronson IA (2001) The investigation and management of the infant with ambiguous genitalia: a surgeon's perspective. Curr Probl Pediatr 31:168–194

Aaronson IA, Cremin BJ (1984) Intersex. In: Aaronson IA, Cremin BJ (eds) Clinical pediatric uroradiology. Churchill Livingstone, Edinburgh, pp 380–395

Alibek S, Cavallaro A, Aplas A et al (2009) Diffusion weighted imaging of pediatric and adolescent malignancies with regard to detection and delineation: initial experience. Acad Radiol 16:866–871

American College of Radiology (2005) American College of Radiology practice guideline for pediatric sedation/analgesia. Res 42:519–525. http://www.acr.org/SecondaryMainMenuCategories/quality_safety/guidelines/iv/pediatric_sedation.aspx. Accessed November 2009

Anesthesiology (1999) Practice guidelines for preoperative fasting and the use of pharmacologic agents to reduce the risk of pulmonary aspiration: application to healthy patients undergoing elective procedures: a report by the American Society of Anesthesiologist Task Force on Preoperative Fasting. Anesthesiology 90:896–905

Bandhu S, Gunabushanam G, Kriplani A et al (2006) Congenital vesicovaginal fistula with partial vaginal agenesis. Clin Radiol 61:630–633

Bellah RD, Rosenburg HK (1991) Transvaginal ultrasound in a children's hospital: is it worthwhile? Pediatr Radiol 21:570–574

Bhalla S, Siegel MJ (2002) Multislice computed tomography pediatrics. In: Silverman PM (ed) Multislice computed tomography: a practical approach to clinical protocols. Lippincott Williams & Wilkins, Philadelphia, pp 231–282

Bryant AE, Laufer MR (2004) Fetal ovarian cysts: incidence, diagnosis and management. J Reprod Med 49:329–337

Bulas DI, Ahlstrom PA, Sivit CJ et al (1992) Pelvic inflammatory disease in the adolescent: comparison of transabdominal and transvaginal sonographic evaluation. Radiology 183:435–439

Chambrier ED, Claudine Heinrichs C, Avni FE (2002) Sonographic appearance of congenital adrenal hyperplasia in utero. J Ultrasound Med 21:97–100

Chaubal N, Dighe M, Shah M et al (2003) Calcified meconium: an important sign in the prenatal sonographic diagnosis of cloacal malformation. J Ultrasound Med 22:727–730

Chung T, Hoffer FA, Lund DP (1996) Transrectal drainage of deep pelvic abscesses in children using combined transrectal sonographic and fluoroscopic guidance. Pediatr Radiol 26:874–878

Connolly B, Racadio J, Towbin R (2006) Practice of ALARA in the pediatric interventional suite. Pediatr Radiol 36:S163–S167

Coté CJ, Wilson S, Work Group on Sedation (2006) American Academy of Pediatrics, American Academy of Pediatric Dentistry. Guidelines for monitoring and management of pediatric patients during and after sedation for diagnostic and therapeutic procedures: an update. Pediatrics 118:2587–2602

Cremin BJ (1974) Intersex states in young children: the importance of radiology in making a correct diagnosis. Clin Radiol 25:63–73

de Amorim e Silva CJT, Mackenzie A, Hallowell LM et al (2006) Practice MRI: reducing the need for sedation and general anaesthesia in children undergoing MRI. Australas Radiol 50:319–323

Dhombres F, Jouannic JM, Brodaty G et al (2007) Contribution of prenatal imaging to the anatomical assessment of fetal hydrocolpos. Ultrasound Obstet Gynecol 30:101–104

Donnelly LF (1997) Commentary: oral contrast medium administration for abdominal CT reevaluating the benefits and disadvantages in the pediatric patient. Pediatr Radiol 27:770–772

Fedele L, Portuese A, Bianchi S, Zanconato G, Raffaelli R (1999) Transrectal ultrasonography in the assessment of congenital vaginal canalization defects. Hum Reprod 14:359–362

Frush DP (2005) Evidence-based principles and protocols for pediatric multislice computed tomography. In: Knollman F, Coakley FV (eds) Multislice CT principles and protocols. Elsevier, Philadelphia, pp 179–201

Frush DP, Bisset GS, Hall SC (1996) Pediatric sedation in radiology: the practice of safe sleep. Am J Roentgenol 167:1381–1387

Gervais DA, Hahn PF, O'Neill MJ et al (2000) CT-guided transgluteal drainage of deep pelvic abscesses in children: selective use as an alternative to transrectal drainage. Am J Roentgenol 175:1393–1396

Haber HP, Mayer EI (1994) Ultrasoundevaluation of uterine and ovarian sizeform birth to puberty. Pediatric Radiol24:11-13

Grattan-Smith P, Bowdler JD, MacMahon RA (1966) Genitography—the radiological investigation of the intersex patient. Australas Radiol 10:236–239

Harned RK, Strain JD (2001) MRI-compatible audio/visual system: impact on pediatric sedation. Pediatr Radiol 31:247–250

Karcaaltincaba M, Oguz B, Haliloglu M (2009) Current status of contrast-induced nephropathy and nephrogenic systemic fibrosis in children. Pediatr Radiol 39:S382–S384

Kihara M, Sato N, Kimura H, KamiyamaM, Sekiya S, Takano H (2001) Magneticresonance imaging in the evaluation ofvaginal foreign bodies in a young girl.Arch Gynecol Obstet 265:221–222

Leyendecker JR, Barnes CE, Zagoria RJ (2008) MR urography: techniques and clinical applications. Radiographics 28:23–46

Nidecker AC, Humphry A (1978) Peritoneal calcification in a neonate with imperforate hymen. J Can Assoc Radiol 29:277–279

Omar HA (2000) Management of labial adhesions in prepubertal girls. J Pediatr Adolesc Gynecol 13:183–185

Orsini LF, Salardi S, Pilu G, Bovicelli L, Cacciari E (1984) Pelvic organs inpremenarcheal girls: real-timeultrasonography. Radiology 153:113-116

Pajkrt E, Petersen OB, Chitty LS (2008) Fetal genital anomalies: an aid to diagnosis. Prenat Diagn 28:389–398

Pappas JN, Donnelly LF, Frush DP (2000) Reduced frequency of sedation of young children with multisection helical CT. Radiology 215:897–899

Pereira JK, Chait PG, Miller SF (1996) Deep pelvic abscesses in children: transrectal drainage under radiologic guidance. Radiology 198:393–396

Pressdee D, May L, Eastman E et al (1997) The use of play therapy in the preparation of children undergoing MR imaging. Clin Radiol 52:945–947

Rosenberg D, Sweeney JA, Gillen JS et al (1997) Magnetic resonance imaging of children without sedation: preparation with simulation. J Am Acad Child Adolesc Psychiatry 36:853–859

Scanlan KA, Pozniak MA, Fagerholm M et al (1990) Value of transperineal sonography in the assessment of vaginal atresia. Am J Roentgenol 154:545–548

Scottish Intercollegiate Guidelines Network (2004) Safe sedation of children undergoing diagnostic and therapeutic procedures. A national clinical guideline. Guideline number 58. Revised April 2004. http://www.sign.ac.uk/guidelines/fulltext/58/index.html. Accessed November 2009

Selke AC, Cowley CE (1978) Calcified intraluminal meconium in a female infant with imperforate anus. Am J Roentgenol 130:786–788

Shellock FG (2009) The reference manual for magnetic resonance safety, implants and devices: 2009 edition. Biomedical Research Publishing Group, Los Angeles

Shopfner CE (1964) Genitography in intersexual states. Radiology 82:664–674

Son le T, Thang le C, Hung le T et al (2009) Single ectopic ureter: diagnostic value of contrast vaginography. Urology 74:314–317

Strauss K (2007) ALARA in pediatric fluoroscopy. J Am Coll Radiol 4:931–933

Teele RL, Share JC (1997) Transperineal sonography in children. Am J Roentgenol 168:1263–1267

Tristan TA, Eberlein WR, Hope JW (1956) Roentgenologic investigation of patients with heterosexual development. Am J Roentgenol Radium Ther Nucl Med 76:562–568

Warne S, Chitty LS, Wilcox DT (2002) Prenatal diagnosis of cloacal anomalies. BJU Int 89:78–81

Willis CE, Slovis TL (2004) The ALARA concept in pediatric CR and DR: dose reduction in pediatric radiographic exams—a white paper conference executive summary. Pediatr Radiol 34:S162–S164

Winderl LM, Silverman RK (1995) Prenatal diagnosis of congenital imperforate hymen. Obstet Gynecol 85:857–860

Wright NB, Smith C, Rickwood AM et al (1995) Imaging children with ambiguous genitalia and intersex states. Clin Radiol 50:823–829

Wu MH, Huang SC, Lin YS, Lin MF,Chou CY (1995) Intravaginal foreignbody retained for a long duration. Int J Gynecol Obstet 50:193–195

Embryology of the Female Reproductive Tract

Andrew Healey

Contents

1 **Introduction** 21

2 **Embryology of the Female Genitourinary Tract** 22
2.1 Development of the Gonads 22
2.2 Relationship Between the Early Fetal Genital and Urinary Systems 25
2.3 Development of the Fallopian Tubes Uterus, Cervix and Vagina 26
2.4 Development of the Lower Genital Tract 28
2.5 Development of the External Genitalia 28
2.6 Development of the Female Genital Accessory Glands 30
2.7 Embryological Vestigial Structures (Wolffian Vestiges) 30

3 **Conclusion** 30

References 30

Abstract

The development of the normal female reproductive tract is a complex process. The indifferent gonad differentiates to the ovary. The mesonephros, Wolffian and Müllerian ducts differentiate in an orchestrated manner to form the uterus, vagina and lower urinary tract. Disordered differentiation can result in congenital abnormalities affecting the female reproductive tracts, renal tract and lower intestines. A number of rudimentary structures can persist and be encountered in clinical practice, most commonly these are derived from the Wolffian ducts. This chapter provides an overview of the embryology of the female genital tract relevant to the multidisciplinary team caring for young females presenting with illnesses related to the reproductive system.

Abbreviations

AMH Anti-Müllerian hormone
UGS Urogenital sinus

1 Introduction

The development of the human reproductive tract, urinary system and distal gastrointestinal tract is intertwined sharing a close temporal and spatial relationship. Knowledge of the normal development and anatomy of the gynaecological tract is critical to the understanding of the timing and nature of a variety of paediatric gynaecological conditions. Malformations of the gynaecological tract are associated with

A. Healey (✉)
Department of Paediatric Radiology, Alder Hey NHS Foundation Trust, Liverpool, L12 2AP, UK
e-mail: andrew.healey@alderhey.nhs.uk

G. Mann et al. (eds.), *Imaging of Gynecological Disorders in Infants and Children*, Medical Radiology. Diagnostic Imaging, DOI: 10.1007/174_2010_128,

disorders of the renal tract and lower intestines. Rudimentary structures from the immature genitourinary tract may persist and be encountered in clinical practice particularly those from the mesonephric (Wolffian) ducts.

This chapter provides an overview of the embryology of the female genital tract relevant to the multidisciplinary team caring for young females presenting with illnesses related to the reproductive system.

Table 1 Summary of key phases of fetal genital tract development

Phase of genital development	Time (weeks of gestation)
Indifferent gonadal phase	4–6
Gonadal differentiation	7
Ductal differentiation	9–11
External genitalia differentiation	10–12

2 Embryology of the Female Genitourinary Tract

In females the genital organs comprise of gonads, reproductive ducts and external genitalia. Gonadal differentiation occurs before the end of the embryonic period. Both the reproductive ducts and external genitalia differentiate before the end of the first trimester. Development of the female genital tract continues in utero. The gonads descend in utero in girls. The main events critical to the in utero development of the female gynaecological tract are summarised in Table 1. Maturation of the genital tract is continuous during childhood through to puberty. The postnatal development of the reproductive tract is discussed in Normal Pubertal Development and Growth.

2.1 Development of the Gonads

2.1.1 Indifferent Gonadal Phase

The gonads develop from primitive germ cells, the mesothelium of the posterior abdominal wall and adjacent mesenchyme. Gonadal development begins in the fifth fetal week. The mesothelium medial to the mesonephros of the developing kidneys thickens, yielding the paired gonadal (urogenital) ridges (Fig. 1a). Transient epithelial finger-like structures, referred to as the primary sex cords, form and extend into the supporting mesenchyme. The gonadal ridges remain similar in both male and female fetuses until the seventh week. The indifferent (undifferentiated) gonads are located inside the Wolffian body on the medial aspect of the urogenital ridge, either side of the spine.

The primitive or primordial germ cells are the precursors of oocytes or spermatozoa. The primitive germ cells are evident from around the fourth fetal week and migrate from the yolk sac of the embryo along the dorsal mesentery of the hindgut to the mesenchyme of the gonadal ridges by the sixth week and incorporate into the primary sex cords (Fig. 1b). The primary sex cords are not well developed in the female embryo but do extend to the medulla of the future ovary and form the rete ovarii, a transient structure. The primary sex cords regress by the eighth week.

The genotype and chromosomal sex of a fetus is determined at conception. The mammalian fetus begins life with an undifferentiated gonad referred to as the indifferent gonad. The indifferent gonad comprises an inner medulla and outer cortex. The cortex contains the precursors of the ovarian parenchyma and the medulla the ovarian stroma. The presence of primitive germ cells is critical to normal ovarian development. Absence of the primitive germ cells will yield sterile gonads lacking follicles which will contain only stroma.

2.1.2 Gonadal Sexual Differentiation

The fetus has bipotential sexual development for the first 3 months of life. The phenotype depends on the presence of sex chromosomes and the prevailing biochemical and hormonal milieu. The default sex phenotype is female in the presence of two X-chromosomes. Under the influence of two X-chromosomes the cortex of the indifferent gonad is much better developed in the female embryo than the male. The cortex gives rise to the secondary sex cords (cortical cords) which extend from the surface epithelium to the mesenchyme (Fig. 1c). The secondary sex cords sustain and regulate ovarian cortical follicular development. The undifferentiated gonads persist until around the tenth week, at which time the ovaries first become identifiable. A male fetus will

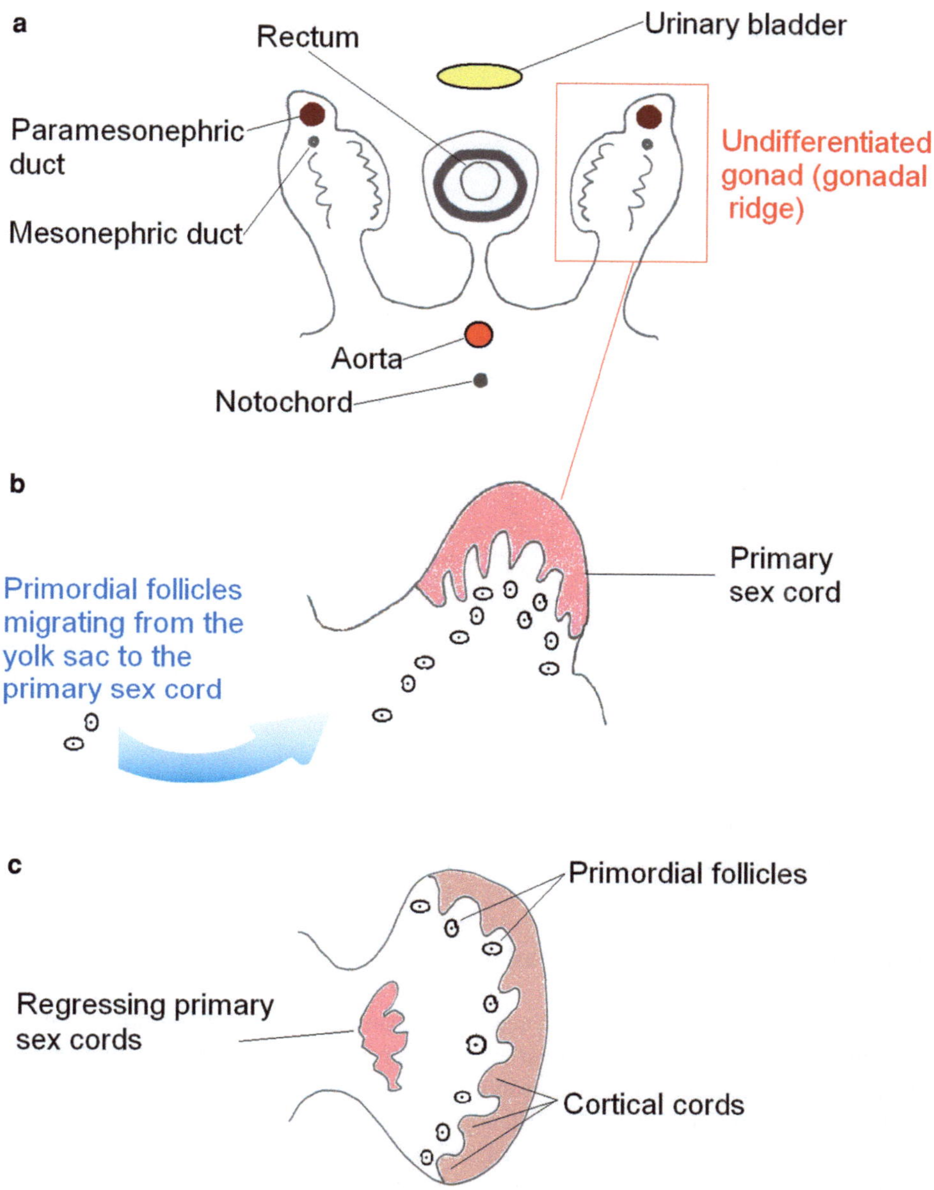

Fig. 1 Development of the ovaries from the undifferentiated (indifferent) gonads: **a** The indifferent gonads appear as primitive longitudinal streaks in the intermediate mesoderm adjacent to the mesonephros. **b** Magnified view of the undifferentiated gonad during 5–6 fetal weeks. The primordial follicles develop in the yolk sac and migrate to the gonadal ridge and are sustained by the primary sex cords. **c** The primary cords are transitory and regress by 8 weeks. The cortical (secondary cords) maintain ovarian follicular development. The ovaries are identifiable by 10 weeks.

develop in the presence of a Y-chromosome which encodes the SRY protein. The SRY protein enables testicular differentiation and the production of androgens including testosterone. The medulla of the indifferent gonad in males differentiates into the testis, the cortex involutes giving rise to vestigial remnants. In addition to the SRY protein and androgens a third factor is required for male development, anti-Müllerian hormone (AMH). AMH prevents female genital ductal differentiation. An immature female will develop in the absence of these three factors. Further maturation of the immature female is contingent upon

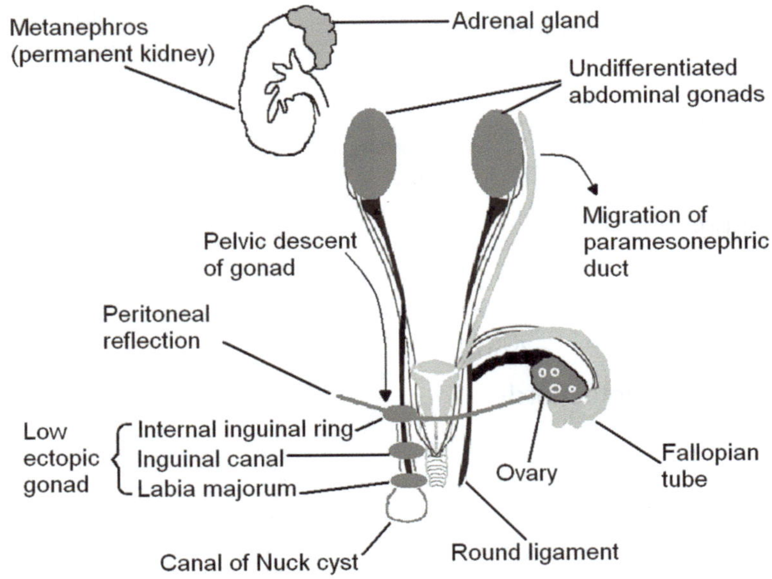

Fig. 2 Pelvic descent of the ovary. The fetal abdominal ovary usually descends into the pelvis as depicted (*left side* of pelvis) lying in close approximation to the fimbrial portion of the lateral aspect of the paramesonephric duct (future fallopian tube). Maldescent of the ovary occurs when the ovary lies above the pelvic brim. Rarely the ovary may be located in the inguinal canal or more inferiorly at the labium majorum (*right hand side* of pelvis). The canal of Nuck is a potential space which results from a patent evagination of the peritoneum to the labium majorum

the influence of oestrogens. Disorders of sexual differentiation are discussed further in Disorders of Sex Development.

2.1.3 Development of the Ovaries (Gonadal Differentiation)

As the cortical cords develop the primitive germ cells are incorporated in the mesenchyme of the ovaries. Gonadal differentiation takes place in the second month of fetal life. The primitive germ cells differentiate under the influence of placental gonadotropins. The germ cells migrating to the genital ridge undergo successive mitotic divisions whilst in contact with the coelomic epithelium differentiating into several million oogonia. By 4–5 fetal months, the primitive follicles organise within the fetal ovarian cortex. By 5–6 months gestation the ovaries contain 6–7 million primordial follicles. At this time, the primordial follicles are enveloped by a layer of epithelial cells, and are referred to as primary oocytes. The fate of an oocyte is determined once meiosis begins and no further mitotic division is possible thereafter. The vast majority of oocytes eventually degenerate over time; the remaining oogonia enter a dormant state referred to as meiotic arrest (first phase of meiosis). First meiosis will not complete until the onset of ovulation. Ovulatory follicles complete meiotic differentiation. At birth, between 2 and 4 million follicles remain. Around 400,000 follicles are present at menarche (Baker 1963). Ovarian follicles undergo varying rates of maturation and involution. The vast majority remain quiescent and eventually involute by apoptosis, but can remain dormant for decades.

2.1.4 Pelvic Descent of the Ovaries

As described previously, the indifferent gonads lie medial to the urogenital ridges at around the seventh fetal week. The ovaries in part undergo descent from the posterior abdominal wall into the pelvis due to the marked growth of the upper abdomen relative to the pelvis. By the third month the maturing ovaries descend into the pelvis guided by the gubernaculum into the ovarian fossae (Fig. 2). The gubernaculum is a peritoneal fold which attaches the caudal aspect of the ovary to the uterus, eventually forming the utero-ovarian (Fig. 3) and round uterine ligaments. Maldescent of the ovaries, although rare, may occur anywhere from the paraspinal posterior abdominal wall to the pelvic brim. Ovarian maldescent results from a short mesovarium and infundibulopelvic ligament and elongation of the utero-ovarian (ovarian)

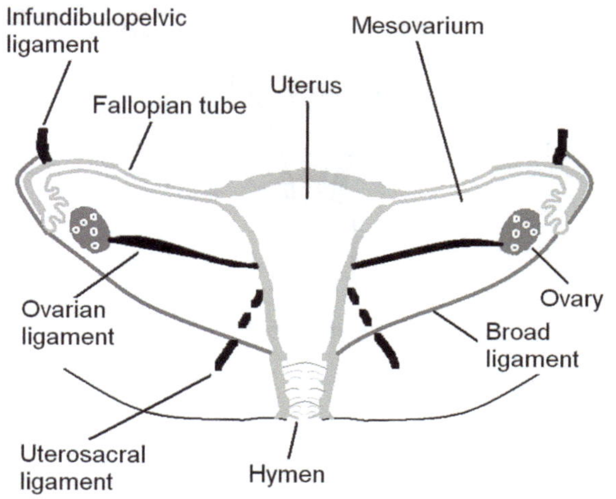

Fig. 3 The pelvic ligaments in the postnatal female

ligament (Verkauf and Bernhisel 1996). On cross-sectional imaging the position of an ectopic ovary may be traced along the course of its vascular pedicle. The ovaries are classically thought to be located in the adnexae/ovarian fossae. A recent study has shown the typical location of the ovaries in girls from birth to 18 years to be found in the lateral aspect of the pelvis, close to the anterior superior iliac spines, just below the iliac crests and umbilicus, and above the pubic symphysis (Bardo et al. 2009). Supernumerary ovary is an extremely rare entity in which a third ovary complete with follicles arises from a separate primordium.

2.2 Relationship Between the Early Fetal Genital and Urinary Systems

A brief description of the embryology of the human kidneys is necessary in order to outline their

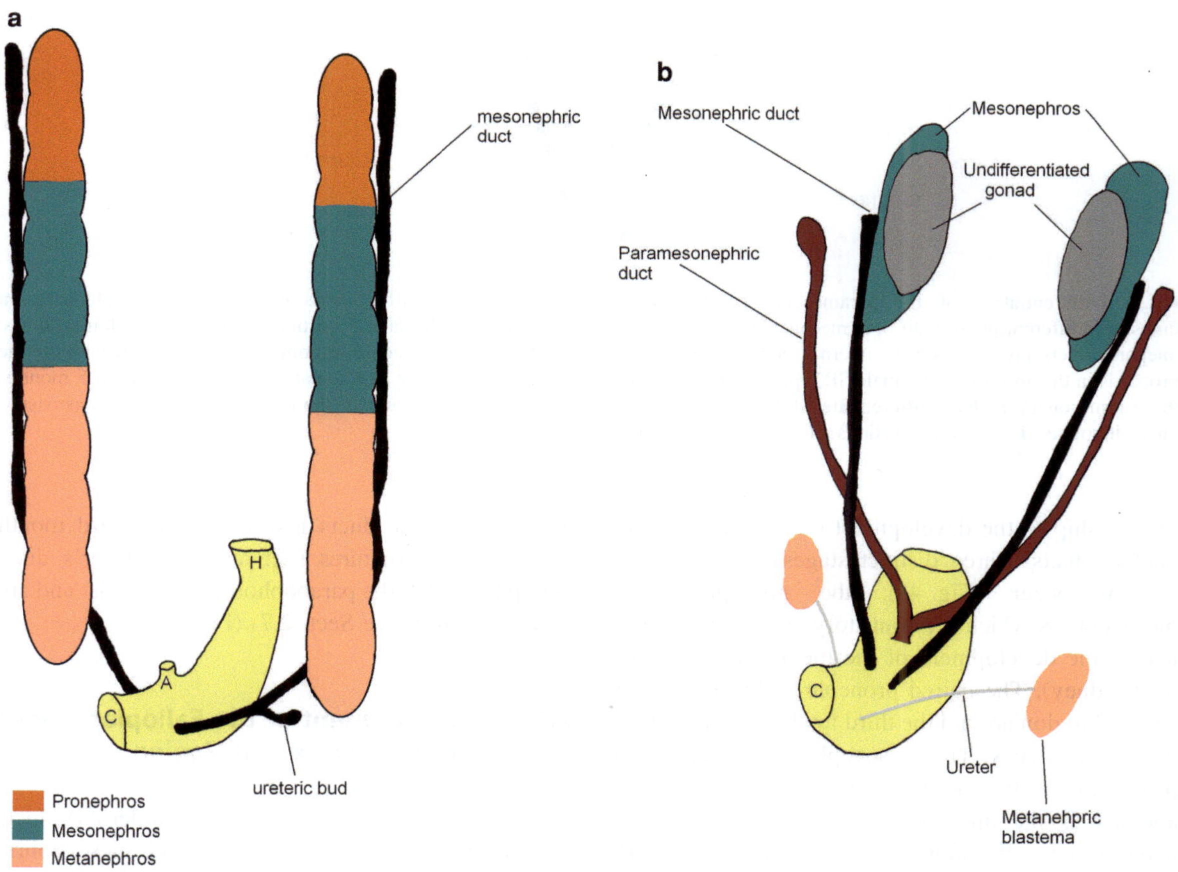

Fig. 4 The embryonic genitourinary tract at **a** 4 weeks and **b** between 6–8 weeks

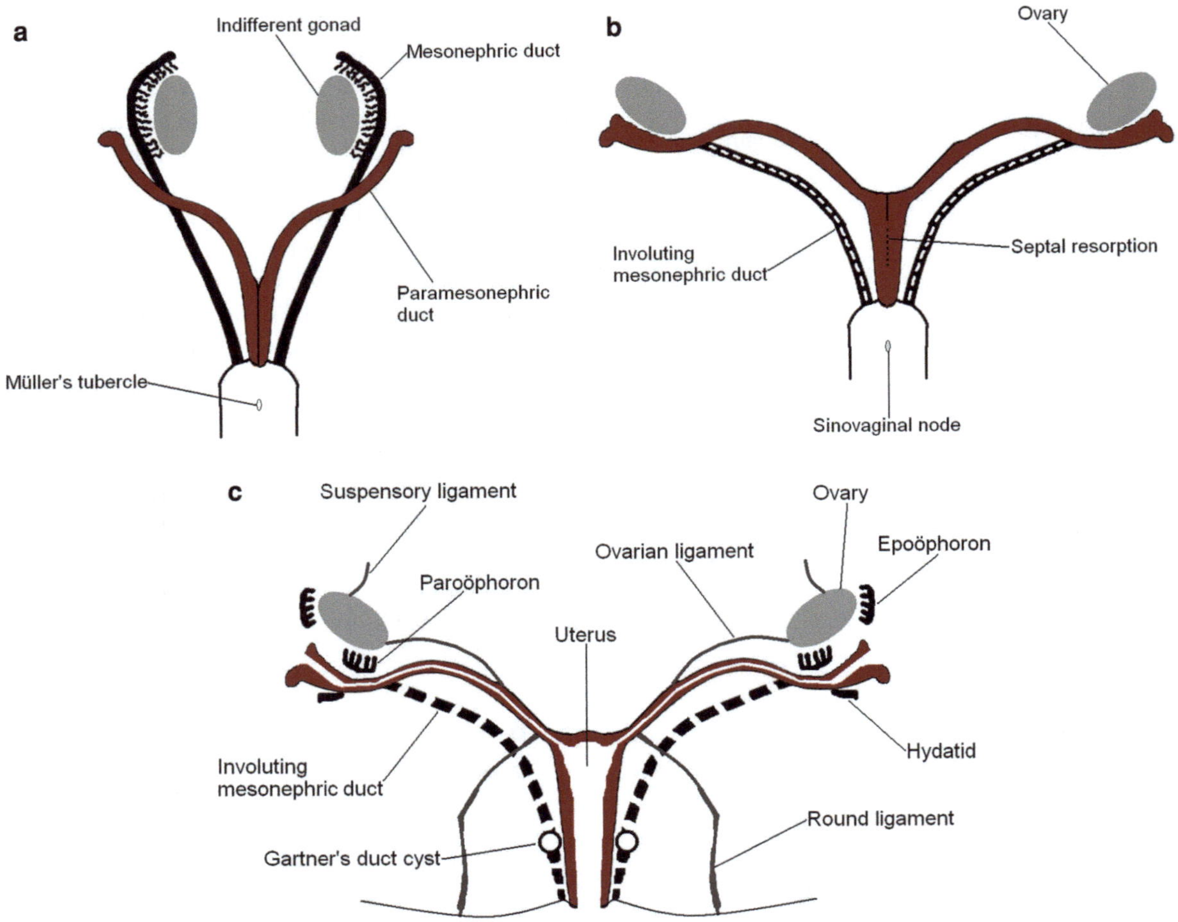

Fig. 5 Differentiation of the paramesonephric (Müllerian) ducts: **a** Indifferent phase with both mesonephric and paramesonephric ducts present. Female internal genital development proceeds in the absence of the male SRY protein. **b** At 7 weeks the paramesonephric ducts differentiate whilst the mesonephric ducts involute. The medial portions of the paramesonephric ducts fuse to form the uterus and upper vagina (lateral fusion 9–11 weeks), the lateral portions give rise to fallopian tubes. Müllerian organogenesis is complete by 5 months with uterine septal resorption. **c** The female internal genitalia at 5 months. Occasionally remnants of the mesonephric duct may persist

relationship to the development of the female reproductive ducts. Three distinct stages of renal development occur (Fig. 4a): the pronephros and mesonephros which are transitory structures but critical to the development of the metanephros (permanent kidney). The paired pronephros develops in the cervical region around the third fetal week and regress by the fifth week. The mesonephros form below the pronephros in the thoracic region in the fourth week and act as the interim kidneys. The paired mesonephric ducts (Wolffian duct) drain the mesonephros into the cloaca ventral to the laterally placed nephrogenic cords (Fig. 4b). In females the mesonephros and mesonephric ducts involute by the third month but vestigial structures such as the Gartner's duct, epoophoron and the paraoophoron may persist and are described later (see Sect. 2.7) (Fig. 5c).

2.3 Development of the Fallopian Tubes Uterus, Cervix and Vagina

In females the paramesonephric (Müllerian) ducts arise from the mesoderm lateral to the mesonephric ducts in the seventh week as focal invaginations of the coelomic epithelium on the upper pole of each

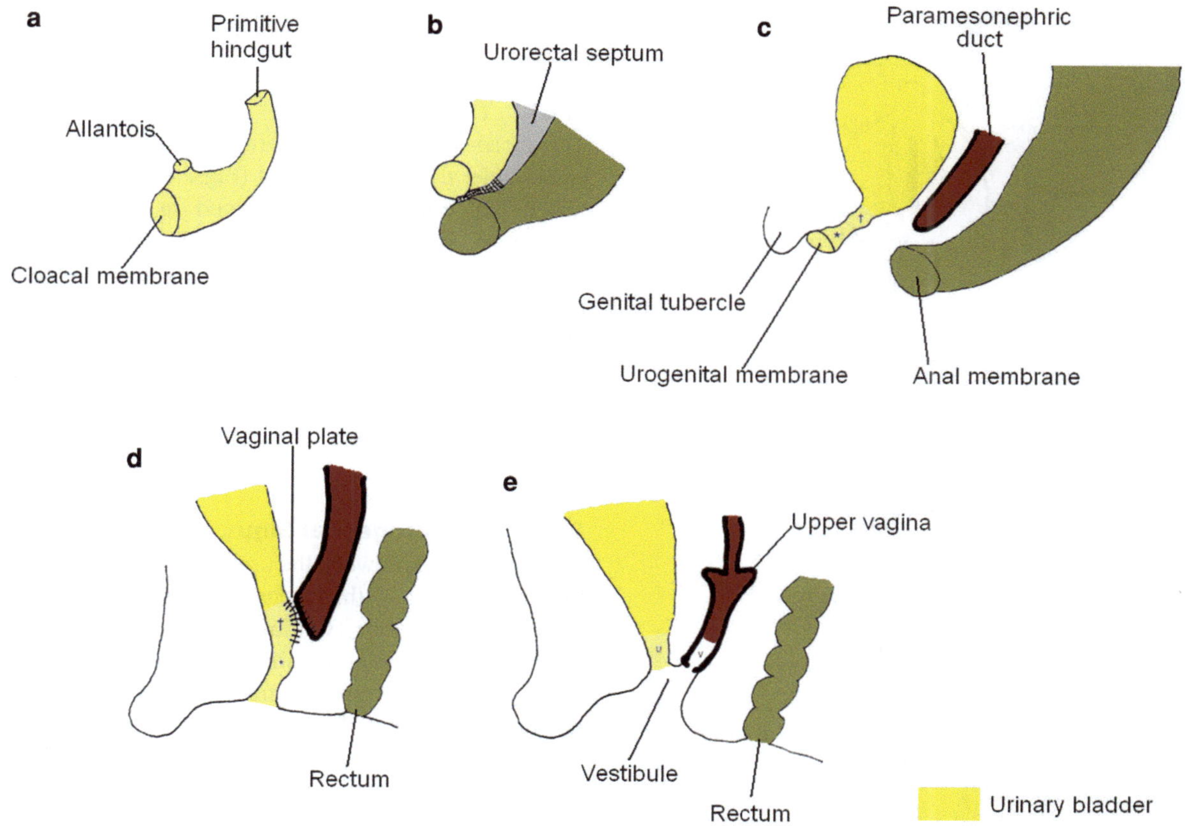

Fig. 6 Division of the cloaca and differentiation of the female lower genitourinary tract. **a** The cloaca. **b** The partition of the cloaca into anorectal and urogenital compartments by the descent of the urorectal septum (4–6 weeks). **c** The formation of the genital tubercle and urogenital sinus (UGS). The phallic (*) and cranial (†) portions of the pelvic UGS form the vaginal vestibule and female urethra, respectively. **d** Canalisation of the vagina at the vaginal plate onto the UGS (vertical fusion). **e** The definitive vaginal vestibule

mesonephros. The paired mesonephric and paramesonephric ducts represent the indifferent stage of the fetal internal genital canal systems. The paramesonephric ducts are the precursors of the uterus, fallopian tubes, cervix and upper vagina.

The paramesonephric ducts grow caudally, coursing lateral to the urogenital ridges. In the eighth week the paired paramesonephric ducts lie medial to the mesonephric ducts. The paramesonephric ducts fuse to form a confluence. This process is referred to as Müllerian organogenesis and represents the initial stage in the development of the upper two-thirds of the vagina, the cervix, uterus and both fallopian tubes (Fig. 5a). The cranial end of the fused ducts yields the future uterus which contains mesoderm that will form the uterine endometrium and myometrium. The unfused cranial ends of the paramesonephric ducts assume a funnel shaped configuration and remain open to the future peritoneal cavity as the fimbrial portions of the fallopian tubes. The caudal end of the fused ducts will form the upper two-thirds of the vagina.

Lateral fusion of the paramesonephric ducts occurs between the seventh and ninth weeks when the lower segments of the paramesonephric ducts fuse. At this stage a midline septum is present in the uterine cavity, this usually regresses at around 20 weeks but can persist (Fig. 5b). Vertical fusion occurs in the eighth week when the lower most fused paramesonephric ducts fuse with the ascending endoderm of the sinovaginal bulb. The lower third of the vagina is formed as the sinovaginal node (bulb) canalises.

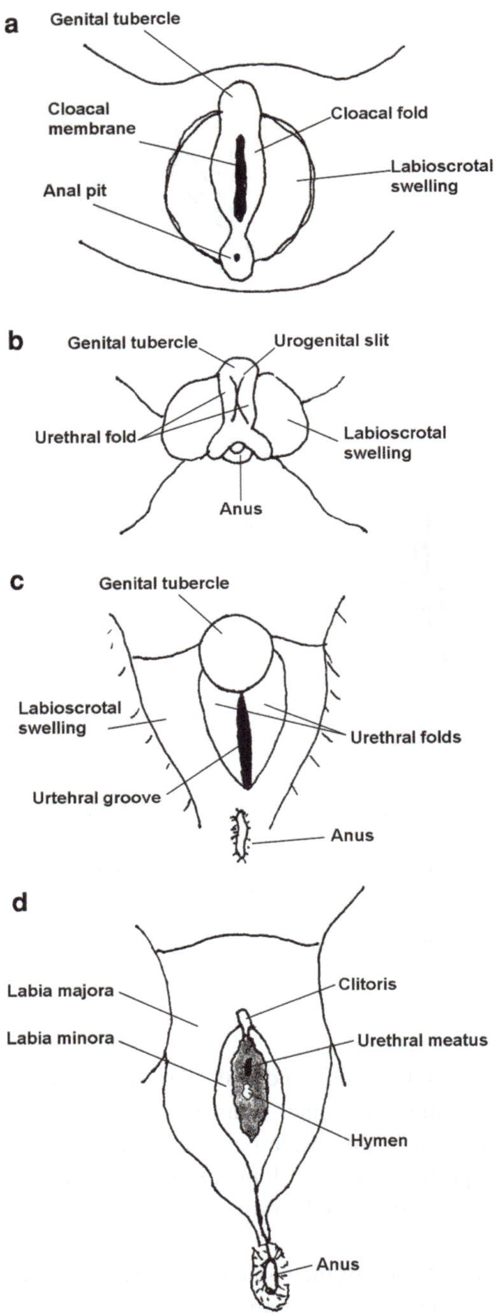

Fig. 7 Differentiation of the female external genitalia. Stages of development at **a** 4 weeks (indifferent stage), **b** 6–7 weeks **c** 9–11 weeks and **d** 12 weeks (full differentiation)

The sinovaginal node inserts into the urogenital sinus at Müller's tubercle. The hymen, a membrane separating the vagina from the urogenital sinus develops and is normally perforated by birth.

2.4 Development of the Lower Genital Tract

2.4.1 The Cloaca

The cloacal membrane is formed in the third fetal week under the umbilical cord (Figs. 4a and 6a). The lower abdominal wall is formed as the cloacal membrane becomes more caudally displaced by adjacent proliferating mesenchyme. By the fifth week the cloacal membrane is delimited laterally by the cloacal folds which fuse anteriorly to give rise to an anlage referred to as the genital tubercle which is formed earlier in the fourth week (see Sect. 2.5.1). The cloacal membrane remains imperforate at this time.

2.4.2 The Urogenital Sinus

During the seventh week the urorectal septum fuses to the inner surface of the cloacal membrane dividing it to form the anterior (ventral) urogenital membrane and the posterior anal membrane dividing the rectum proper from the urogenital tract (Fig. 6b). The urogenital membrane perforates and free communication between the amniotic cavity and the primary urogenital sinus is established. The folds surrounding the urogenital membrane are now referred to as the urethral folds and those around the anus the anal folds.

2.4.3 Differentiation of the Urogenital Sinus

The primary urogenital sinus develops into the definitive urogenital sinus (UGS). The UGS consists of a caudal phallic portion and a pelvic portion (Fig. 6c). The urethral groove and phallic (distal) portion of the UGS enlarge to form the vaginal introitus (vestibule) (Fig. 6d). This is closed off externally by the urogenital membrane which perforates in the seventh week. The narrow pelvic (proximal) segment of the definitive urogenital sinus contributes to the short distal female urethra and lower third of the vagina (Fig. 6e).

2.5 Development of the External Genitalia

The external genitalia remain sexually undifferentiated until around the seventh fetal week. During the tenth week distinct sexual characteristics appear with complete differentiation occurring around the twelfth week.

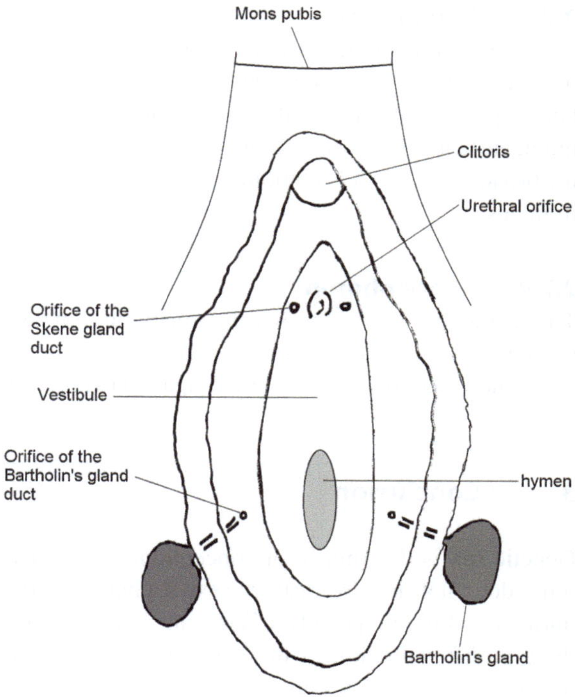

Fig. 8 Anatomy of the vestibular glands and ducts: The position of the greater vestibular glands (Bartholin's) and the lesser vestibular (Skene) or periurethral glands

2.5.1 Indifferent External Genitalia

In the fourth week the genital tubercle results from mesenchymal proliferation and a protophallus ventral to the cloacal membrane begins to develop. During the sixth week, the urethral groove and anal pit form resulting in focal depressions along the cloacal membrane (Fig. 7a). The primary urethral (urogenital) folds surround the primary urethral groove. The genital or labioscrotal swellings form lateral to the urethral folds.

In the seventh week, the cloacal membrane involutes and the primary urethral groove becomes continuous with the definitive urogenital sinus. The secondary urethral groove forms as a result of deepening and widening the primary urethral groove in the eighth week. The external genitalia begin display sexual differentiation during the tenth week (Fig. 7c).

2.5.2 Female External Genitalia

In girls the unfused parts of the labioscrotal (genital) swellings give rise to the labia majora, the folds fuse anteriorly to form the mons pubis and anterior labial commissure, and posteriorly the posterior labial commissure. The urethral folds fuse posteriorly to form the frenulum of the labia minora. The unfused

Table 2 Vestigial remnants and postnatal derivatives of the genitourinary tract

Embryonic structure	Female	Male homologue
Gonad	Ovary	Testis
Cortex	Ovarian follicles	Seminiferous tubules
Medulla	Rete ovarii	Rete testis
Gubernaculum	Ovarian ligament and round ligament of uterus	Gubernaculum
Mesonephric tubules	Epoophoron, paroophoron	Ductuli efferentes
Mesonephric duct	Appendix vesiculosa, duct of epoophoron, duct of Gartner	Appendix of epididymis, duct of epididymis, ductus deferens, ejaculatory duct and seminal vesicles
Paramesonephric duct	Hydatid of Morgagni, uterine tube, uterus	Appendix of testis
Urogenital sinus	Urethra, vagina urethral, paraurethral and greater vestibular glands	Urethra, prostatic utricle, prostate and bulbourethral glands
Sinus tubercle	Hymen	Seminal colliculus
Phallus	Clitoris	Penis
Urogenital folds	Labia minora	Ventral aspect of penis
Labioscrotal swellings	Labia majora	Scrotum

Adapted from Moore and Persaud (1998) with permission from Elsevier publishers LTD urethral (urogenital) folds give rise to the labia minora. The unfused genital swellings enable the urogenital sinus to open into the anterior (urethral) part of the vagina and the vaginal vestibule. The genital tubercle becomes the clitoris and is recognisable by the fourteenth week (Fig. 7d).

2.6 Development of the Female Genital Accessory Glands

The accessory urethral glands including the lesser vestibular or paraurethral glands (Skene) and urethral glands arise from the urogenital sinus from endodermal (epithelial) buds growing into the urethral mesenchyme (Fig. 8). The paired greater vestibular glands (Bartholin) form in the 12th week and empty into the vaginal vestibule.

2.7 Embryological Vestigial Structures (Wollfian Vestiges)

In early fetal life the mesonephric Wolffian and paramesonephric ducts co-exist. The mesonephric ducts regress in a female, but remnants of the mesonephric duct typically persist. Their importance relates to the potential for the development of pathology. The mesonephric remnants in a female are reviewed here and summarised in Table 2.

2.7.1 Gartner's Duct

The Gartner's ducts are paired remnants of the mesonephric duct that may give rise to Gartner's duct cysts and are typically located in the broad ligament (Fig. 5c).

2.7.2 Canal of Nuck

The canal of Nuck is a virtual space and is the female analogue of the processus vaginalis in the male, if patent it is abnormal and forms a pouch of peritoneum in the labia majorum (Fig. 2).

2.7.3 Epoophoron

The epoophoron (Fig. 5c) is the most cranial part of the mesonephric duct remnant. It is situated in the lateral portion of the broad ligament and may communicate with the Gartner's ducts more inferiorly in the broad ligament. It is homologous to the epididymis in males.

2.7.4 Paraoophoron

The paraoophoron is also a mesonephric remnant analogous to the paradidymis in males. It is usually positioned medially in each broad ligament (Fig. 5c).

3 Conclusion

Genetic sex is determined at conception. The female fetus does not acquire distinct sexual characteristics until the indifferent gonads differentiate to ovaries and there is differentiation of the external genitalia. The development of the uterus and vagina requires integrated differentiation of the paramesonephric and mesonephric ducts in close relation the development of the excretory system. This interdependence accounts for the association of anomalies of the female genital system, urinary tract and more complex cloacal malformations.

References

Baker TG (1963) A quantitative and cytological study of germ cells in the human ovaries. In: Proceedings of the Royal Society of London, Series B. 158:417–433

Bardo DM, Black M, Schenk K, Zaritzky MF (2009) Location of the ovaries in girls from newborn to 18 years of age: reconsidering ovarian shielding. Pediatr Radiol 39:253–259

Moore KL, Persaud TVN (1998) The urogenital system. In: Moore KL, Persaud TVN (eds) The developing human. Clinically oriented embryology, ed 6. WB Saunders, Philadelphia, pp 303–347

Verkauf BS, Bernhisel M (1996) Ovarian maldescent. Fertil Steril 65:189–192

Disorders of Sex Development

Justin H. Davies, Pat S. Malone, and Jo Fairhurst

Contents

1	**Introduction**	32
2	**Development of the Reproductive Systems**	33
2.1	Sex Determination	33
2.2	Sex Differentiation	33
3	**Genital Duct Development**	34
3.1	Male Genital Duct Development	34
3.2	Female Genital Duct Development	34
3.3	Urogenital Sinus	35
4	**External Genital Development**	35
5	**Disorders of Sex Development**	35
6	**Initial Clinical Evaluation of a Newborn with a Disorder of Sex Development**	35
7	**Radiological Evaluation of a Newborn with a Disorder of Sex Development**	36
7.1	Initial Assessment and Diagnosis	36
8	**The Role of Imaging in Delayed Diagnosis or Later Assessment**	38
9	**46,XX Disorders of Sex Development**	39
9.1	Congenital Adrenal Hyperplasia	39
10	**46,XY Disorders of Sex Development**	42
10.1	Defects in Testis Determination	42
10.2	Imaging of 46,XY Disorders of Sex Differentiation	43
10.3	Defects in Androgen Biosynthesis	43
11	**Defects in Androgen Action**	44
11.1	Androgen insensitivity syndromes	44
11.2	5α-Reductase Deficiency	46
12	**Congenital Hypopituitarism**	47
13	**Ovotesticular Disorders of Sex Development**	47
13.1	Imaging of Ovotesticular DSD	48
14	**Management of Disorders of Sex Development**	48
References		49

Abstract

The contribution of imaging in disorders of sex development is not confined to the diagnosis of the underlying condition. Imaging has an important role in assisting pre-operative planning where surgery is contemplated, in identifying the location of occult gonads and in assessment of suspected complications of these conditions, including malignant transformation. In each of these scenarios, close collaboration with paediatric endocrinologists and paediatric surgeons is essential if an appropriate management strategy is to be adopted, as imaging is of greatest value where the radiologist is aware of the context in which it is performed.

Abbreviations

DSD	Disorders of sex development
AMH	Anti-Müllerian Hormone

J. H. Davies (✉)
Department of Paediatric Endocrinology, Southampton University Hospital Trust, Southampton, UK
e-mail: justin.davies@suht.swest.nhs.uk

P. S. Malone
Department of Paediatric Urology, Southampton University Hospital Trust, Southampton, UK

J. Fairhurst
Department of Paediatric Radiology, Southampton University Hospital Trust, Southampton, UK

G. Mann et al. (eds.), *Imaging of Gynecological Disorders in Infants and Children*, Medical Radiology. Diagnostic Imaging, DOI: 10.1007/174_2010_81, © Springer-Verlag Berlin Heidelberg 2012

SRY	Sex determining region of the Y chromosome
AR	Androgen receptor
21-OHD	21-hydroxylase deficiency
AMH	Anti-Müllerian hormone
AMHR	Anti-Müllerian hormone receptor
US	Ultrasound
CT	Computed Tomography
MRI	Magnetic Resonance Imaging
TUM	Total Urogenital Mobilisation
INSL3	Insulin-like 3
T	Testosterone
DHT	Dihydrotestosterone
SF-1	Steroidogenic factor 1
WT-1	Wilm's tumour-1
SOX-9	SRY box 9
DAX-1	Dosage-sensitive sex reversal-adrenal hypoplasia congenita critical region on the X chromosome gene 1
StAR	steroidogenic acute regulatory
LH	Luteinising hormone
TFT	Thyroid function tests
FSH	Follicle stimulating hormone
DHEAS	Dehydroepiandrosterone sulfate
HCG	Human chorionic gonadotropin
MHz	Megahertz
LHRH	Luteinising hormone releasing hormone
17-hydroxy-progesterone	17-OH progesterone
AR	Androgen receptor
MCUG	Micturating Cystourethrogram
PAIS	Partial Androgen Insensitivity Syndrome
AIS	Androgen Insensitivity Syndrome
CAIS	Complete Androgen Insensitivity Syndrome
CAH	Congenital Adrenal Hyperplasia
LGR8	Leucine-rich repeat-containing G-protein-coupled receptor 8
ACTH	Adrenocorticotropic Hormone
GH	Growth hormone
AVP	Arginine vasopressin

1 Introduction

The contribution of imaging in disorders of sex development is not confined to the diagnosis of the underlying condition. Imaging has an important role in assisting pre-operative planning where surgery is contemplated, in identifying the location of occult gonads and in assessment of suspected complications of these conditions, including malignant transformation. In each of these scenarios, close collaboration with paediatric endocrinologists and paediatric surgeons is essential if an appropriate management strategy is to be adopted, as imaging is of greatest value where the radiologist is aware of the context in which it is performed.

Recently, there has been a change to the nomenclature of the various descriptions of genital anomalies (Table 1) (Hughes et al. 2006). This was necessary following advances in molecular genetics and evolving ethical considerations together with concerns voiced by patient advocacy groups. Terms such as pseudohermaphroditism, intersex and sex reversal and other gender-based labels are controversial and may be perceived to be pejorative. Furthermore, such terms may be confusing to both health professionals and parents, with the potential for diagnostic confusion.

Thus, the term 'disorders of sex development (DSD)' is now used, and is defined as congenital conditions in which development of chromosomal, gonadal or anatomical sex is atypical (Hughes et al. 2006).

Radiological evaluation of the reproductive system requires an understanding of the embryology and anatomy of the genital tracts, the influence of sex chromosomes on gonad development and hormonal influences on genital development.

Table 1 Revised nomenclature for disorders of sex development (Hughes et al. 2006)

Previous	Revised 2006
Intersex	Disorders of sex development (DSD)
Male pseudohermaphrodite Undervirilisation of an XY male Undermasculinisation of an XY male	46,XY DSD
Female pseudohermaphroditism Overvirilisation of an XX female Masculinisation of an XX female	46,XX DSD
True hermaphrodite	Ovotesticular DSD
XX male or XX sex reversal	46,XX testicular DSD
XY sex reversal	46,XY complete gonadal dysgenesis

2 Development of the Reproductive Systems

Reproductive development is a complex process that begins at 5 weeks gestation and is completed 14 years later when fertility is achieved during puberty. The majority of cases of DSD present in the neonatal period as genital ambiguity. Less commonly girls may present in infancy with inguinal hernia and more rarely they may present as non-isosexual puberty or in adulthood as primary amenorrhoea and infertility. Reproductive development is governed by the processes of sex determination and sex differentiation.

2.1 Sex Determination

Sex determination depends on the sex chromosome complement of the embryo and is established by multiple molecular events that direct the development of germ cells, their migration to the urogenital ridge and the formation of either a testis (in the presence of a Y chromosome) or an ovary (in the absence of a Y chromosome and the presence of a second X chromosome) (Maclaughlin and Donahoe 2004; Federman 2004). In males and females the indifferent gonad develops from the genital ridge under the control of various factors (Fig. 1). Primordial germ cells originate in the yolk sac and migrate through the mesentery of the hind gut to reach the urogenital ridge by 6–8 weeks gestation (Federman 2004). Thus, genetic sex is determined at conception and controls the differentiation of the gonad.

Testis-determining genes, such as the SRY gene, are important for the development of the bipotential gonad to a testes. In the absence of testes-determining genes, ovarian development will occur. The maintenance of ovarian development is an active process which depends on the presence of primordial germ cells. Primary oocytes undergo several cycles of meiotic division before undergoing meiotic arrest.

2.2 Sex Differentiation

Sex differentiation enables the sex-specific response of tissues to hormones produced by gonads after they have differentiated in a male or female pattern.

2.2.1 Male Sex Differentiation

Testicular differentiation and testosterone production occurs by 9 weeks gestation. Male sex differentiation involves the development of the internal genitalia, the urogenital sinus and external genitalia, and is partly under endocrine regulation. The Leydig cells of the testes synthesise testosterone from 9 weeks gestation, which mediates development of the vas deferens, epidydymis and seminal vesicles by stabilising the Wolffian ducts (Ahmed and Hughes 2002). Dihydrotestosterone, a metabolite of testosterone, causes masculinisation of the genital anlage to form the external male genitalia, the penis and scrotum. Leydig cells also synthesis insulin-like 3 which promotes transabdominal migration of the testes prior to scrotal descent. From 9 weeks gestation, an increase in testosterone production is critical subsequent masculinising the internal and external genitalia (Ahmed and Hughes 2002). The Sertoli cells of the testes synthesise anti-Müllerian hormone (AMH), which binds to its receptor on Müllerian ducts, to prevent this structure developing into the uterus, fallopian tubes and upper part of the vagina. Furthermore, the testes themselves exert a paracrine effect on adjacent tissues and cause Wolffian duct development and regression of Müllerian structures.

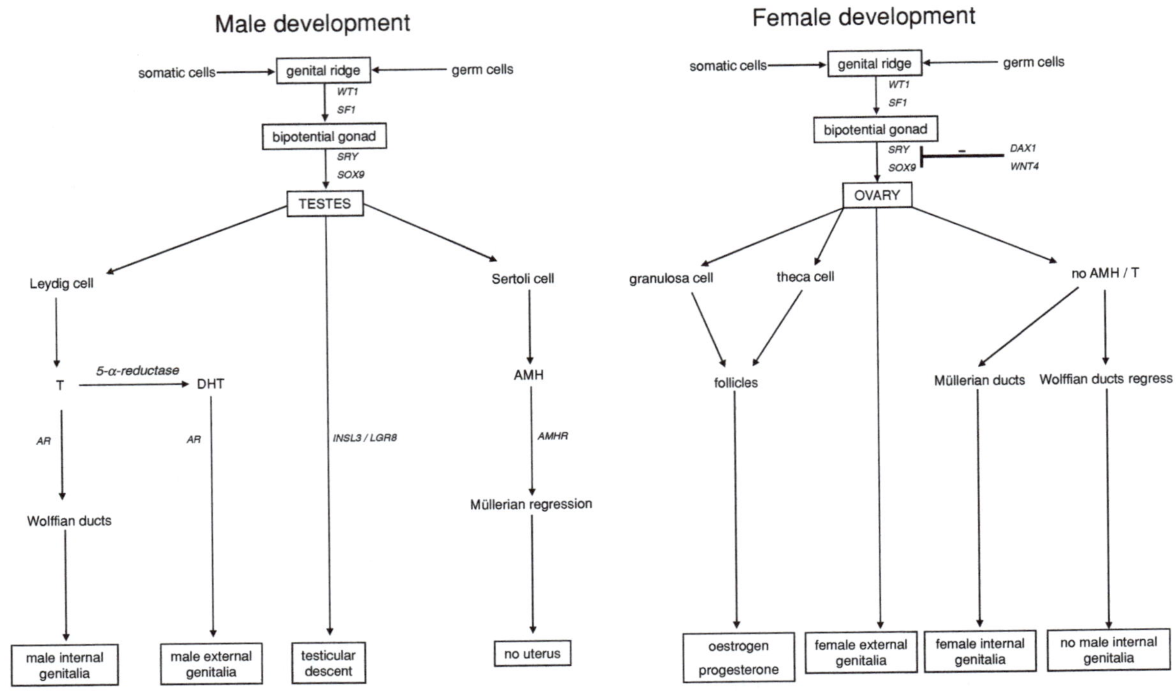

Fig. 1 Sex determination and sex differentiation. *AR* androgen receptor, *AMH* anti-Müllerian hormone, *AMHR* anti-Müllerian hormone receptor, *INSL3* insulin-like 3, *T* testosterone, *DHT* dihydrotestosterone, *SF-1* steroidogenic factor 1, *SRY* sex-determining region of the Y chromosome, *WT-1* Wilm's tumour-1, *DAX-1* dosage-sensitive sex reversal-adrenal hypoplasia congenita critical region on the X chromosome gene 1, SOX-9 SRY box 9

2.2.2 Female Sex Differentiation

Although there are no known ovarian-determining genes, ovarian differentiation and germ cell meiosis occurs by 11–12 weeks gestation (Federman 2004). Female differentiation of the foetus will occur unless there is expression of specific genes and hormones that control testicular differentiation and the subsequent development of male internal and external genitalia.

3 Genital Duct Development

The development of internal genitalia is an important component of sex differentiation and may be abnormal in DSD. At 7 weeks gestation, a foetus has two genital duct systems: Wolffian ducts (with the potential for male development) and Müllerian ducts (with the potential for female development). In the absence of male-inducer factors, the foetus has a natural tendency towards female differentiation.

3.1 Male Genital Duct Development

Functional testes in utero, with the ability to release testosterone and AMH, are critical for controlling the subsequent internal genital duct development in males. Testosterone, secreted by the Leydig cells causes stabilisation of Wolffian duct development. The testes also exert a paracrine effect on adjacent tissues and promote local differentiation of the Wolffian system and involution of the Müllerian ducts. The Wolffian ducts will develop into the epidydymis, vas deferens, ejaculatory ducts and seminal vesicles. The Sertoli cells of the testes release AMH which leads to involution of Müllerian structures.

3.2 Female Genital Duct Development

In the absence of a testis, the Wolffian system involutes and the Müllerian ducts develop. These form the fallopian tubes and fuse in the midline to give rise to the corpus and cervix of the uterus and upper third of the vagina.

3.3 Urogenital Sinus

The development of the urogenital sinus differs greatly between the two sexes. The anatomy of the urogenital sinus may be abnormal in some forms of DSD and the degree to which the anatomy is altered may influence the subsequent surgical procedure.

During weeks 4–7 of fetal development, the urorectal septum divides the cloaca into the anorectal canal and the primitive urogenital sinus. The primitive urogenital sinus constitutes three components: (1) the upper and largest part—the urinary bladder, (2) the pelvic part of the urogenital sinus, which in males gives rise to the prostatic and membranous parts of the urethra and (3) the definitive urogenital sinus (Thomas 2009).

In the presence of androgens, the definitive urogenital sinus narrows to form the posterior urethra. In the male, the prostate gland and bulbourethral glands of Cowper are formed as outbuddings of the urethra. In the absence of androgens the definitive urogenital sinus develops into the lower two-thirds of the vagina and the urethra which are separated to form two distinct structures. Outgrowths form the paraurethral glands of Skene and the vestibular glands of Bartholin.

4 External Genital Development

Male and female external genitalia develop from a common anlage. At 6 weeks gestation this is composed of a genital tubercle and urethral folds flanked by genital swellings. The genital tubercle elongates to form a phallus and in females into the clitoris and in the male into the glans penis. The urethral folds fuse to form the corpus spongiosum and penile urethra in the male, and in the female the urethral folds develop into the labia minora. Labioscrotal folds develop from the genital swellings and fuse in the midline to form the scrotum and the ventral part of the penis in the male, and remain separate to form the labia majora in the female (Thomas 2009).

The development of the anlage and the urogenital sinus is under the control of dihydrotestosterone (DHT) which is synthesised locally by 5α-reductase from circulating testosterone.

5 Disorders of Sex Development

The causes of disorders of sexual differentiation can be classified clinically as 46,XX DSD, 46,XY DSD and ovotesticular DSD (Table 2). The commonest cause of ambiguous genitalia at birth is 46,XX DSD caused by Congenital Adrenal Hyperplasia (CAH) from 21-hydroxylase deficiency, which results in a masculinised female phenotype. In the majority of cases of 46,XY DSD, however, no cause is identified.

Even though genital anomalies occur in 1 in 4,500 births, the presentation of DSD is not confined to the newborn period. Non-isosexual development (virilisation of a phenotypic female) may occur at puberty with 17β-hydroxysteroid dehydrogenase deficiency, 5α-reductase deficiency, late-onset congenital adrenal hyperplasia and partial androgen insensitivity.

6 Initial Clinical Evaluation of a Newborn with a Disorder of Sex Development

Often a baby with ambiguous genitalia is born at a local hospital so initial management is at a distance. The need to define a baby's gender is treated as a semi-emergency. The investigative process itself often causes distress to the family and there may be adverse effects on the parent–infant interaction. The parents should be told how long it will be before results will be available. Parents will often require guidance regarding information disclosure to the wider family. Information should be given to the family in a consistent manner and appropriate to their levels of understanding and sensitive to their cultural and religious background. Adrenal insufficiency may be associated with some forms of DSD and appropriate monitoring should be put in place.

The aim is to achieve a gender assignment as soon as possible. Prior to discharge a management plan, further investigations and follow-up should be arranged. The diagnosis may not be established prior to gender assignment. The management of these infants should be by a multidisciplinary team including paediatric endocrinologists, urologists, radiologists, geneticists, psychologists and biochemists.

A thorough history and examination should be undertaken which may give insight into the aetiology of the genital anomaly (Table 3). It is not possible to

Table 2 Clinical classification and aetiology of disorders of sex development

46,XX disorder of sex development
Congenital adrenal hyperplasia
21-Hydroxylase deficiency
11β-Hydroxylase deficiency
3β-Hydroxysteroid hydrogenase deficiency
Placental aromatase deficiency
Adrenal tumours
Ovarian tumours
Transplacental passage of maternal androgens, e.g. danazol administration, luteoma of pregnancy
Ovotesticular DSD
46,XY disorder of sex development
1. *Failure in testes determination*
Gonadal dysgenesis
XO/XY mosaicism
Mutations in:
WT-1
SF-1
SOX-9
DAX-1
SRY
2. *Failure in androgen biosynthesis*
StAR protein deficiency
3β-Hydroxysteroid hydrogenase deficiency
17,20 Desmolase deficiency
17β-OH-dehydrogenase deficiency
Leydig cell hypoplasia (LH deficiency or LH receptor defect)
Secondary to hypopituitarism
3. *Failure in androgen action*
Androgen insensitivity syndrome
5α-Reductase deficiency
Ovotesticular disorder of sex development
XX
XY
XX/XY

assign gender on the basis of clinical evaluation alone, and radiological and biochemical investigations in these individuals are usually required. A discriminatory approach to the investigation of newborns with ambiguous genitalia is essential (Ogilvy-Stuart and Brain 2004) and is guided by the history and examination and also the age of the baby (Table 4).

7 Radiological Evaluation of a Newborn with a Disorder of Sex Development

7.1 Initial Assessment and Diagnosis

7.1.1 Ultrasonography

Initial imaging assessment of an infant with ambiguous genitalia should always include ultrasound. The aim of imaging at this stage is to determine the presence, morphology and location of any gonads and whether there is a uterus evident. The identification of a uterus in the context of ambiguous genitalia indicates the presence either of an ovary, dysgenetic testis or absent 'gonads'.

Assessment of adrenal size may also be valuable, whilst bearing in mind that normal adrenal glands are prominent at this age. Ultrasound is made easier in the neonatal period by the relative prominence of any uterine or ovarian tissue secondary to stimulation by maternal hormones. Use of an intermediate frequency curvilinear probe is sufficient for initial evaluation although a 10–12-MHz linear transducer often allows detailed analysis of the sonographic architecture of the gonads.

As with any pelvic ultrasound examination at this age, it is advisable to start with assessment of the pelvis via transvesical scanning, to avoid the pitfall of losing the opportunity to use the bladder as a window when the infant voids—a regular occurrence when a cold ultrasound probe is applied to the abdomen. A trans-perineal approach may help to locate ectopic gonads, and assessment should also include the renal and suprarenal areas. When undertaking imaging studies at this stage it is preferable to avoid the terms 'testis' and 'ovary' and refer instead to 'gonads'.

The normal sonographic appearance of the testis in the newborn period is that of an oval structure of homogenous echogenicity which is slightly less than that generally seen in the adult. The mediastinum testis (a fold of the tunica albuginea) may be appreciated as an echogenic band running longitudinally through the testis: apart from this the testis is essentially featureless (Fig. 2).

Neonatal ovaries may be similarly featureless, presenting an identical appearance to testicular tissue,

Table 3 Clinical evaluation of ambiguous genitalia

History
Maternal medication during pregnancy, maternal virilisation during pregnancy, previous miscarriages, if available: prenatal karyotype (amniocentesis), phenotype on foetal ultrasound scan
Family history: consanguinity, family history of neonatal deaths (undiagnosed adrenal insufficiency), ambiguous genitalia, infertility, absent puberty/amenorrhoea, adrenal failure, hernia repair in girls
Examination
Size of clitoris/phallus, degree of labial fusion, position of urethra/urogenital sinus, degree of hypospadias, are gonads palpable? (check inguinal canals); examination of anus; signs of hypopituitarism (midline defects, hypoglycaemia, hypocortisolism, prolonged jaundice); features of adrenal insufficiency: excess pigmentation, weight loss, cardiovascular instability; features of Turner's syndrome may be seen in mosaicism or partial gonadal dysgenesis

Table 4 Investigation of ambiguous genitalia

Day 1 of life
Karyotype
Daily electrolytes and glucose daily to monitor for adrenal insufficiency
USS pelvis to determine presence of Müllerian structures and gonads in labial folds
After day 2 of life
17-OH progesterone, consider 11-deoxycorticosterone
Testosterone, DHEAS, androstenedione
LH, FSH
TFT
Plasma renin activity, aldosterone
Urine for steroid metabolites
Consider,
Short synacthen test
Three-day HCG test if undermasculinised male
LHRH test if suspected hypopituitarism
Clinical photography

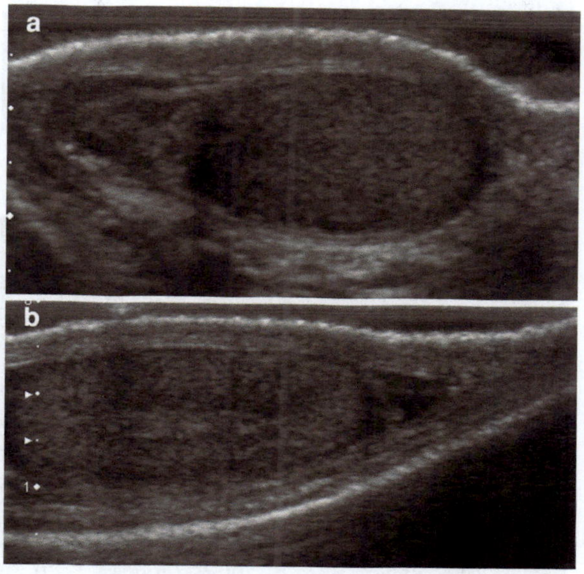

Fig. 2 Sonographic appearance of normal neonatal testis. **a** Oval structure of homogenous echogenicity. **b** The mediastinum testis is visible as an echogenic band running longitudinally through the testis

although there are often some ovarian follicles visible in the immediate postnatal period, which aid in distinguishing the nature of the gonad (Fig. 3).

7.1.2 Genitography

Genitography is most commonly employed in the early postnatal period in infants with DSD. Here, the aim of imaging is to demonstrate the configuration of the urethra, the anatomy of any urogenital sinus and the presence of any fistulous connections between the genital tract, bladder or rectum. This may confirm the presence of a vagina and cervical impression, demonstrate the length of any common channel and the site at which the vagina and urethra unite, and may elucidate more complex malformations.

Several approaches can be used to maximise the chance of demonstrating the anatomy in full: if there is a common perineal opening or two perineal orifices, a 4F- or 6F-feeding tube can be advanced followed by injection of contrast under fluoroscopic control. Depending on what structure is cannulated and the calibre of any communicating sinus, it may be possible to demonstrate the entire anatomy of the urogenital tract at MCUG. If the bladder is entered and the voiding study does not delineate the genital components, it can be useful to piggy-back a second catheter over the first and enter any communicating structures. A similar approach may allow cannulation of the bladder where the first catheter preferentially enters

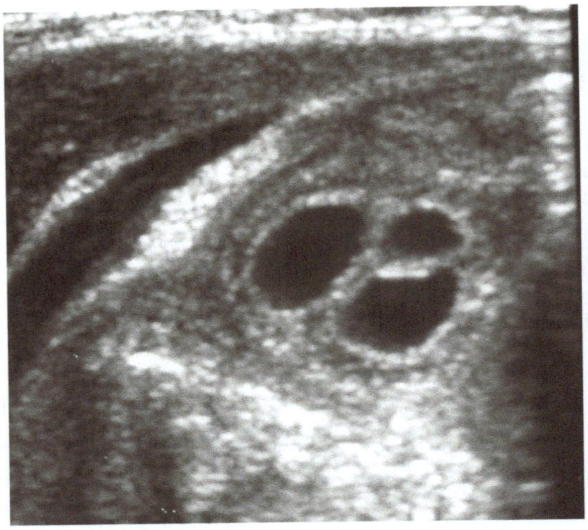

Fig. 3 Sonographic appearance of normal neonatal ovary

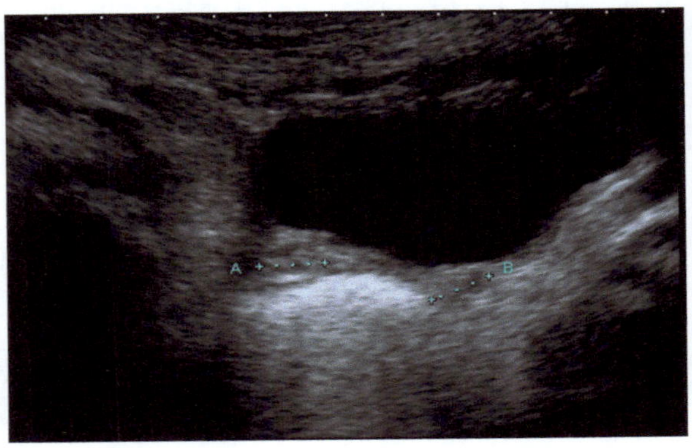

Fig. 4 Streak ovaries. Bilateral dysgenic ovarian tissue is just visible on transverse ultrasound of the pelvis

the vagina. Alternatively, the use of an inflated Foley catheter balloon on the perineal surface may create an adequate seal to permit retrograde injection of contrast at sufficient pressures to delineate any patent channel. It is important to explore all perineal openings.

8 The Role of Imaging in Delayed Diagnosis or Later Assessment

DSDs not associated with ambiguous genitalia not infrequently present well beyond the neonatal period. The chief role of ultrasound in the post-neonatal patient is in determining the location of undescended or occult testes and assessing the possible cause of primary amenorrhoea. Ultrasound may also identify streak gonads

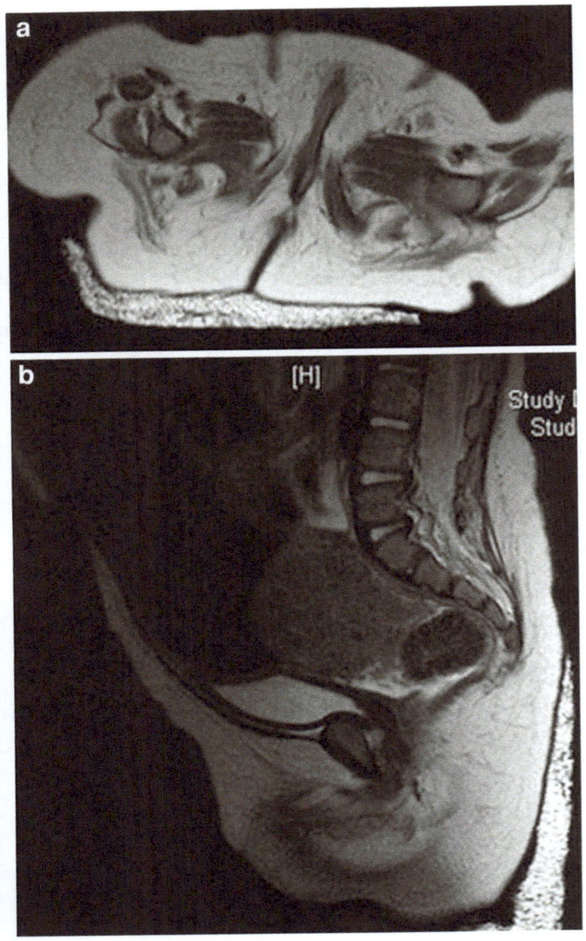

Fig. 5 T2-weighted MRI in a patient with ambiguous genitalia. **a** Axial, **b** sagittal midline and paramidline: the external genitalia were difficult to categorise, but no convincing Müllerian structures were identified. No gonads were seen on MRI or US, but there was a suggestion of prostatic tissue below the bladder base

(Fig. 4), or mixed gonadal tissue as in the case of ovotestes in ovotesticular DSD. Magnetic resonance imaging (MRI) has been shown to be of considerable value in cases where ultrasound is unable to elucidate the anatomy, although intra-abdominal testes and streak gonads remain challenging to image (Biswas et al. 2004).

In addition to demonstrating anatomy of ambiguous genital structures (clitoral hypertrophy vs. micropenis, for example), MRI can be used to assess adrenal size, the presence of occult uteri (Fig. 5) and associated renal anomalies. It is also of considerable value in the assessment of the hypothalamic–pituitary axis in suspected hypopituitarism.

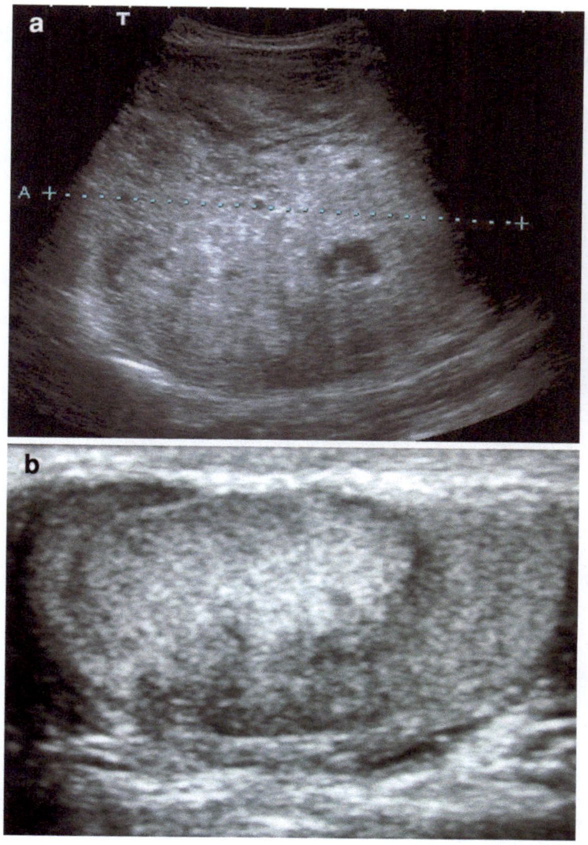

Fig. 6 Gonadoblastoma. **a** Delayed presentation of gonadal dysgenesis—this patient presented with an abdominal mass. Ultrasound demonstrates a well-defined mass (between callipers) of heterogeneous echotexture confirmed as a gonadoblastoma on histology. **b** Well-defined intratesticular echogenic focus identified in a patient with mixed gonadal dysgenesis

Occasionally the radiologist is called upon to image a patient with suspected malignant complication of DSD. This usually manifests as malignant change in a dysgenic gonad. Ultrasound is again the initial imaging modality of choice, and may demonstrate the heterogeneous echotexture of a gonadoblastoma (Fig. 6) or echogenic foci in the reproductive tract representing calcification in the early stages of malignant change. Denys–Drash syndrome (an autosomal dominant condition typically manifesting with nephropathy, Wilm's tumour and DSD) is included in the list of conditions where regular ultrasound is recommended for Wilm's tumour screening (Rao et al. 2008).

Computed tomography is not advocated in the assessment of patients with suspected disorders of sex development, but patients may present with adrenal enlargement as an incidental finding on abdominal imaging (Fig. 7).

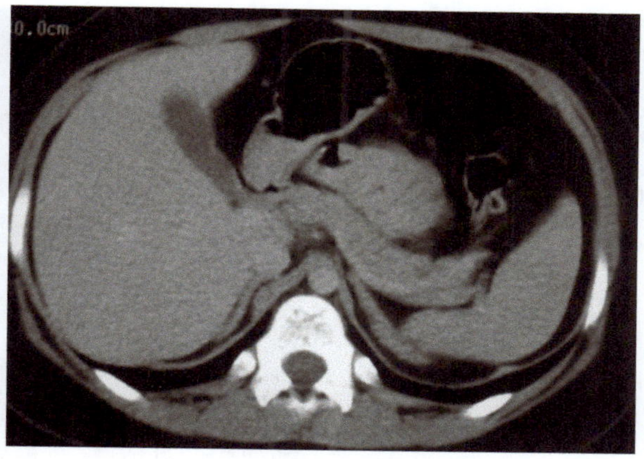

Fig. 7 Non-contrast CT demonstrating bilateral adrenal hyperplasia

9 46,XX Disorders of Sex Development

These disorders lead to virilisation of a 46,XX foetus.

9.1 Congenital Adrenal Hyperplasia

Congenital adrenal hyperplasia (CAH) describes a group of autosomal recessive disorders of cortisol synthesis (Merke and Bornstein 2005). More than 95% of cases are due to 21-hydroxylase deficiency (21-OHD) which is characterised by cortisol deficiency, androgen excess with variable aldosterone deficiency. The incidence of 21-OHD in the UK is approximately 1 in 10–15,000 births. 21-OHD is the commonest cause of ambiguous genitalia and this disorder will be discussed further.

The 21-hydroxylase gene is located on chromosome 6p21.3 and 1–2% of affected individuals result from spontaneous mutations. Most patients are compound heterozygotes. The phenotype shows a range of severity and is typically classified as classic (the severe form) and non-classic (the mild or late-onset form) (Merke and Bornstein 2005). Classic CAH is subclassified as salt-losing or non-salt losing (simple virilising), reflecting the degree of aldosterone deficiency. Individuals with non-classic CAH have manifestations of hyperandrogenism, generally later

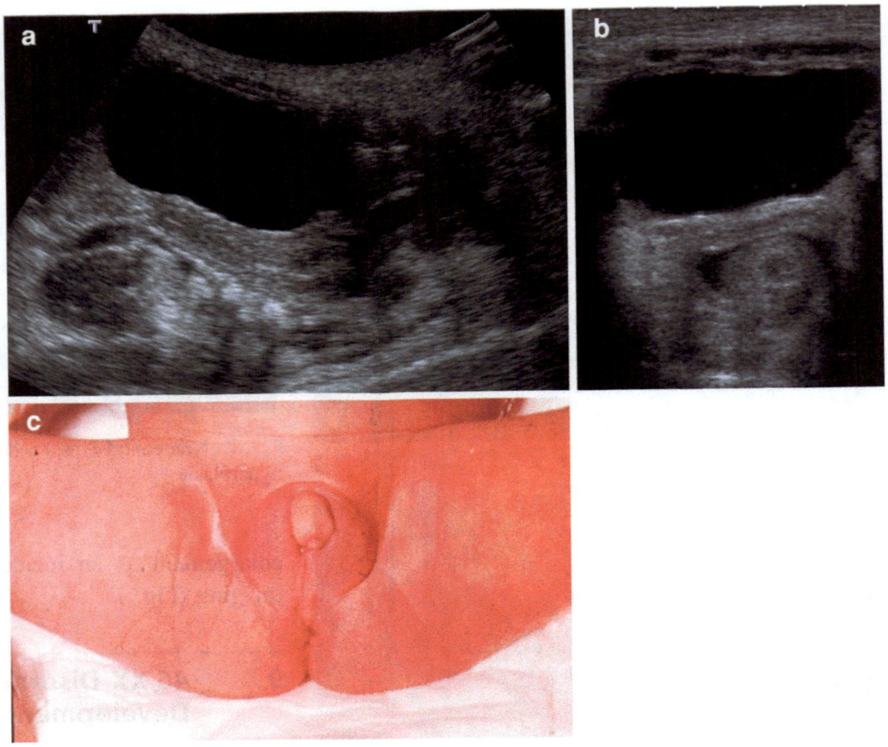

Fig. 8 Sagittal (**a**) and transverse (**b**) ultrasound of uterus in neonate with congenital adrenal hyperplasia (**c**) external appearance of a virilised female with CAH

in childhood or in early adulthood and this does not present as a DSD.

9.1.1 Clinical Features of 21-Hydroxylase Deficiency

Female infants with classic CAH typically have varying degrees of ambiguous genitalia at birth from exposure to high concentrations of androgens in utero. Characteristic findings vary from enlarged clitoris, partly fused and rugose labia majora to a fully virilised female with apparent male external phenotype but with no palpable gonads. A urogenital sinus in place of a distinct urethra and vagina is seen in the more severely affected. The internal female structures (uterus, fallopian tubes, upper vagina and ovaries) are normal and there are no Wolffian ducts. Male infants do not present as a DSD and may have no signs of CAH at birth, except subtle hyperpigmentation and possible penile enlargement, and the age at diagnosis varies according to the degree of aldosterone deficiency. Boys with the salt-losing form typically present at 7–14 days with a salt-losing crisis, whereas in girls ambiguous genitalia leads to earlier diagnosis and treatment.

9.1.2 Imaging Features of Congenital Adrenal Hyperplasia

Infants presenting with clinically suspected CAH are likely to require urgent imaging, as a prompt diagnosis is vital to prevent life-threatening complications of salt-wasting. Expected sonographic findings in CAH include normal neonatal uterus and ovaries in girls and normal testes in boys (Fig. 8). The adrenal glands may be enlarged: this can be difficult to appreciate in the neonate where the adrenal glands are normally prominent. The upper limit of normal for neonatal adrenal size has been defined as a limb width no greater than 4 mm. The demonstration of a lobulated or cerebriform surface has also been found to be of value in identifying adrenal hyperplasia (Al-Alwan et al. 1999) (Fig. 9).

Genitography is of value in demonstrating the degree of masculinisation of a 46,XX female genital tract: most commonly contrast delineates the vagina communicating with the distal portion of the urethra beyond which they jointly form a common channel, the urogenital sinus. This extends to the base of the phallus. A cervical impression may be noted at the apex of the vagina, and is a useful finding in confirming the presence of a uterus (Fig. 10). The urogenital sinus is

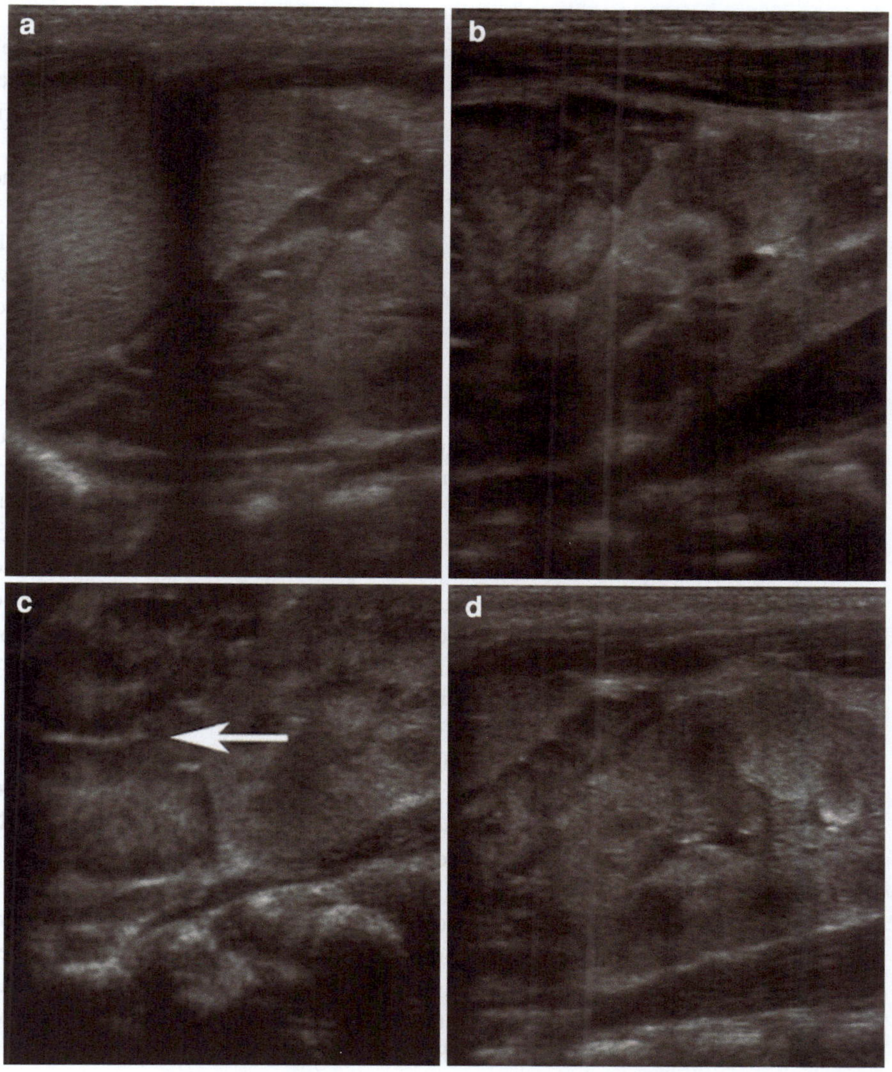

Fig. 9 Adrenal ultrasound in congenital adrenal hyperplasia. **a** The adrenal has a smooth outline, but limb width exceeds 4 mm. **b** Marked adrenal enlargement: the adrenal gland is larger than the adjacent kidney. **c** and **d** Demonstrate cerebriform and lobular margins—a helpful finding in CAH

of varying length depending on the level at which the vagina joins the urethra and the degree of phallic enlargement. Demonstration of the exact length and relationships of the urogenital sinus is of particular value in planning reconstructive surgery: the higher the connection between vaginal canal and urethra, the greater the risk of damage to the external urethral sphincter during vaginoplasty (Fig. 11).

9.1.3 Surgery in Congenital Adrenal Hyperplasia

It is important to classify the degree of virilization in order to plan the surgical approach and to compare the outcomes following various operative procedures. Previously this used the Prader classification, which simply graded the degree of virilisation of the external genitalia but gave no information on the urogenital confluence, which is vital when planning surgery. Some experts then described the urogenital confluence as being 'high' or 'low' which was of some help but with the modern operative procedures being influenced by actual distances a newer classification was required. Rink et al. (2005) have developed a user friendly classification that provided the urologist with all the data required to plan surgery and assess outcomes. This is the PVE classification; P represents the phallus and two measurements are given, the stretched length and the width; V represents the urogenital

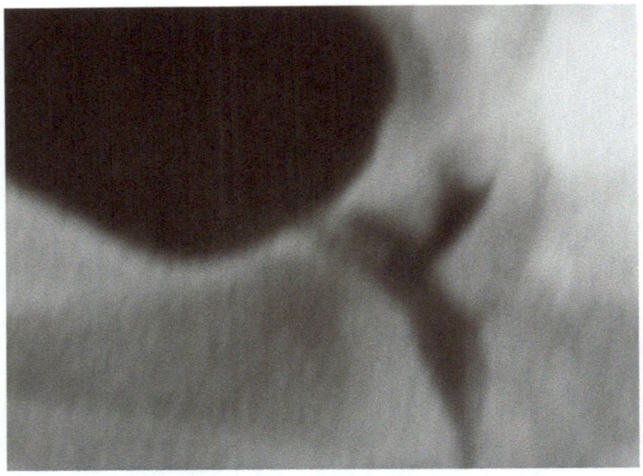

Fig. 10 Genitogram in an infant with CAH showing a long common channel (urogenital sinus) with a small vagina. A cervical impression is clearly visible at the apex of the vagina

confluence and two measurements are given, the distance from the confluence to the bladder neck and from the confluence to the perineal opening; E represents the external genitalia and is classified using the previously described Prader number. P and E are obviously clinical assessments but some diagnostic investigations are required for V. These are the sinogram and endoscopy. Therefore, when a sinogram is performed it is extremely helpful if the site of the confluence to the perineum is noted and the distance from the confluence to the bladder neck and the perineal opening is measured. Similar information is required from sinograms for other structural anomalies such as persistent cloaca and isolated urogenital sinus (see Structural Abnormalities of the Female Reproductive Tract). If the distance from the confluence to the perineum is <3 cm, surgical reconstruction in the form of a total urogenital mobilisation (TUM) is the procedure of choice.

9.1.4 21-Hydroxylase Deficiency and Adrenal Rest Tumours

In prenatal life, the adrenal gland develops in close proximity to the gonads, and separation of both does not evolve until the adrenal groove becomes prominent. Prior to this, adrenal cortical tissue may become adherent to the gonad. This aberrant adrenal tissue may then descend with the testes or ovary (Dahl and Bahn 1962; Symonds and Driscoll 1973) and is responsive to ACTH (Stikkelbroeck et al. 2001).

Adrenal rest tumours are ACTH-dependent and usually develop during periods of sustained elevation of plasma ACTH levels and may result from inadequate glucocorticoid dosing or non-compliance with treatment, although they have been observed with satisfactory treatment. There may be palpable lumps on the testes which may lead to a misdiagnosis of a Leydig cell tumour and unnecessary testicular biopsy and orchidectomy. However, features like young age, bilateral presence of tumours, absence of metastases and decreased size with glucocorticoid may lead to investigation confirming the diagnosis of CAH. In most patients the diagnosis of CAH is made before the tumours become manifest. They have a fairly typical appearance on ultrasound scan (Barwick et al. 2005) where the adrenal rests are seen as well-defined, hypoechoic, vascular rounded foci clustered around the mediastinum testis (Fig. 12). The tumours have a direct adverse effect on testicular function and fertility (Martinez-Aguayo et al. 2007) and may regress when glucocorticoid treatment is instituted or intensified.

10 46,XY Disorders of Sex Development

These disorders cause varying degrees of male undermasculinisation, from glandular hypospadias, micropenis, ambiguous genitalia to an external female phenotype. There are many different causes and the aetiology can be subdivided as defects in testes determination, androgen biosynthesis and androgen action (Table 2).

10.1 Defects in Testis Determination

These disorders result from failure of sex determination either by abnormal development of the bipotential gonad from the genital ridge, or from abnormal Sertoli or Leydig cell development from the bipotential gonad. The result is gonadal dysgenesis. These gonads have a high risk for malignant transformation (15–35%) (Hughes et al. 2006).

When both gonads are streaks there is a female external phenotype and thus 46,XY complete gonadal dysgenesis and complete sex reversal (previously known as Swyer syndrome). There is a high risk of

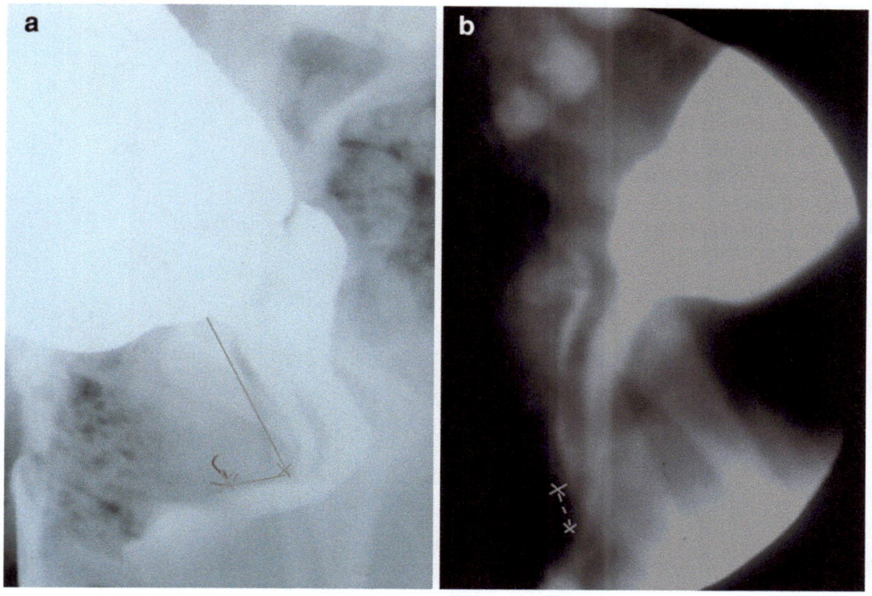

Fig. 11 Variation in length of urogenital sinus (see also Fig. 10). **a** Intermediate length urogenital sinus: genitogram showing measurements from bladder neck to confluence and from confluence to perineal opening. **b** Short length

gonadoblastoma and germinoma in streak gonads and early surgical removal is usually recommended.

Partial gonadal dysgenesis (associated with a 46,XY karyotype) or mixed gonadal dysgenesis (associated with 45,XO/46,XY chromosomal mosaicism) may lead to ambiguous genitalia. Inadequate AMH production from poor Sertoli cell function leads to Müllerian remnants which may be detected by ultrasound. In the persistent Müllerian duct syndrome (from AMH deficiency or AMH resistance) Müllerian remnants may be identified coincidentally when the patient is undergoing routine surgery for undescended testis, the external genitalia will be normal. In other disorders, reduced Leydig cell function leads to incomplete masculinisation from severe hypospadias, clitoromegaly to complete sex reversal. Some of these disorders may be associated with other features that are important to consider, such as adrenal insufficiency (SF-1 mutations) and Wilm's tumours (WT-1 mutations and Denys–Drash syndrome).

10.2 Imaging of 46,XY Disorders of Sex Differentiation

The findings at genitography in mixed gonadal dysgenesis generally resemble those in CAH, with a vagina of varying size communicating with the urethra to form a urogenital sinus. Occasionally complex anomalies may be delineated (Fig. 13). Sonography may demonstrate a unilateral testis, which is usually incompletely descended and often intra-abdominal. A streak gonad is usually present on the other side, and may occasionally be demonstrated with ultrasound, although the majority of streak gonads are not identified on either ultrasound or MRI (Biswas et al. 2004).

The sonographic approach when searching for the testis should include careful scrutiny of the inguinal canal, anterior thigh and abdominal contents. MRI should be the next step if a testis cannot be found with ultrasound: even though the detection rate remains below 100% for intra-abdominal testes, this is still better than a blind surgical approach (Kanemoto et al. 2005).

10.3 Defects in Androgen Biosynthesis

These disorders result in abnormalities of sex differentiation. Defects in the synthesis of androgen production cause undermasculinisation and sex reversal of the male infant. Many are enzyme defects of adrenal steroid biosynthesis. Sertoli function is usually unaffected and Müllerian structures are thus absent. Adrenal insufficiency is a feature in many of these disorders.

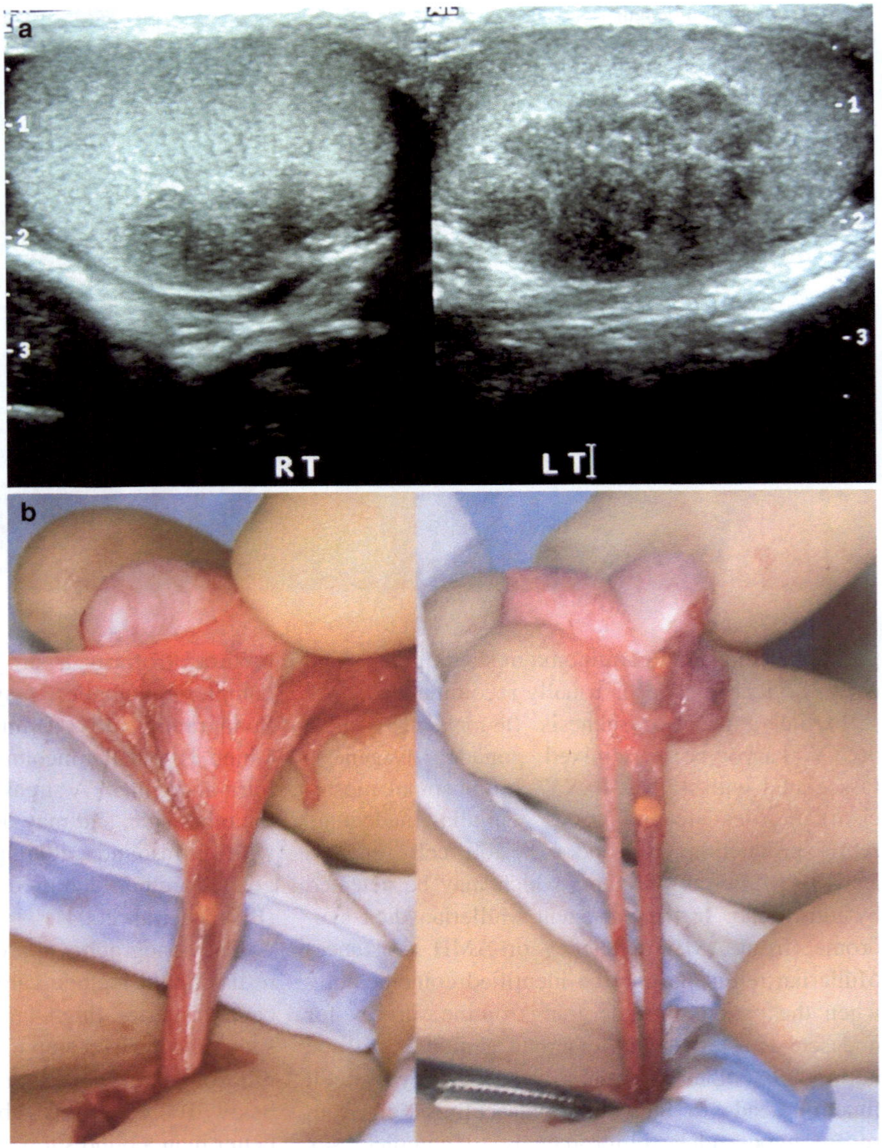

Fig. 12 **a** Ultrasound of testicular adrenal rests: longitudinal scans of both testes show well-defined hypoechoic lesions bilaterally. These have slightly lobulated margins and some internal echogenic 'septa'. **b** Macroscopic appearance of adrenal rest tumours

11 Defects in Androgen Action

11.1 Androgen insensitivity syndromes

Androgen insensitivity syndrome (AIS) results from target tissue resistance to androgen action from mutations in the androgen receptor (AR) gene or from post-receptor abnormalities. AIS is estimated to be present in 1:20,000–64,000 male births. The gene for the AR is on the X chromosome and maps to Xq11–q12. The AR binds testosterone and has an even greater affinity for DHT.

Affected individuals have a 46,XY karyotype. The clinical manifestations vary from normal female external genitalia (complete AIS) to varying degrees of male undermasculinisation (partial AIS) (Fig. 14). The testes function normally and production of AMH from Sertoli cells in utero prevents the development of Fallopian tubes, uterus and upper third of the vagina. Leydig cells produce testosterone and serum levels are often in the male adult range. The Wolffian

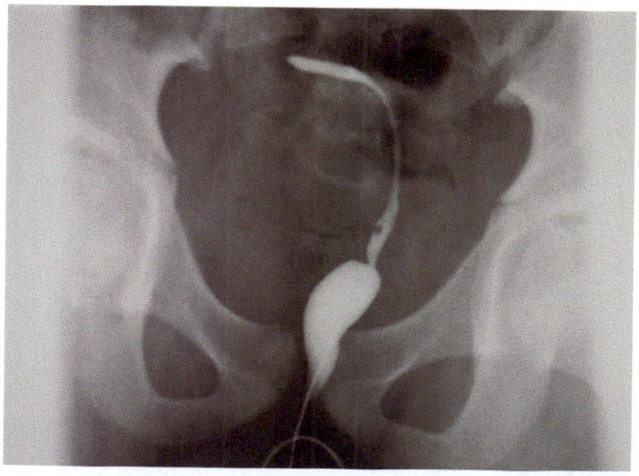

Fig. 13 Patient with confirmed left-sided scrotal testis and right streak ovary. A catheter was passed at cystoscopy into an opening in the verumontanum and contrast injection showed a uterine structure and blind-ending Fallopian tube. Laparotomy confirmed the presence of a uterus communicating with the verumontanum. The Fallopian tube and streak ovary were removed

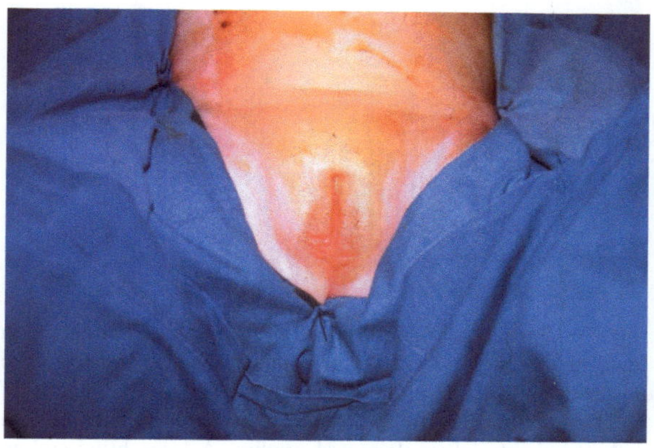

Fig. 14 Partial androgen insensitivity syndrome. There is severe undermasculinisation

structures are present but often underdeveloped and there is no prostate or seminal vesicles. The gonads may be intra-abdominal and have a low risk of malignant transformation (<2%) in complete AIS, whereas the risk is increased in partial AIS (50%) (Hughes et al. 2006).

11.1.1 Complete Androgen Insensitivity Syndrome

Individuals with complete androgen insensitivity syndrome (CAIS) have a 46,XY karyotype with a normal female external phenotype. Most are diagnosed early when inguinal hernias or inguinal or labial swellings in an apparently female infant are found to be testes, and inguinal hernias are observed in up to 90% of cases of CAIS. Some have suggested that the incidence of AIS in female infants with hernias are as high as 12%, and a karyotype should be performed in such individuals (Viner et al. 1997; Ahmed et al. 2000). The clitoris has a normal female appearance, there is a blind vaginal pouch and often slightly hypoplastic labia majora. The testes may have a normal appearance on ultrasound scan but histology shows hypoplastic seminiferous tubules. The testes may be intra-abdominal or palpable in the inguinal region or labioscrotal folds. A later presentation of CAIS is during puberty with primary amenorrhoea and absent pubic and axillary hair. Breast development is normal as the elevated testosterone levels are aromatised to oestrogens. As adults, there is a normal female habitus, and both sexual orientation and gender identity are unaffected. Testes have a low malignant potential and are often removed in early adulthood. Vaginal dilators may be required if the vagina is inadequate for sexual intercourse.

11.1.2 Partial Androgen Insensitivity Syndrome

Individuals with partial androgen insensitivity syndrome (PAIS) have a 46,XY karyotype with a broad spectrum of clinical severity of undermasculinisation (Fig. 14). In the most severe form, individuals have clitoromegaly and labioscrotal folds and posterior labial fusion. At the other extreme the genitalia are male but small or there may be a coronal hypospadias. During puberty, sparse sex hair and gynaecomastia may develop and in adulthood, spermatogenesis and fertility may be impaired.

11.1.3 Imaging in Androgen Insensitivity Syndrome

Sonography fails to detect a uterus or ovaries, but undescended testes may be found in the labia, inguinal canal or higher along the line of descent (Fig. 15). As with mixed gonadal dysgenesis, accurate localisation of the gonads is important as there is a risk of malignancy.

In PAIS, patients are more likely to present earlier with ambiguous genitalia. Where the phenotype is predominantly female the imaging findings resemble those in complete androgen insensitivity, with

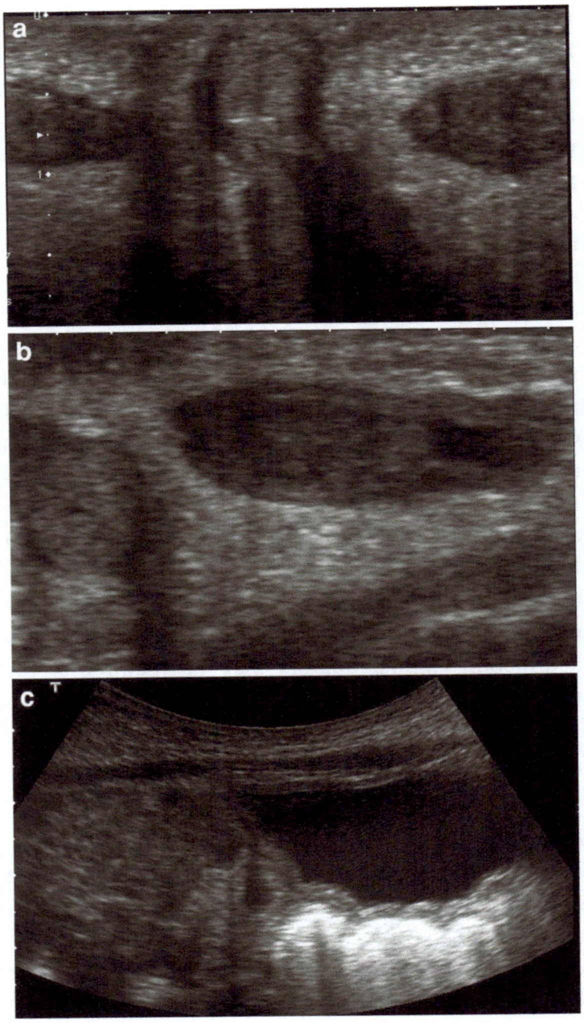

Fig. 15 Androgen insensitivity syndrome. Neonate with female external genitalia. **a**, **b** Transverse and longitudinal ultrasound of the labia reveals bilateral gonads. **c** Pelvic ultrasound shows absence of uterus

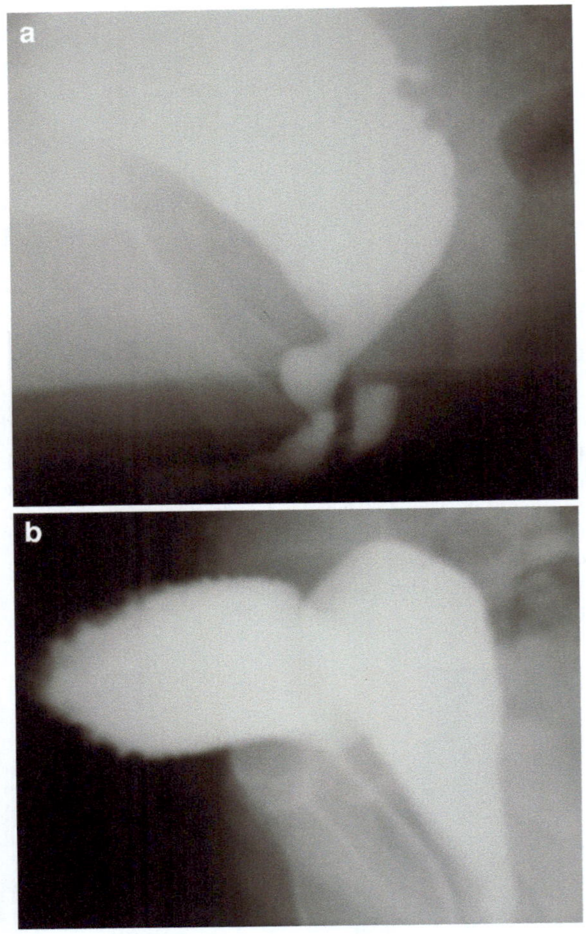

Fig. 16 Partial androgen insensitivity syndrome. Patients with male phenotype. **a** A small utriculus is seen arising from the posterior urethra: the urethra is elongated and predominantly of male configuration. **b** Contrast is seen in the bladder, with a catheter visible in an elongated urethra. A large blind-ending pouch is seen behind the bladder, arising from the posterior urethra. There is no evidence of a cervical impression on the apex of this utriculus

absence of uterus and ovaries, but Wolffian duct remnants can be seen on contrast studies, together with a degree of elongation of the urethra. Where the phenotype is predominantly male, sonography again fails to demonstrate ovaries or uterus, but contrast studies are likely to show a blind-ending vaginal pouch (utricle) connecting to the posterior urethra. Importantly, there is no cervical impression on this pseudovagina (Fig. 16).

11.2 5α-Reductase Deficiency

Testosterone is converted locally by 5α-reductase to the more potent DHT that promotes the development of the male external genitalia from the common anlage. Fusion of the labioscrotal folds is a DHT-dependent process. Mutations in the SRD5A2 gene lead to 5α-reductase deficiency. Affected individuals have varying degrees of external undermasculinisation but

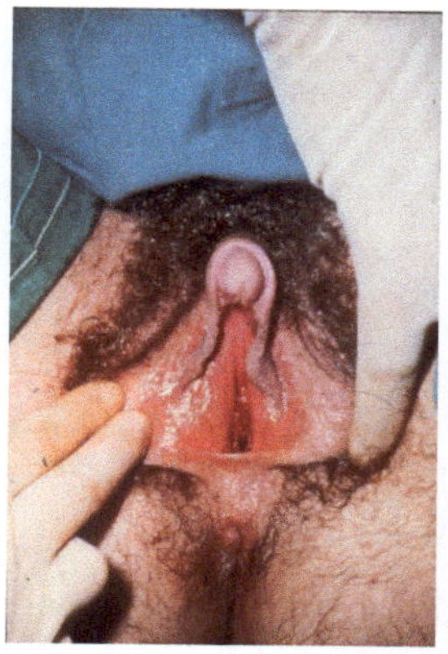

Fig. 17 5α-Reductase deficiency. This 46,XY individual was raised female and virilised with clitoromegaly during puberty

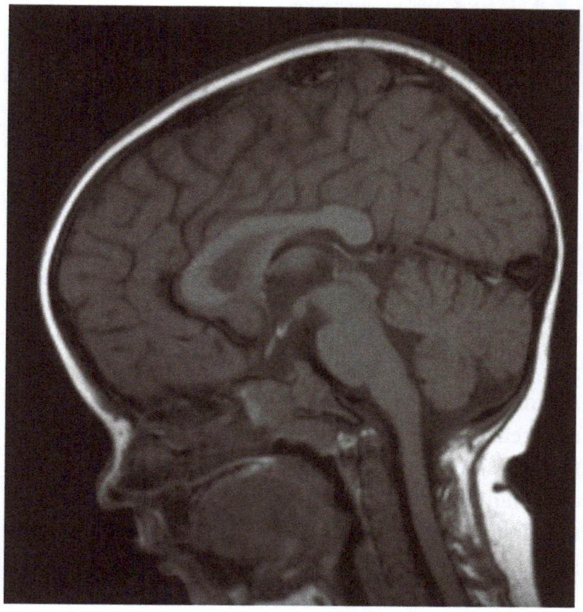

Fig. 18 Sagittal T1-weighted MRI. The pituitary 'bright spot' is ectopic and the hypothalamic stalk is elongated

occasionally micropenis or hypospadias are the only features (Sinnecker et al. 1996). Müllerian structures are absent as Sertoli cell function is normal. The incidence of 5α-reductase deficiency is increased in the Dominican republic, New Guinea, Turkey and Egypt. It is a cause of non-isosexual puberty, i.e. where a 46,XY individual, with female external genitalia or severe undermasculinisation during childhood then subsequently virilises during puberty (Fig. 17).

12 Congenital Hypopituitarism

Genital abnormalities may be associated with other midline abnormalities such as hypopituitarism. Abnormalities of gonadotrophin (LH and FSH) secretion in utero may lead to a reduction of testosterone production and present in the newborn period with hypoplastic genitalia with undescended testes and a micropenis. Other features of wider pituitary dysfunction may be present such as prolonged jaundice and adrenal insufficiency (ACTH deficiency), hypoglycaemia (ACTH and GH deficiency) and diabetes insipidus (AVP deficiency). MRI is of value in identifying ectopic pituitary tissue and hypothalamic anomalies (Fig. 18). Hypopituitarism may occur as part of septo-optic dysplasia with features such as absent septum pellucidum on cranial ultrasound.

13 Ovotesticular Disorders of Sex Development

Affected individuals have both testicular and ovarian tissue that is well differentiated. If the gonad contains ovarian tissue with follicles and testicular tissue with seminiferous tubules, the gonad is an ovotestis which is a histological diagnosis. These gonads often have a soft consistency. The commonest karyotype is 46,XX (70%) and the next commonest is 46,XX/46,XY (20%). An ovotestis may release excessive androgens leading to virilisation of an infant with female external genitalia, conversely inadequate testosterone production leads to undermasculinisation in the infant with male external genitalia.

Ovotestes may become clinically apparent at puberty when the hypothalamic–pituitary–gonadal axis becomes active. FSH release at this time stimulates follicular development in the ovotestis and there may be a clinical presentation with a new testicular lump and pain from ovulation. The ovotestes have the potential to release oestradiol and cause feminisation, such as gynaecomastia, in a phenotypic male.

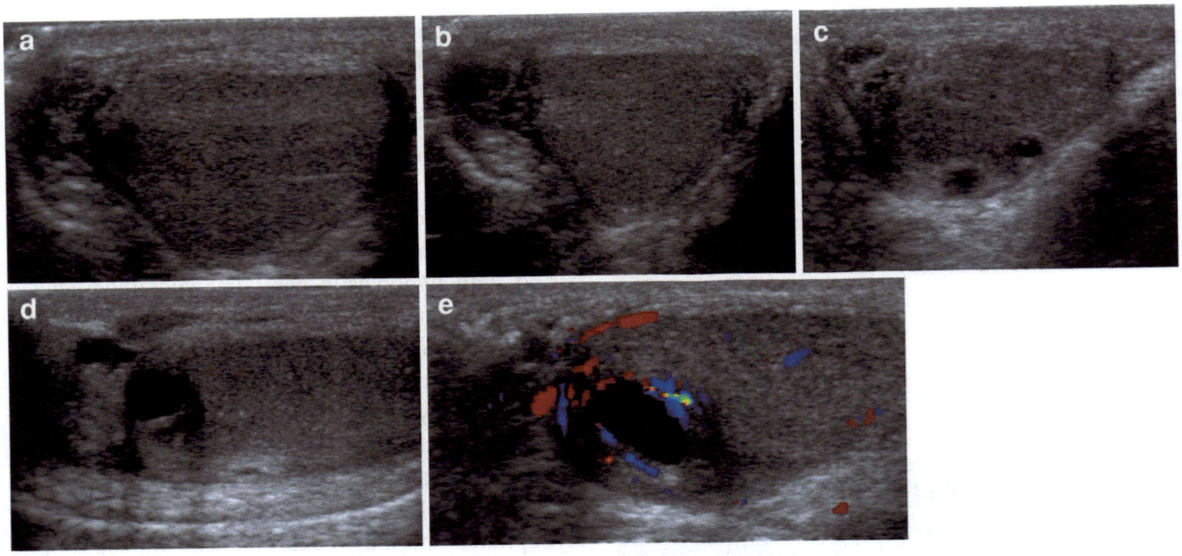

Fig. 19 Ultrasound of ovotestis. **a**, **b** Pre-pubertal study shows a gonad with typical testicular appearance, with the exception of the suggestion a small cluster of cysts at the upper pole. **c** At puberty several small cysts become visible in the periphery of the gonad. **d**, **e** Sonography during an episode of testicular pain demonstrates several large anechoic, avascular areas representing enlarging follicular cysts

13.1 Imaging of Ovotesticular DSD

Imaging in this condition concentrates on determining the type of gonadal tissue present on each side. The majority of patients will have one ovotestis, where the gonad contains elements of both ovarian and testicular tissue, and a testis or ovary on the other side. Less commonly patients have an ovary on one side and a testis on the other, and still less frequently there are ovotestes on both sides. The sonographic appearance of an ovotestis is variable: in infancy and early childhood the ovarian component may be difficult to appreciate, and it may be impossible to differentiate between a testis and ovotestis. This often becomes more obvious approaching puberty when ovarian follicles become evident (Fig. 19). A uterus is almost always present. There is also great variability in appearance of the external genitalia and inguinal herniae containing gonads are a common feature.

14 Management of Disorders of Sex Development

Initially the baby should be admitted to the neonatal unit for observation and monitored for manifestations of adrenal insufficiency such as hypoglycaemia and salt-wasting. The aim is to assign gender as early as possible, which involves consultation of the parents with a paediatric endocrinologist, paediatric urologist and a psychologist. The need to establish a diagnosis should not delay gender assignment. The infant is referred to as 'your baby' until gender is assigned though some parents prefer to use a non-gender-specific name during this time. Surgery is appropriate in the first year of life for 46,XX DSD, whereas hypospadias repair is usually undertaken between 12 and 18 months of age. A view is emerging that feminising surgery for undermasculinised males may be inappropriate in terms of the potential for fertility and psychological and adverse sexual health in adulthood.

At the outset, the family should be informed of the plan for any medical and surgical interventions that may be needed over the coming years. When counselling families regarding gender assignment it is important to be sensitive to the wider social and cultural implications this may have within different communities. The criteria for consideration of gender assignment include the diagnosis, presence of female structures, adequacy of phallic tissue, potential for fertility and the parental wishes and cultural aspects.

These individuals require life-long follow-up. There is now a move for affected individuals to be seen in a dedicated regional DSD service. During childhood and adolescence regular contact with medical services is required to address ongoing issues of growth, medication administration, psychosexual development, fertility and surgical outcomes. Diagnosis and karyotype disclosure to the patient must be handled sensitively and is usually planned over a number of discussions with input from parents and the DSD team. Individuals with a DSD have disparate health needs, and input from many different specialties is usual. Historically, this group have frequently been lost to follow-up at the time of transfer to adult services despite their ongoing complex health needs. Thus, transition to adult services should be planned carefully and with close coordination between paediatric and adult health professionals.

References

Ahmed SF, Hughes IA (2002) The genetics of male undermasculinization. Clin Endocrinol (Oxf) 56:1–18

Ahmed SF, Cheng A, Dovey L, Hawkins JR, Martin H, Rowland J, Shimura N, Tait AD, Hughes IA (2000) Phenotypic features, androgen receptor binding, and mutational analysis in 278 clinical cases reported as androgen insensitivity syndrome. J Clin Endocrinol Metab 85:658–665

Al-Alwan I, Navarro O, Daneman D, Daneman A (1999) Clinical utility of adrenal ultrasonography in the diagnosis of congenital adrenal hyperplasia. J Pediatr 135:71–75

Barwick TD, Malhotra A, Webb JAW, Savage MO, Reznek RH (2005) Embryology of the adrenal glands and its relevance to diagnostic imaging. Clin Radiol 60:953–959

Biswas K, Kapoor A, Karak AK, Kriplani A, Gupta DK, Kucheria K, Ammini A (2004) Imaging in intersex disorders. J Pediatr Endocrinol Metab 17:841–845

Dahl EV, Bahn RC (1962) Aberrant adrenal cortical tissue near the testis in human infants. Am J Pathol 40: 587–598

Federman DD (2004) Three facets of sexual differentiation. N Engl J Med 350:323–324

Hughes IA, Houk C, Ahmed SF et al (2006) Consensus statement on management of intersex disorders. LWPES Consensus Group; ESPE Consensus Group. Arch Dis Child 91:554–563

Kanemoto K, Hayashi Y, Kojima Y, Maruyama T, Ito M, Kohri K (2005) Accuracy of ultrasonography and magnetic resonance imaging in the diagnosis of non-palpable testis. Int J Urol 12:668–672

MacLaughlin DT, Donahoe PK (2004) Sex determination and differentiation. N Engl J Med 350:367–378

Martinez-Aguayo A, Rocha A, Rojas N, García C, Parra R, Lagos M, Valdivia L, Poggi H, Cattani A (2007) Chilean Collaborative Testicular Adrenal Rest Tumor Study Group. Testicular adrenal rest tumors and Leydig and Sertoli cell function in boys with classical congenital adrenal hyperplasia. J Clin Endocrinol Metab 92:4583–4589

Merke DP, Bornstein SR (2005) Congenital adrenal hyperplasia. Lancet 365:2125–2136

Ogilvy-Stuart AL, Brain CE (2004) Early assessment of ambiguous genitalia. Arch Dis Child 89:401–407

Rao A, Rothman J, Nichols KE (2008) Genetic testing and tumour surveillance for children with cancer predisposition syndromes. Curr Opin Paediatr 20:1–7

Rink RC, Adams MC, Misseri R (2005) A new classification for genital ambiguity and urogenital sinus anomalies. BJU Int 95:638–642

Sinnecker GH, Hiort O, Dibbelt L, Albers N, Dörr HG et al (1996) Phenotypic classification of male pseudohermaphroditism due to steroid 5 alpha-reductase 2 deficiency. Am J Med Genet 63:223–230

Stikkelbroeck NM, Otten BJ, Pasic A, Jager GJ, Sweep CG, Noordam K, Hermus AR (2001) High prevalence of testicular adrenal rest tumours, impaired spermatogenesis, and Leydig cell failure in adolescents and adult males with congenital adrenal hyperplasia. J Clin Endocrinol Metab 86:5721–5728

Symonds DA, Driscoll SG (1973) An adrenal cortical rest within the fetal ovary: report of a case. Am J Clin Pathol 60:562–564

Thomas WS (2009) Langman's medical embryology, 11th edn. Lippincott Williams and Wilkins, Baltimore

Viner RM, Teoh Y, Williams DM, Patterson MN, Hughes IA (1997) Androgen insensitivity syndrome: a survey of diagnostic procedures and management in the UK. Arch Dis Child 77:305–309

Gynaecological Disorders in the Neonate and Young Child

Gurdeep S. Mann and Angela T. Byrne

Contents

1	**Introduction**	52
2	**Neonatal Ovarian Cysts**	52
3	**Complex Neonatal Ovarian Cyst and Adnexal Torsion**	54
4	**Congenital Obstruction of the Gynaecological Tract**	55
5	**Cloacal Anomalies**	56
6	**Interlabial Mass**	59
6.1	Gynaecological Causes	59
6.2	Urological Causes	59
6.3	Diagnostic Work-up	60
7	**Labial Masses**	60
8	**Vaginal Discharge**	62
9	**Conclusion**	63
References		63

G. S. Mann (✉)
Department of Radiology,
Alder Hey Children's Hospital NHS Foundation Trust,
Liverpool, UK
e-mail: gurdeep.mann@alderhey.nhs.uk

G. S. Mann
Department of Radiology,
Liverpool Women's Hospital NHS Foundation Trust,
Liverpool, UK

A. T. Byrne
Department of Radiology,
British Columbia Children's Hospital,
University of British Columbia,
Vancouver, BC, Canada

Abstract

Improvements in antenatal imaging have resulted in greater detection of genitourinary pathology in the female fetus such as ovarian cyst, hydrocolpos and cloacal malformation. Postnatal US imaging follow-up is initially indicated in these children and will contribute significantly to the subsequent management plan, including the timing and nature of imaging follow-up. US is the first line investigation for a suspected abdominopelvic mass, inguinal hernia or labial mass. This chapter will review the role of diagnostic imaging in the neonate or young child with suspected ovarian or genital tract pathology.

Abbreviations

DSD	Disorders of sex development
NOC	Neonatal ovarian cyst
β-hCG	Beta Human Chorionic Gonadotropin
US	Ultrasound
LH	Luteinising hormone
HPO	Hypothalamic-Pituitary-Ovarian
FSH	Follicle stimulating hormone
IVC	Inferior vena cava
CT	Computed Tomography
MRI	Magnetic Resonance Imaging
UGS	Urogenital sinus
VACTERL	Vertebral, Anorectal, Cardiac, Esophageal, Renal, Limb defects
F	French
MR	Magnetic Resonance
DMSA	Dimercaptosuccinic acid
MAG-3	Mercapto-acetyltriglycine
AIS	Androgen Insensitivity Syndrome

G. Mann et al. (eds.), *Imaging of Gynecological Disorders in Infants and Children*, Medical Radiology. Diagnostic Imaging, DOI: 10.1007/174_2011_435,

1 Introduction

Ongoing developments in antenatal imaging have resulted in improved detection of genitourinary pathology in the female fetus. Antenatally detectable conditions include ovarian cysts (Bryant and Laufer 2004), hydrocolpos (Winderl and Silverman 1995; Dhombres et al. 2007), cloacal malformations Warne et al. (2002a, b), ambiguous external genitalia (Pajkrt et al. 2008) and congenital adrenal hyperplasia (Chambrier et al. 2002). Postnatal US imaging follow-up is indicated in these children and will contribute significantly to subsequent management. US is the first line investigation for a suspected abdomino-pelvic mass, inguinal hernia, labial mass or congenital anatomical anomaly. This chapter will review the role of diagnostic imaging in the neonate or young child with suspected ovarian or genital tract pathology.

2 Neonatal Ovarian Cysts

An ovarian cyst is defined by its size and ultrasound characteristics. The diameter of an ovarian microcyst, also referred to as a 'follicle', does not exceed 10 mm. Ovarian follicles are seen throughout childhood and are a normal finding. An ovarian macrocyst, also referred to as an 'ovarian cyst' is defined by a diameter exceeding 10 mm.

Ovarian cysts are common in infancy. The reported incidence of antenatally diagnosed, clinically significant ovarian cysts is around 1 in 2,500 live births (Bryant and Laufer 2004). Ovarian cysts are the most common cause of antenatally sonographically diagnosed abdominopelvic cystic mass in the female fetus (Fig. 1). Approximately 20% of newborn girls have ovarian cysts which exceed 10 mm in diameter (Vogtlander et al. 2003). During the last trimester fetal gonadotropin (LH and FSH) levels fall, but rise following delivery, only to fall again at three months of age. The postnatal rise in gonadotropins is attributed to immaturity of the hypothalamic-pituitary-ovarian (HPO) axis, this is also referred to as an immature gonadostat. Once the gonadostat responds to the negative feedback from the postnatal fall in the levels of sex hormones—mainly oestrogens, FSH and LH levels fall to prepubertal levels. Most neonatal ovarian cysts result from disordered folliculogenesis.

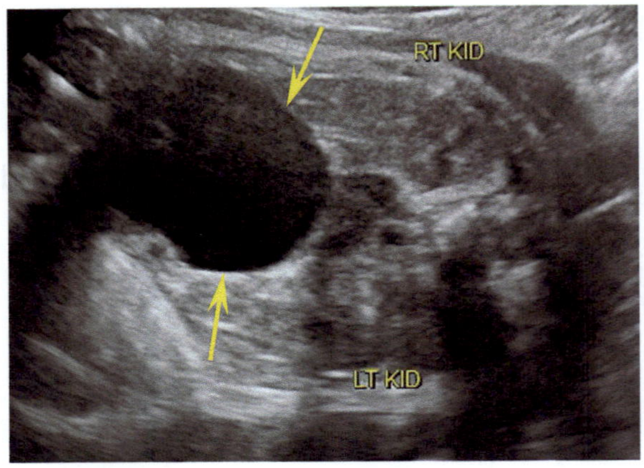

Fig. 1 Fetal ovarian cyst. Transverse section through the fetal pelvis (female) at 36 weeks gestation showing an anechoic ovarian cyst (*arrows*)

Table 1 Pelvic mass lesions arising from the female neonate

Cystic mass	Solid mass
Hydrocolpos	Sacrococcygeal teratoma
Ovarian cyst	Neuroblastoma
Urinary bladder	Pelvic kidney
Ureteric dilatation	Adnexal torsion
Adnexal torsion	Haemorrhagic ovarian cyst
Enteric duplication cyst	
Meconium pseudocyst	
Cloacal malformation	
Urachal cyst	
Omental cyst	
Mesenteric cyst	
Neuroenteric cyst	
Lymphangioma	
Anterior meningomyelocele	

Postnatal US is essential in the follow-up and characterisation of an antenatally detected cystic mass. The most common palpable pathological cystic lesion in the neonatal abdomen is a hydronephrotic kidney. In a female neonate, an ovarian cyst must always be considered as a cause of an abdominopelvic cystic mass unless both ovaries have been demonstrated. The differential for neonatal abdominal or pelvic cystic masses are summarised in Table 1 and includes mesenteric, omental, urachal or duplication cyst.

The US appearances of an uncomplicated neonatal ovarian cyst (NOC) are fairly typical. Simple cysts are unilocular, anechoic elliptical or spherical lesions,

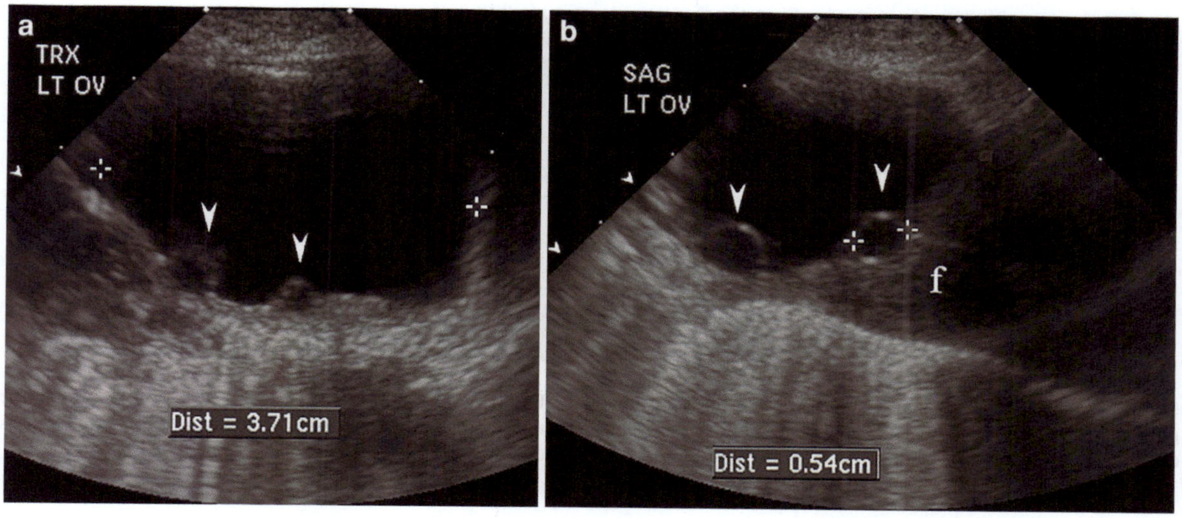

Fig. 2 Neonatal ovarian cyst. **a** Transverse and **b** longitudinal US images showing a left ovarian cyst in a newborn girl adjacent to the uterine fundus (*f*). Small daughter cysts are demonstrated in the periphery (*arrowheads*) and are a specific feature of cysts of ovarian origin

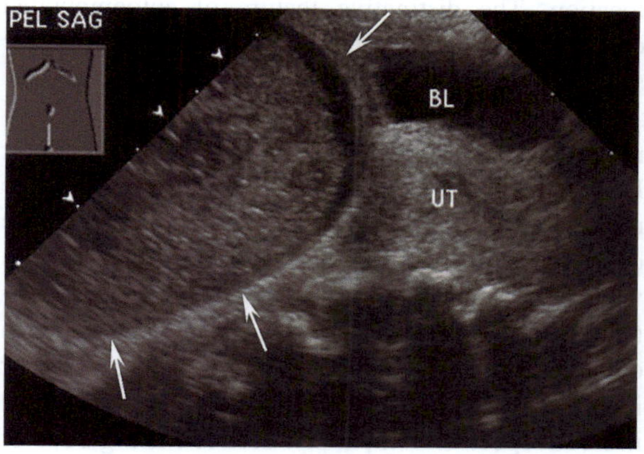

Fig. 3 Intestinal duplication cyst in a newborn female. Longitudinal US image showing a cyst with echogenic content lined by the characteristic double-wall sign (*arrows*) also referred to as gut signature. Uterus (*UT*), urinary bladder (*BL*)

with a uniform barely perceptible wall (Fig. 2a). Where present, a small 'daughter cyst' (Fig. 2b) in the wall of the primary cyst is a specific sign suggestive of an ovarian cyst (Lee et al. 2000). Duplication cysts have typical features, the so-called 'double-wall sign' (Fig. 3), due to the layered appearance of enteric mucosa and the hypoechoic muscularis in the duplication cyst wall in around half of cases. The double-wall sign has also been described in two cases of ovarian torsion (Godfrey et al. 1998). Omental cysts can bleed and may be indistinguishable from complex ovarian cysts. An omental cyst should be considered in a female infant with a complex cystic mass where both ovaries are visualised (Enriquez et al. 2005). The diagnostic criteria for a NOC include:

- Confirmation of female sex
- Identification of normal gastrointestinal and urinary tract structures
- Identification of a thin-walled cystic structure located off the midline (Bryant and Laufer 2004).

The incidence of NOC increases with rising placental chorionic gonadotropin levels in complicated pregnancies with a large placenta such as in diabetes mellitus, rhesus incompatibility and pre-eclampsia (Akin et al. 2010). Ovarian hyperstimulation in preterm babies results from immaturity of the gonadostat mechanism. FSH and LH levels in infants continue to increase until the maturation of the gonadostat mechanism, cysts may enlarge in the first three months of life. Following this, the influence of maternal and placental oestrogens and β-hCG wanes, and most NOC resolve spontaneously. NOC are also associated with endocrinopathies including fetal hypothyroidism and congenital adrenal hyperplasia, the latter due to 21-hydroxylase deficiency or 11-β-hydroxylase deficiency (Akin et al. 2010).

The management of most NOC is expectant and conservative. Serial ultrasound follow-up is all that is required until the cyst regresses and involutes spontaneously. There are no consensus guidelines as to the management of large, growing or complex ovarian cysts (Fig. 4). The decision to intervene must be

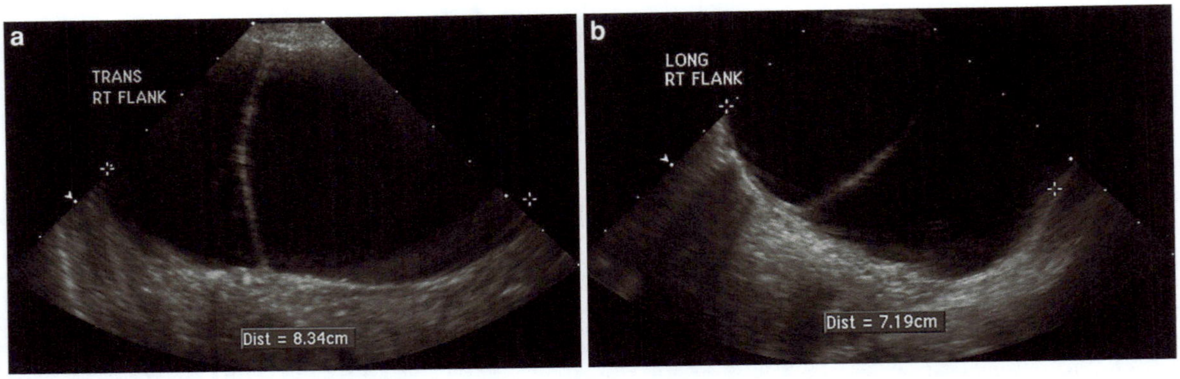

Fig. 4 Giant neonatal ovarian cyst. **a** Transverse and **b** longitudinal US images showing a large ovarian cyst (between callipers). A single thin-walled septa is demonstrated, this finding does not imply the presence of a complex cyst in the absence of any other findings. Colour Doppler US was unremarkable

based on cyst size, US characteristics and clinical symptoms. Symptomatic cysts merit intervention. NOC when sufficiently large may result in bowel or urinary tract obstruction, IVC compression or rarely life-threatening respiratory compromise (Muller-Leisse et al. 1992). Severe complications include shock from cyst haemorrhage, ascites, peritonitis and adhesions from perforation, and incarceration in ovarian inguinal herniae. Criteria for management have been established at several individual centres; however, controversy over conservative versus surgical therapy remains. Percutaneous ultrasound-guided cyst aspiration and evacuation should be reserved for large anechoic cysts >5 cm in diameter which have traditionally been considered at higher risk of torsion (Strickland 2002). Cyst fluid content should be evaluated for oestrogen levels to confirm the cyst is of ovarian origin (Widdowson et al. 1998). Laparoscopic cystectomy with preservation of ovarian tissue is safe and preferable to more invasive surgery.

3 Complex Neonatal Ovarian Cyst and Adnexal Torsion

NOC can occasionally present as complex lesions secondary to haemorrhage and/or antenatal torsion. Complex cysts show specific characteristics such as a fluid-debris level, septa of variable thickness, echogenicity mimicking a solid appearance (Fig. 5), retracting clot, fibrotic mural nodule and calcification (Nussbaum et al. 1988). A single cyst septum should not be considered diagnostic of a complex cyst. The risk of antenatal torsion has traditionally been considered higher when associated with larger ovarian cysts. These cysts may rupture or very rarely autoamputate and migrate from the usual pelvic location. The distinctive feature of autoamputated cysts is the detection of a freely mobile mass or the so-called '*wandering tumour*' (Koike et al. 2009).

Primary malignant ovarian neoplasms in the neonatal ovary are all but non-existent in the literature. Benign ovarian tumours such as germ cell tumours are recognised in infants but are so rare that a haemorrhagic ovarian cyst or torsion should be still considered even when a neonatal ovarian mass appears solid. Traditionally a surgical diagnosis has been indicated where a complex neonatal ovarian mass does not resolve or increases in size (Fig. 6). Enriquez et al. (2005) found in a retrospective comparison between two groups of neonates with complex ovarian cyst, comparing conservative imaging surveillance management with those undergoing surgical treatment, that those in the surgical group almost all received oophorectomy or salpingo-oophorectomy. In the conservatively managed group a progressive decrease in cyst size was more evident on follow-up imaging after the age of three months. Involution of the cyst occurred in most patients between 3 and 15 months of age, with or without evidence of involution of the gonad.

Approximately 10% of cases occur neonatally or in utero. In all cases a lead point such as an ovarian cyst, teratoma or tumour should be actively sought as the underlying cause. Outside the infantile period the likelihood of a lead point is low and increases with age. The paediatric adnexa are more mobile than in

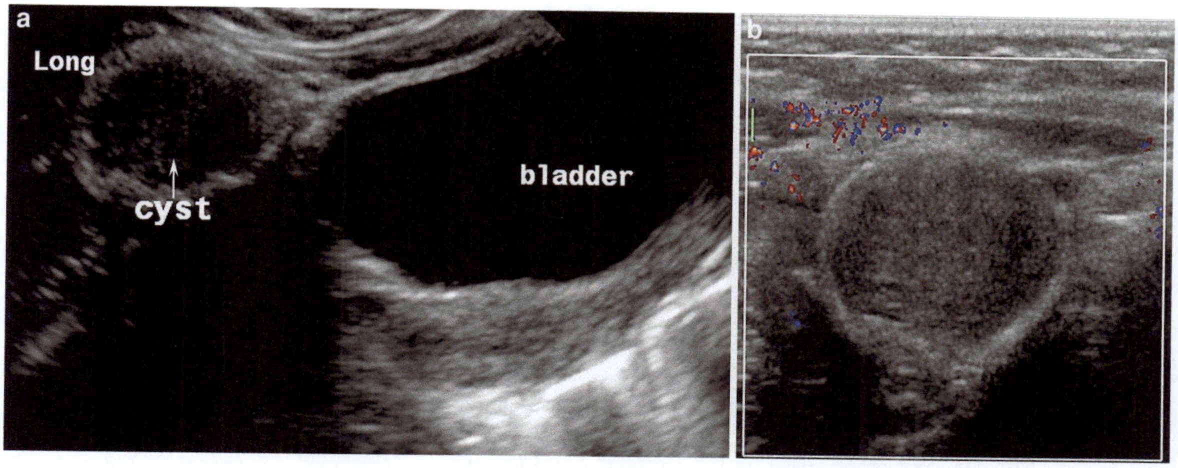

Fig. 5 Complex ovarian cyst. Postnatal US of an antenatally detected pelvic cyst. **a** On grayscale imaging the cyst contains uniform intermediate echoes simulating the appearances of a solid lesion. **b** High-resolution colour Doppler image reveals no internal or capsular flow. The contralateral ovary was normal. This lesion involuted on imaging follow-up, the ipsilateral ovary was never seen on subsequent imaging implying ovarian torsion

adults. Developmental abnormalities such as an absent mesosalpinx or redundant fallopian tube predispose to twisting of normal adnexa which is a more common finding in children.

It must be noted however that these appearances are fairly non-specific.

Amputation of a torsed ovary has been described and is characterised by the finding of a cystic mass with a partially calcified mural nodule (Currarino and Rutledge 1989). Rarely bowel obstruction may result from adhesions caused by a torsed necrotic ovary (Jeanty et al. 2010). In the neonate the presence of an adnexal cyst with a fluid-debris level has been used to define a complicated cyst either resulting from haemorrhage and/or torsion (Nussbaum et al. 1988).

4 Congenital Obstruction of the Gynaecological Tract

Congenital obstruction of the gynaecological tract may present in infancy. The underlying causes in young children are the same as in older children and include imperforate hymen, transverse vaginal septum, severe genital outflow tract stenosis, and cervical or vaginal atresia. Mucoid secretions from the cervical and uterine glands stimulated in utero by maternal oestrogens, or blood from postnatal oestrogen withdrawal can accumulate in the vagina (hydrocolpos) and uterus (hydrometrocolpos) proximal to the level of obstruction. Rarely this may be associated with a urogenital sinus (UGS) or cloacal malformation (Blask et al. 1991).

Clinically the infant may present with an abdominopelvic mass. The palpable mass is due to the obstructed fluid-filled vagina lying between the rectum and urinary bladder (Fig. 7). This may be of sufficient size to cause bowel or urinary tract obstruction. Respiratory compromise may rarely occur due to mass effect. The accumulated genital secretions can cause eversion of the obstructing vaginal membrane or septum resulting in an interlabial mass.

US in the vast majority of cases is usually sufficient to make the diagnosis in uncomplicated presentations. The imaging findings are similar to those in older children. A cystic pelvic mass is demonstrated between the rectum and urinary bladder representing the distended vagina. The uterus may also show distension. The fluid content is often anechoic; however, a fluid-debris level is not uncommon. Local mass effect may compress the ureters and imaging should document the renal upper tracts. Pelvic vascular compression can induce lower limb oedema. The presence of associated congenital anomalies should alert to the presence of either vaginal atresia, or a mid or high transverse septum. In complex cases such as vaginal atresias, where associated spinal or genital tract malformations are suspected US of the spine is performed to exclude a spinal dysraphism. Contrast studies are required in UGS and cloacal malformations.

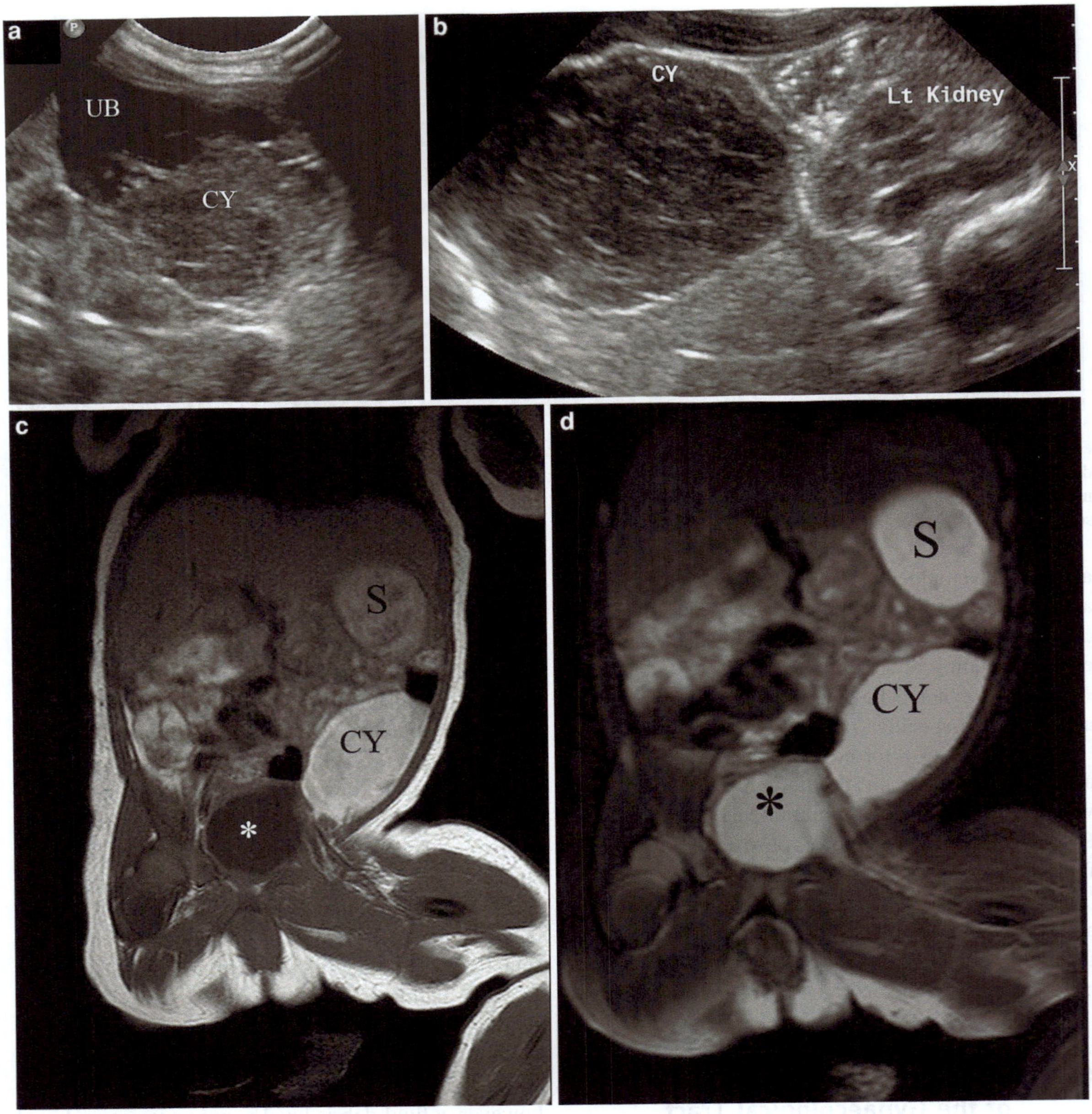

Fig. 6 Antenatal ovarian torsion. **a–b** Day four of life postnatal US imaging of an antenatally detected complex pelvic cyst. **a** Transverse and **b** longitudinal US images of the cyst (*CY*) which shows similar appearances to Fig. 5. **c** Coronal T1W TSE and **d** T2W-SPAIR fat-suppressed imaging at four weeks showing the persisting *left* adnexal cyst (*CY*), stomach (*S*), urinary bladder (*). This was surgically proven to be ovarian torsion, the ipsilateral fallopian tube was atretic, no lead point was identified. The contralateral ovary and tube were normal

5 Cloacal Anomalies

The cloaca is the common channel for urine, genital secretions and faecal residue in the terminal portion of the fetal hindgut. Failure of the cloaca to partition into the urethra, vagina and rectum results in a persisting cloaca. The characteristic antenatal US features for cloacal anomalies include fetal ascites, hydronephrosis, increasing cystic pelvic mass and progressively worsening oligohydramnios (Ohno et al. 2000). Stenotic cloacae or fistulae between genitourinary

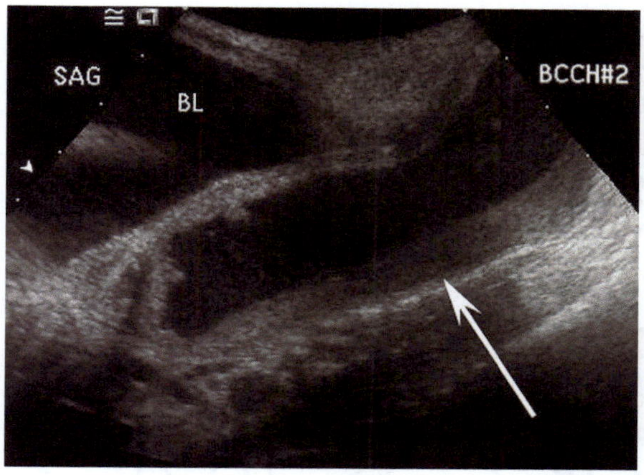

Fig. 7 Hydrocolpos. Longitudinal US in a newborn showing a distended vagina containing a fluid-debris level between the rectum and urinary bladder. Hydrocolpos (*arrow*) is a marker of genital outflow tract obstruction and can be seen genital tract atresias and stenoses, imperforate hymen, vaginal membranes and septa, or as part of complex malformations such as cloacal malformations

structures and the rectum may bring meconium into contact with urine resulting in meconium calcification (Warne et al. 2002a).

Persisting cloacae represent the most severe form of anorectal malformation and are seen exclusively in girls. Cloacal malformations are rare with an incidence of 1 in 50,000 newborns (Warne et al. 2002b). A female infant with an imperforate anus, single perineal orifice and normal abdominal wall should immediately alert the clinician to the presence of a cloacal malformation. The external genitalia may appear rudimentary with absent labia or a hypertrophied clitoris and simulate a disorder of sexual differentiation (Warne et al. 2011). Clinical examination may reveal a palpable mass from a hydrocolpos.

A number of clinical classifications exist for describing the subtypes of cloacal malformation, the spectrum of radiological appearances have been summarised by Jaramillo et al. (1990) (Fig. 8). The least severe form is referred to as an incomplete cloaca with two perineal openings with a persisting urogenital sinus opening adjacent to an anteriorly placed anus (Fig. 8a). In a posterior cloacal malformation a persisting urogenital sinus opens in the anterior wall of the rectum or orthotopic anus (Fig. 8b). According to Jaramillo et al. (1990) the classification of the cloacal malformations is defined according to the urinary-cloacal or urinary-rectal communication (Fig. 8c–f).

Vaginal anomalies include duplicated vagina and uterus, unilateral obstruction of one hemivagina, vaginal agenesis, vaginal stenosis or vaginal ectopia (Fig. 9a–d) (Geley and Gassner 2008). A combination of urine, meconium and genital tract secretions may accumulate proximal to an obstruction, this may decompress into the peritoneal cavity via a patent fallopian tube. Admixing of urine and meconium can give rise to meconium enterolith calcifications (Fig. 10) and implies a rectovesical or rectourethral communication with vaginal stenosis or atresia.

Cloacal dysgenesis is associated with a spectrum of other genitourinary malformations including renal agenesis (Stephens and Smith 1986; Hendren 1992), multicystic dysplastic kidney and renal ectopia. Other well recognised malformative associations include VACTERL (Vertebral, Anorectal, Cardiac, Esophageal, Renal, Limb defects), caudal regression and sirenomelia (Mermaid syndrome).

Initial management requires early multidisciplinary involvement with a team including a paediatric urologist, nephrologist, neonatologist, cardiologist and radiologist. The main aim of initial imaging is to confirm the diagnosis and detect serious associated anomalies prior to urgent surgical palliation. Ultrasound of the genitourinary tract should be undertaken in the early neonatal period (day 0–3) to document hydrocolpos, renal upper tract dilatation and any associated anomalies. This coincides with the period of oliganuria in the neonate but should not preclude prompt ultrasound imaging. Cardiac echocardiography forms part of the urgent work-up. A radiograph of the abdomen performed in the first few hours of life will document bowel obstruction and may alert to a fistulous connection between the bowel and vagina or bladder as indicated by the presence of gas in these structures. Radiographs will also demonstrate meconium calcifications, sacral agenesis and pubic diastasis. Ultrasound of the lower spine is desirable and where possible should be undertaken at the time of the abdominal ultrasound. Associated abnormal findings include high position of the conus, tethered cord or lipomyelomeningocele (Fig. 11).

Initial management of the child includes resuscitation with intravenous fluids and commencement of long-term prophylactic antibiotics aiming for prompt bowel decompression with placement of a nasal or oral gastric tube. The latter will exclude a tracheaoesophageal fistula. Early surgical intervention in the

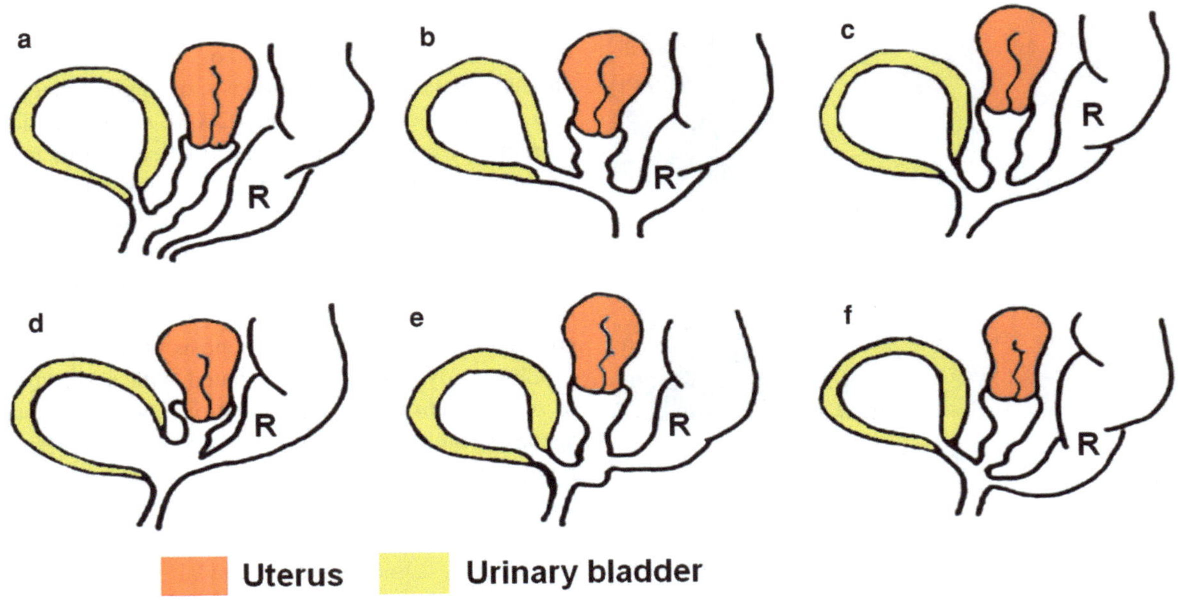

Fig. 8 Schematic diagram illustrating the imaging classification of cloacal malformations (**a**) Incomplete cloacal malformation: with a persisting urogenital sinus adjacent to an anteriorly placed anus, (**b**) Posterior cloacal malformation: the persisting urogenital sinus is orientated posteriorly and opens in the anterior wall of the rectum or anus. According to Jaramillo et al. (1990) the classification of the cloacal malformations is defined according to the urinary cloacal or urinary-rectal communication. **c** Urethrocloacal communication: the patent urethra empties into the proximal aspect of the cloaca, (**d**) Vesicocloacal communication with a rudimentary or absent urethra (**e**) Vaginal communication of the rectum: the rectum drains into the low posterior wall of the vagina, (**f**) Rectal communication with the cloacal common channel. Images Reproduced from (Geley and Gassner 2008) with permission from Springer publishers

neonatal period includes bowel decompression with a diverting colostomy (Levitt and Peña 2005) and drainage of hydrocolpos (Levitt and Peña 2006). Decompression of the urinary tract may require formal tube vesicostomy if catheterisation is not possible. At the time of initial surgery the surgeon can endoscopically evaluate the length of the common channel and may be able to define the unique urethral and vaginal anatomy. In a large case series of surgically managed infants with cloacal malformations, those with a common channel length less than 3 cm were associated with urologic defects in 59% compared to 91% of girls with longer channels in whom surgical repair was often more technically challenging (Peña et al. 2004). Incomplete cloacal malformations may not require urgent intervention.

Subsequent diagnostic imaging is targeted towards identifying precise anatomical relations for pre-operative planning of the definitive surgical repair. It is extremely helpful for the treating urologist or paediatric surgeon to be present at the time of contrast studies. The surgeon can guide the radiologist on the sequence of imaging, in particular which structures must be opacified and in what order, and also assist in the interpretation of the anatomy. Contrast studies require installation of contrast medium via the single perineal orifice using an 8F feeding tube similar to a conventional neonatal voiding cystogram (Fig. 12). A larger catheter may be required for bigger perineal openings. Contrast spill from small additional perineal openings should not be overlooked. Lateral imaging is necessary to depict subtle connections between the rectum, vagina and urinary bladder. Frontal projections are required to confirm duplication anomalies. Simultaneous opacification of the bladder can be achieved via an ultrasound guided percutaneous vesicostomy (Fig. 13), this can also be combined with an antegrade distal colonogram (loopogram). Adequate distension is required to define fistulous connections. Cross-sectional imaging has a role in delineating complex anatomy and can immediately follow conventional opacification of

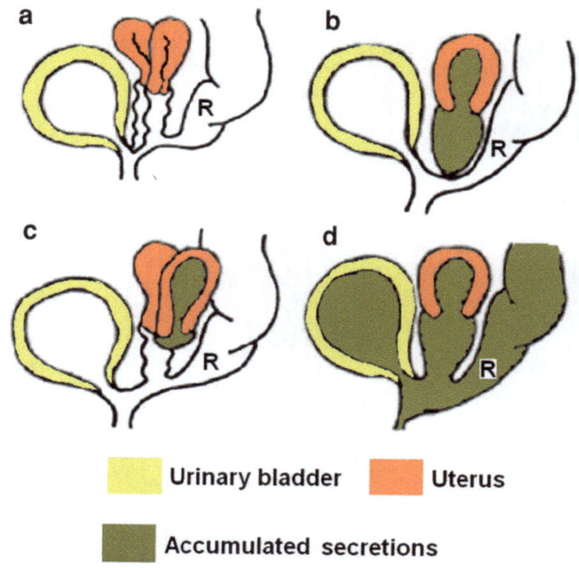

Fig. 9 Schematic diagram illustrating the variants of cloacal malformation and genital anomalies. **a** Bifid vagina and uterus, the rectal fistula enters the base of the septum dividing the vagina. **b** Distal vaginal stenosis or atresia leading to hydrometrocolpos. **c** Bifid uterus and vagina with unilateral obstruction and hydrometrocolpos. **d** Obstruction of the urogenital sinus resulting in distension of the vagina by urine, meconium and genital tract secretions. Images Reproduced from (Geley and Gassner 2008) with permission from Springer publishers

the bladder, distal colon and colpos. Both MRI (Baughman et. al 2007) and CT (Adams et. al. 2006) have been advocated, CT is more widely available and gives high resolution imaging but MR, although more technically challenging is preferable due to the lack of exposure to ionising radiation. MRI of the spine is undertaken in those with abnormal spinal ultrasound and a full work-up of renal tract anomalies includes follow-up ultrasound, and DMSA and MAG-3 scintigraphy where indicated. Definitive surgical repair may involve either total urogenital mobilisation or posterior sagittal anorectourethroplasty aged 6–24 months.

6 Interlabial Mass

Interlabial masses are rare. US is typically requested to characterise the mass and assign the organ of origin. The differential diagnosis of an interlabial mass in the newborn or young girl include gynaecological and non-gynaecological conditions, these are summarised in Table 2. Clinical examination of the interlabial mass is helpful in establishing the correct diagnosis, with particular attention paid to its relation to the urethra. This may require assessment under anaesthesia and correlation with cystourethroscopy.

6.1 Gynaecological Causes

As previously described hydrocolpos and cloacal malformations can present as interlabial masses. Rhabdomyosarcoma of the vagina is the most common malignancy of the genitourinary tract in girls under the age of five years and should be suspected when a mass consisting of grape-like clusters is visualised at the introitus (see Chapters 'Gynaecological Neoplasia' and 'Menstrual Disorders and Vaginal Discharge').

A paraurethral cyst is rare cause of an interlabial mass and may go unnoticed for some time. These may be congenital remnants or acquired inclusion cysts. The paraurethral glands and ducts are rudimentary homologues of the prostate gland, the largest glands are the paired Skene's ducts which secrete into the female urethra. Urothelial cysts (Skene duct cyst) may arise from these ducts. The cyst mass may be palpable and is seen to displace the urethral meatus laterally resulting in a distorted urinary stream.

Labial hypertrophy is another rare cause of an apparent lobulated interlabial mass (Kirks 1983). The causes of true labial masses are summarised in Table 3. Genital prolapse is extremely rare and is usually seen in the first two weeks of life and is associated with myelomeningocele or exceptionally with breech delivery or sacrococcygeal teratoma resection.

6.2 Urological Causes

A prolapsed urethra is a donut shaped mass with urine exiting from a central meatus. An ectopic ureterocele (Fig. 14) is a congenital anomaly which includes cystic dilatation of the terminal portion of the ureter. This presents as a smooth mass which protrudes from the urethral meatus so that urine exits circumferentially (Nussbaum and Lebowitz 1983), this may occasionally obstruct the urinary tract. Approximately 90% of cases with ureterocele are associated with an ipsilateral upper renal tract duplex anomaly.

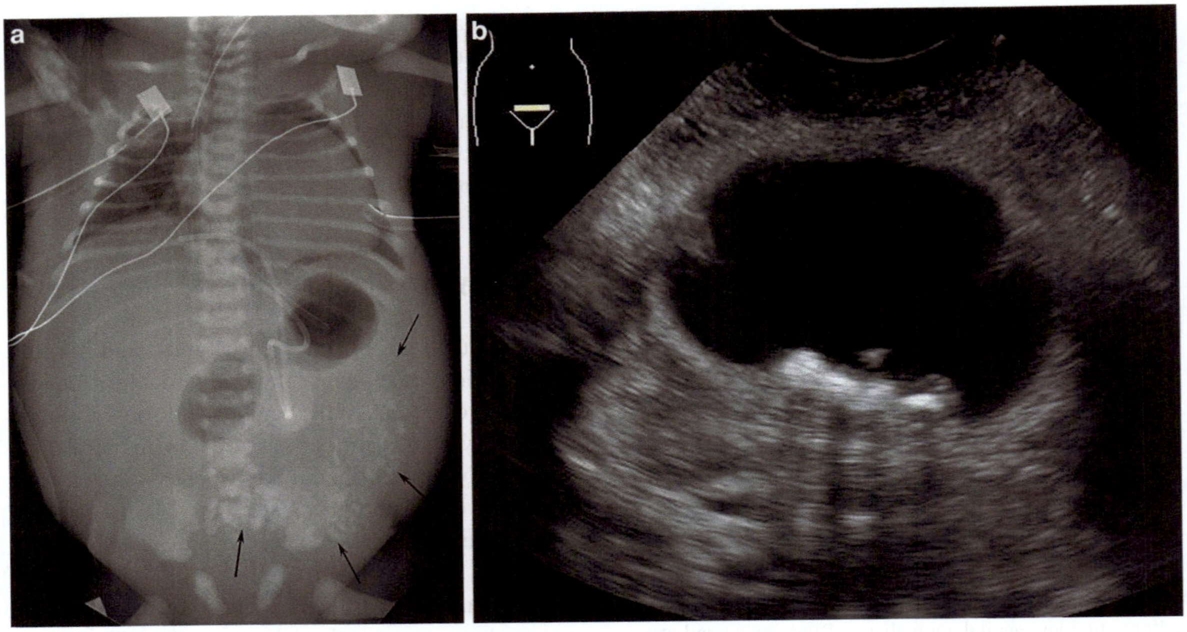

Fig. 10 Cloacal malformation. **a** Frontal radiograph showing an infant with a truncated sacrum and meconium calcifications in the left lower quadrant of the abdomen (*arrows*). **b** Transverse US of the same infant confirming intraluminal calcifications which are seen to cast acoustic shadowing. These were located within a distended viscus which was suspected to be the confluence of the vagina and gastrointestinal tract, posterior to the urinary bladder. Meconium calcifications result from the mixture of meconium and urine and indicate either a cloacal malformation in females or an imperforate anus in males. This infant developed multiorgan failure and was palliated with a percutaneous tube cloacostomy

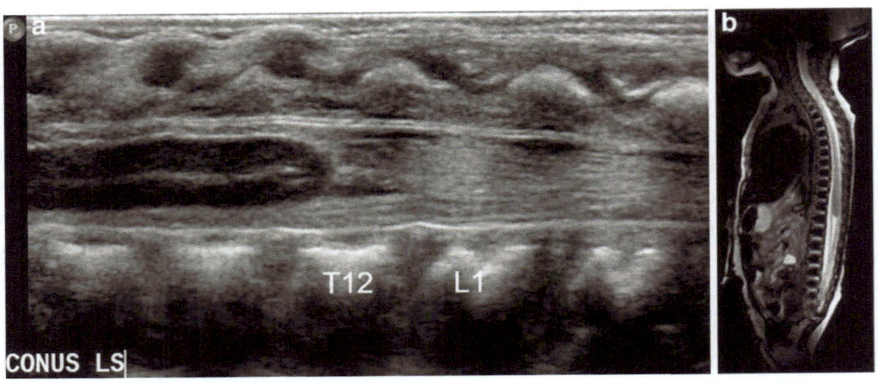

Fig. 11 Cloacal malformation. **a** Longitudinal high-resolution US of the spine showing an abnormal high position to the conus. The morphology of the conus is abnormal and appears blunt or plump. **b** Sagittal T2W MR image of the whole spine confirming partial sacral agenesis and caudal regression

6.3 Diagnostic Work-up

Diagnostic imaging with transabdominal and transperineal ultrasound will help to refine the diagnosis by differentiating between solid and cyst, and define the internal genitourinary anatomy. Occasionally an intravenous pyelogram, voiding cystourethrography and catheter contrast studies will clarify the diagnosis. MRI is indicated in the work-up of rhabdomyosarcoma.

7 Labial Masses

Labial masses are uncommon. They are usually congenital and may be identified on a newborn screening physical examination. Congenital lesions can often present later in life. Acquired labial masses are very rare. The causes of labial masses are summarised in Table 3, and include cliteromegally associated with disorders of sexual differentiation (DSD). Infants with

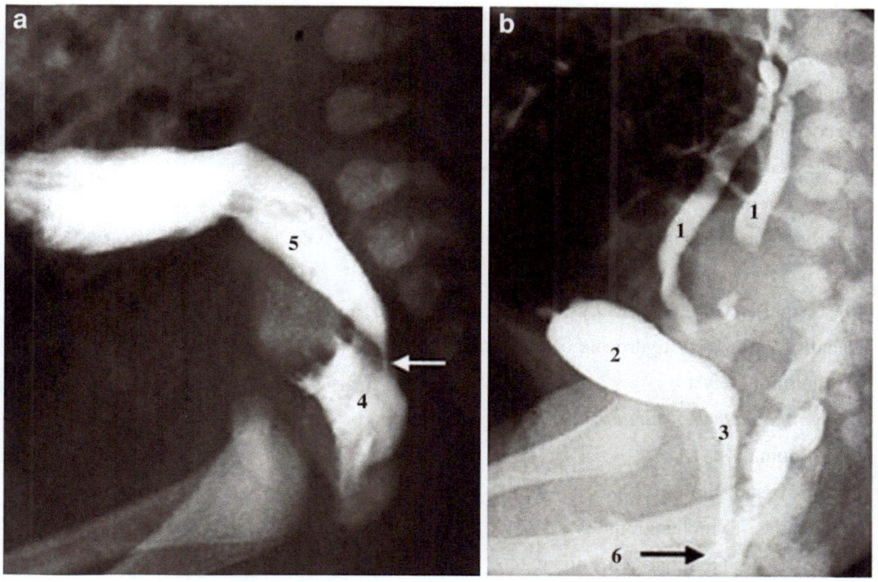

Fig. 12 Cloacal malformation. Catheter contrast studies (**a**) showing a recto-vaginal fistula (*arrow*) and (**b**) urethrocloacal connection with bilateral vesicoureteric reflux. (*1*) Bilateral ureteric reflux (*2*) Urinary bladder (*3*) Urethra (*4*) Vagina (*5*) Rectum (*6*) Cloacal common channel. Reproduced from (Couture 2008) with permission of Springer publishers

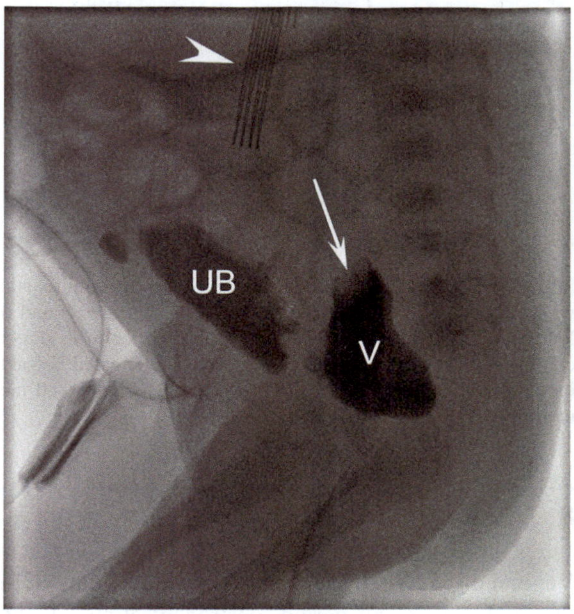

Fig. 13 Cloacal malformation. Lateral view from a contrast series showing instillation of contrast medium in the urinary bladder (*UB*) via a suprapubic catheter in a four month old, no vesicoureteric reflux is demonstrated. Contrast quickly filled the vagina (*V*); a cervical impression is noted (*arrow*). Despite adequate distension of the bladder neither the vesicocloacal fistula nor the common channel could be demonstrated. Contrast administered directly into the single perineal orifice did not provide any additional information. A stoma bag (*arrowhead*) indicates prior defunctioning colostomy. The sacrum is hypoplastic

Table 2 The causes of interlabial masses in young girls

Urological
Prolapsed urethra
Prolapsed ectopic uteroecele
Prolapsed ectopic cecouteroecele
Urethral polyp
Gynaecological
Hydro-(metro)colpos (Imperforate hymen, vaginal septum, vaginal atresia)
Paraurethral cyst (Skene duct cyst, Gartner's duct cyst)
Other cyst (Hymenal cyst, Müllerian remnant cyst, Bartholin duct cyst, Vaginal wall inclusion cysts)
Rhabdomyosarcoma of the vagina (Sarcoma botryoides)
Genital prolapse
Gastrointestinal
Rectal duplication
After Nussbaum and Lebowitz (1983)

DSD are discussed more fully in Chapter 'Disorders of Sex Development'.

Inguinal hernias in girls (Fig. 15) are uncommon but should be managed according to the same principles as infant boys. Non-reducible hernias merit prompt surgical repair, strangulation requires immediate surgical intervention. Most 'girls' identified in

Table 3 The differential for a labial mass

Cliteromegally (Disorders of sexual differentiation—DSD)
Labial hypertrophy
Precocious puberty
Congenital adrenal hyperplasia
Inguinal hernia
Androgen insensitivity syndrome
Embryonic remnant
Mesonephric (Gartner duct) cyst
Canal of Nuck cyst (hydrocele of the canal of Nuck)
Bartholin duct cyst
Benign mesenchymal tumours
Fat: Lipoma
Fibrous tissue: Fibroma
Lymphatics: Lymphangioma
Neural tissue: Granular cell tumour
Hamartoma: Neurofibromatosis
Vascular tissue: Haemangioma
Malignant tumours
Striated muscle: Embryonal rhabdomyosarcoma—Sarcoma botryoides
After Lowry and Guido (2000)

the neonatal period with an androgen insensitivity disorder (AIS) will present with an inguinal hernia. The association of an inguinal hernia containing a gonad in the inguinal canal in a phenotypic female should alert the clinician to the possibility of AIS. The presence of a gonad at the labium majorum is also a recognised finding in AIS (Fig. 16).

A hydrocele of the canal of Nuck (canal of Nuck cyst) is another rare congenital cause of a labial mass. The canal of Nuck in the female is the homologue of the processus vaginalis in the male. The canal of Nuck represents a small evagination of parietal peritoneum which accompanies the round ligament through the inguinal ring into the inguinal canal. This potential space normally obliterates during the first year of life, its persistence is associated with either an indirect inguinal hernia or a hydrocele of the canal of Nuck (Fig. 17). Embryonic remnants of the mesonephric (Wolffian) duct include the Gartner duct cyst. These often present in later life or as incidental finding on imaging.

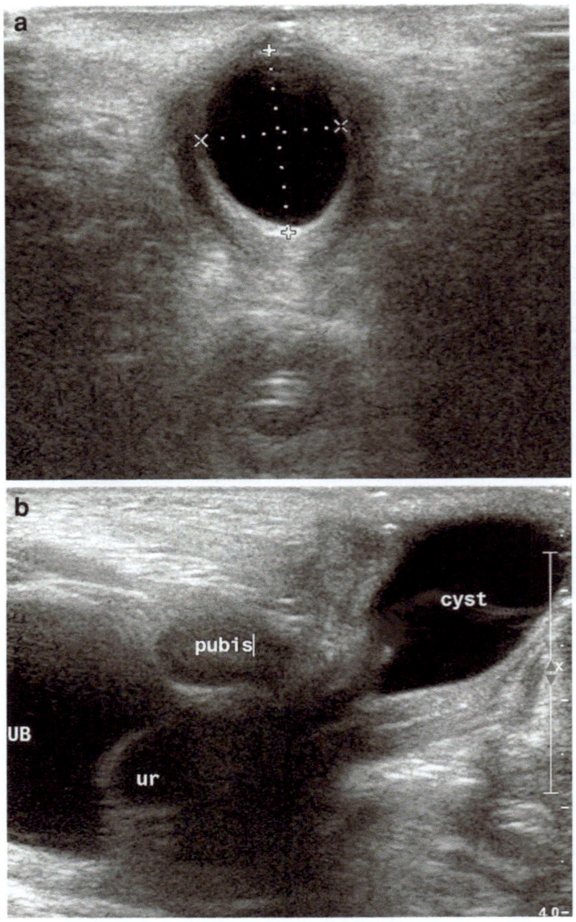

Fig. 14 High-resolution transperineal US of a newborn female with a transilluminable mass at the vulva. **a** Transverse and **b** longitudinal imaging shows a cyst (cecoureterocele) in direct continuity with the urethra, the ureterocele is elongated beyond its orifice by coursing under the bladder (UB) trigone and the urethra (ur)

8 Vaginal Discharge

Vaginal discharge in the neonate is not uncommon. In the early neonatal period oestrogenisation of the genital tract wanes as maternal oestrogen hormonal influence subsides. The effects of oestrogens begin to recede after two weeks (Kass-Wolff and Wilson 2003). Mucoid vaginal discharge, which may be bloody, can be seen in the first two weeks of life and is almost always a benign and self-limiting finding. Any vaginal discharge or bleeding beyond three weeks merits further clinical investigation.

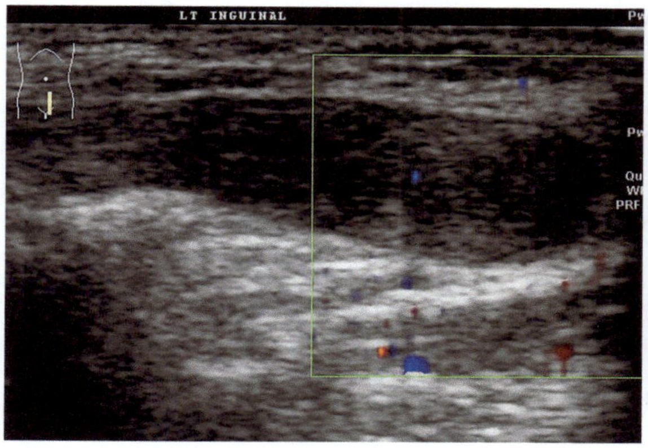

Fig. 15 Indirect inguinal hernia. Longitudinal high-resolution US image showing an inguinal hernia containing a gonad in an infant girl

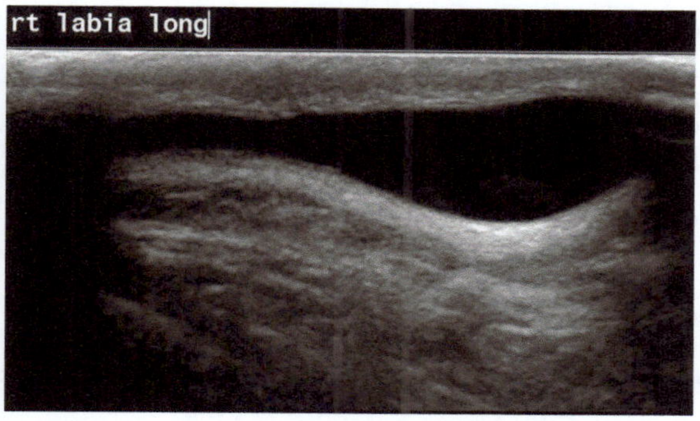

Fig. 17 Canal of Nuck hydrocele. Longitudinal high-resolution translabial US image showing a well-defined tubular cystic structure in the inguinal canal. The superior extent of the cyst is clearly defined. No double-wall sign, peristalsis or bowel content was identified to suggest the presence of bowel

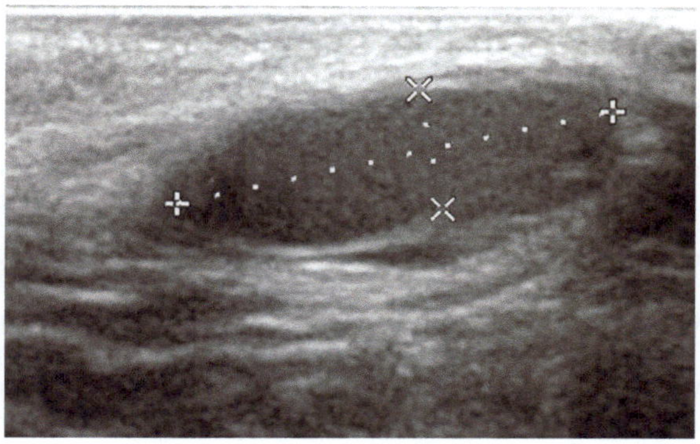

Fig. 16 Labial gonad. Longitudinal high-resolution translabial US image showing a gonad (between callipers) in the labium majora in this two month old infant with complete androgen insensitivity syndrome. Bilateral labial gonads were present but no hernia was demonstrated

9 Conclusion

Antenatally detected disorders and anatomical anomalies in the newborn form the bulk of the gynaecological disorders which require diagnostic imaging work-up in early life. US is ideally suited to imaging the neonate and provides real-time anatomical information with superb soft tissue contrast resolution. US imaging in most cases provides superior information to that achieved with MRI in infants whom typically lack body fat where the signal-to-noise ratio is limited. Contrast studies are indicated for complex anomalies such a cloacal malformations and persisting urogenital sinus.

References

Adams ME, Hiorns MP, Wilcox DT (2006) Combining MDCT, micturating cystography, and excretory urography for 3D imaging of cloacal malformation. Am J Roentgenol 187:1034–1035

Akın MA, Akın L, Ozbek S et al (2010) Fetal-neonatal ovarian cysts-their monitoring and management: retrospective evaluation of 20 Cases and review of the literature J Clin Res Ped Endo 2:28–33

Baughman SM, Richardson RR, Podberesky DJ et al (2007) 3-Dimensional magnetic resonance genitography: a different look at cloacal malformations. J Urol 178:1675–1679

Blask AR, Sanders RC, Gearhart JP (1991) Obstructed uterovaginal anomalies: demonstration with sonography. Part I. Neonates and infants. Radiology 179:79–83

Bryant AE, Laufer MR (2004) Fetal ovarian cysts: incidence, diagnosis and management. J Reprod Med 49:329–337

Chambrier ED, Heinrichs C, Avni FE (2002) Sonographic appearance of congenital adrenal hyperplasia in utero. J Ultrasound Med 21:97–100

Couture A (2008) Fetal Gastrointestinal Tract: US and MRI In: Couture AC, Baud C, Ferran FL, et al (eds) Gastrointestinal tract sonography in fetuses and children, 1st edn. Springer, Berlin, pp 1–84

Currarino G, Rutledge JC (1989) Ovarian torsion and amputation resulting in partially calcified, pedunculated cystic mass. Pediatr Radiol 19:395–399

Dhombres F, Jouannic JM, Brodaty G et al (2007) Contribution of prenatal imaging to the anatomical assessment of fetal hydrocolpos. Ultrasound Obstet Gynecol 30:101–104

Enriquez G, Durán C, Torán N et al (2005) Conservative versus surgical treatment for complex neonatal ovarian cysts: outcomes study. Am J Roentgenol 185:501–508

Geley TE, Gassner I (2008) Lower Urinary Tract anomalies of Uogenital Sinus and Female Genital Anomalies In: Fotter (ed) Paediatric Uroradiology, 2nd edn. Springer, Berlin, pp 137–164

Godfrey H, Abernethy L, Boothroyd A (1998) Torsion of an ovarian cyst mimicking enteric duplication cyst on transabdominal ultrasound: two cases. Pediatr Radiol 28:171–173

Hendren WH (1992) Cloacal malformations: Experience with 105 cases. J Paed Surg 27:890–901

Jaramillo D, Lebowitz RI, Hendren WH (1990) The cloacal malformation: radiologic findings and imaging recommendations. Radiology 177:441–448

Jeanty C, Frayer EA, Page R et al (2010) Neonatal ovarian torsion complicated by intestinal obstruction and perforation, and review of the literature. J Pediatr Surg 45:5–9

Kass-Wolff JH, Wilson EE (2003) Pediatric gynecology: assessment strategies and common problems. Sem Rep Med 21:329–338

Kirks DR (1983) Genital hypertrophy: a neonatal pseudotumor in females. Pediatr Radiol 13:244–245

Koike Y, Inoue M, Uchida K et al (2009) Ovarian autoamputation in a neonate: a case report with literature review. Pediatr Surg Int 25:655–658

Lee HJ, Woo SK, Kim JS, Suh SJ (2000) Daughter cyst sign: a sonographic finding of ovarian cyst in neonates, infants, and young children. Am J Roentgenol 174:1013–1015

Levitt MA, Peña A (2005) Pitfalls in the management of newborn cloacas. Pediatr Surg Int 21:264–269

Levitt MA, Peña A (2006) Management in the newborn period. In: Holschneider AM, Hutson JM (eds) Anorectal malformations in children: embryology, diagnosis, surgical treatment, follow-up, 4th edn. Springer, Berlin, pp 289–292

Lowry DLB, Guido RS (2000) Vulvar mass in the prepubertal child. J Pediatr Adolesc Gynecol 13:75–78

Muller-Leisse C, Bick U, Paulussen K et al (1992) Ovarian cysts in the fetus and neonate: changes in sonographic pattern in their follow-up and management. Pediatr Radiol 22:395–400

Nussbaum AR, Sanders RC, Hartman DS et al (1988) Neonatal ovarian cysts: sonographic-pathologic correlation. Radiology 168:817–821

Nussbaum AR, Lebowitz RL (1983) Interlabial masses in little girls: review and imaging recommendations. Am J Roentgenol 141:65–71

Ohno Y, Koyama N, Tsuda M et al (2000) Antenatal ultrasonographic appearance of a cloacal anomaly. Obstet Gynecol 95:1013–1015

Pajkrt E, Petersen OB, Chitty LS (2008) Fetal genital anomalies: an aid to diagnosis. Prenat Diagn 28:389–398

Peña A, Levitt MA, Hong A, Midulla P (2004) Surgical management of cloacal malformations: a review of 339 patients. J Pediatr Surg 39:470–479

Stephens FD, Smith ED (1986) Classification, identification, and assessment of surgical treatment of anorectal anomalies. Pediatr Surg Int 1:200–205

Strickland JL (2002) Ovarian cysts in neonates, children and adolescents. Curr Opin Obstet Gynecol 14:459–465

Vogtländer MF, Rijntjes-Jacobs EG, van den Hoonaard TL et al (2003) Neonatal ovarian cysts. Acta Paediatr 92:498–501

Warne S, Chitty LS, Wilcox DT (2002a) Prenatal diagnosis cloacal malformation. BJU Int 89:78–81

Warne SA, Wilcox DT, Ransley PG (2002b) Long-term urological outcome in patients presenting with persistent cloaca. J Urol 168:1859–1862

Warne SA, Hiorns MP, Curry J et al (2011) Understanding cloacal anomalies

Winderl LM, Silverman RK (1995) Prenatal diagnosis of congenital imperforate hymen. Obstet Gynecol 85:857–860

Widdowson DJ, Pilling DW, Cook CM (1988) Neonatal ovarian cysts: therapeutic dilemma. Arch Dis Child 63: 737–742

Structural Abnormalities of the Female Reproductive Tract

Paul Humphries

Contents

1	**Introduction**	66
1.1	Classification of Structural Anomalies	66
1.2	Imaging Assessment of Structural Abnormalities	68
1.3	Structural Abnormalities	70
2	**Conclusion**	78
3	**Acknowledgment**	79
References		79

P. Humphries (✉)
University College London Hospital NHS Trust,
235 Euston Road, London, NW1 2BU, UK
e-mail: paul.humphries@uclh.nhs.uk

Abstract

The true incidence of structural abnormalities of the female reproductive tract in paediatric and adolescent patients is difficult to determine. The term "structural abnormality" encompasses a wide spectrum of anatomical anomalies, which, depending on the precise anomalies present, have a varied temporal and clinical presentation. Imaging assessment of these abnormalities often requires a multimodality approach with the methods employed being modified depending on the clinical presentation and age of the patient. Classification of structural genital abnormalities is not standardized, with several different schema proposed. Ultimately good communication between clinical and radiological multidisciplinary team members is vital to ensure that there is unambiguous interpretation of the spectrum of abnormalities in a given patient and best care delivered.

Abbreviations

FLASH	Fast low angle single shot
SE	Spin echo
TSE	Turbospin echo
FISP	Fast imaging with steady-state precession
3D	Three dimensional
US	Ultrasound
MDCT	Multi-detector computed tomography
2D	Two dimensional
MRI	Magnetic resonance imaging
HSG	Hysterosalpingogram
CSF	Cerebrospinal fluid
STIR	Short tau inversion recovery
MRA	Magnetic resonance angiography

G. Mann et al. (eds.), *Imaging of Gynecological Disorders in Infants and Children*, Medical Radiology. Diagnostic Imaging, DOI: 10.1007/174_2010_79,

ASRM	American society of reproductive Medicine
MRKH	Mayer-Rokitansky-Küster-Hauser syndrome
VCUAM	Vagina, Cervix, Uterus, Adenxa and associated Malformations
MURCS	Müllerian duct aplasia, renal aplasia and cervical somite dysplasia
GRESS	Genital renal ear and skeletal syndrome
HWWS	Herlyn–Werner–Wunderlich syndrome
DES	Oestrogen diethylstibisterol

1 Introduction

The true incidence of structural abnormalities of the female reproductive tract in paediatric and adolescent patients is difficult to determine. The term "structural abnormality" encompasses a wide spectrum of anatomical anomalies, which, depending on the precise anomalies present, have a varied temporal clinical presentation. The vast majority of female genital tract structural abnormalities do not present until after the expected onset of menstruation. At the time of expected menarche there may be abdominal or pelvic pain, which may be cyclical when there is an obstructed system present. Such pain may be the clinical complaint even in the presence of menstruation if an abnormality is unilateral. Primary amenorrhoea can be seen when there is agenesis of the uterus. Failure to conceive or maintain a pregnancy is often the presentation in young adults. Female neonates with a cloacal anomaly or urogenital sinus (UGS) may present with an abdominal mass, neonatal sepsis or respiratory distress (Nazir et al. 2006). Cloacal anomaly may also be diagnosed antenatally, although this is challenging (Subramanian et al. 2006).

Owing to several different classification systems, varied patient populations and different methods of describing abnormalities, the reported incidence of female genital malformations varies widely, quoted as being between 0.1 and 5% of the general female population (Byrne et al. 2000; Marten et al. 2003; Nahum 1998; Raga et al. 1997). If one considers women with subfertility and recurrent miscarriage, the incidence increases markedly, up to 35% in the latter group (Salim et al. 2003).

1.1 Classification of Structural Anomalies

The classification of structural reproductive system anomalies is complex, with several different schema available and different ideologies behind each. The overall classification of a congenital anomaly may be based on a multidisciplinary palette of investigations, including clinical examination, ultrasound (which may be either transabdominal, transperineal, transrectal or transvaginal, depending on the age and developmental appropriateness of each method), contrast studies, MRI, laparoscopy and laparotomy.

1.1.1 American Society of Reproductive Medicine Classification

The simplest means by which Müllerian system abnormalities can be classified via description of the abnormal embryological development observed, for example failure of organogenesis leading to uterine agenesis; failure of lateral fusion leading to a variable degree of separation of the uterus, cervix and upper vagina, depending on severity; failure of vertical fusion leading to a transverse vaginal septum and failure of septal resorption leading to septate uterus. The most widely utilised schema is that of The American Society of Reproductive Medicine (ASRM) (1988), based upon the work of Buttram and Gibbons (1979), which classifies Müllerian anomalies into seven groups according to clinical presentation and foetal prognosis and is largely based upon the uterine findings (Fig. 1). Despite its wide utilisation there are limitations to the ASRM schema, chiefly that complex cases that do not fit neatly into one of the classes cannot be adequately described using the system. There is a temptation when reporting such abnormalities to ascribe a 'best fit class' for the constellation of abnormalities present, which should be avoided as an exact description of the anatomic abnormalities is needed in order to plan the most appropriate care for the patient.

1.1.2 Clinico-embryological Classification

The limitations of the ASRM schema have led to alternative methods of describing reproductive tract abnormalities. A clinico-embryological classification has been proposed by Acien et al. (1992, 2004) in which the precise embryological origin of each component is considered to explain the overall anomaly and guide treatment.

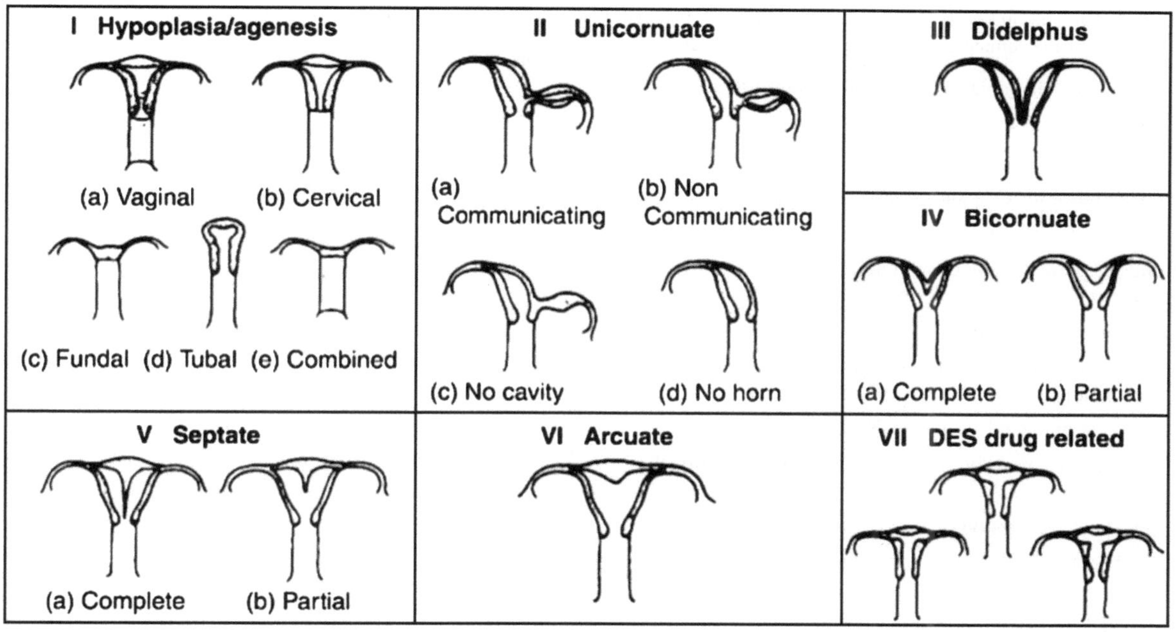

Fig. 1 American Society of Reproductive Medicine Classification of Müllerian anomalies. Reprinted by permission from the American Society of Reproductive Medicine (1988)

The embryological classification proposed by Acien et al. is based upon laboratory studies, case reports and the authors own case series, particularly complex anomalies that require a more rounded explanation than that afforded by the ASRM classification system, with an emphasis on the embryological interaction between the mesonephric (Wolffian) and the paramesonephric (Müllerian) ducts.

Particular importance is given to the Wolffian duct acting as a promoter of normal Müllerian duct development, and a dual embryological origin of the vagina, with the Wolffian duct contributing in addition to the Müllerian tubercle. Acien's clinico-embryological classification proposes that defective Wolffian development leads to a combination of renal absence, uterovaginal duplication with an ipsilateral blind ending vagina. There may be an associated ectopic vaginal ureteric insertion. The ipsilateral uterus may or may not communicate with the contralateral side and therefore may or may not be obstructed. If there is failure of an entire urogenital ridge, either agenesis or hypoplasia, there will be complete absence of the kidney, ovary, fallopian tube, uterus, cervix and vagina on that side, with contralateral unicornuate uterus.

Acien considers isolated Müllerian abnormalities separately: Müllerian duct anomalies (uterine abnormalities), Müllerian tubercle (cervico-vaginal abnormalities and transverse vaginal septum) and combined duct/tubercle anomalies (uni or bilateral Mayer–Rokitanski–Kuster–Hauser syndrome) grouped together. Cloacal/UGS abnormalities either alone or in combination with the above complete this classification system (Table 1).

1.1.3 VCUAM Classification

As the above clinico-embryological classification system is reliant on a good understanding of the complex embryology of the female reproductive system in order to characterise specific abnormalities, the clinical utility of the system is felt by some authors to be difficult (Oppelt et al. 2007) and an alternative staging system has been proposed, the so-called VCUAM (Vagina, Cervix, Uterus, Adenxa and associated Malformations) classification (Oppelt et al. 2005). The VCUAM system, which is based upon a combination of clinical examination, laparoscopy and imaging, evaluates each of the anatomical structures in turn, assigning a 'stage' depending on the abnormality present (Table 2). The advantage of this system is that any constellation of abnormalities can be described accurately and comprehensively. The disadvantage is that there are 56,700 possible

Table 1 Clinical and embryological classification of the malformations of the female genital tract—Acien et al. (2004)

1. Agenesis or hypoplasia of a whole genital ridge
a. Unicornuate uterus
b. Contralateral uterine agenesis
c. Contralateral tubal and ovarian agenesis
d. Contralateral renal agenesis
2. Mesonephric anomalies with absence of Wolffian duct opening into the urogenital sinus
a. Uterovaginal duplicity
b. Blind hemivagina with ipsilateral renal agenesis presenting as
i. Large unilateral haematocolpos
ii. Gartner's pseudocyst on the anterolateral wall of the vagina
iii. Partial resorption of intervaginal septum
iv. Unilateral vaginal agenesis with or without communication between the hemiuteri
3. Isolated Müllerian anomalies
a. Müllerian ducts: uterine malformations
b. Müllerian tubercle: cervico-vaginal atresia and segmental anomalies, i.e. transverse vaginal septum
c. Both Müllerian ducts and tubercle: Mayer–Rokitansky–Kuster–Hauser syndrome
4. Anomalies of the urogenital sinus: cloacal anomalies, urogenital anomalies
5. Malformative combinations: Wolffian, Müllerian and cloacal anomalies

combinations of findings, which may limit the clinical utility of the system.

In practical terms, a good dialogue between clinical and radiological colleagues is vital to ensure that both groups understand what is being described when cases are being discussed, regardless of the classification system used.

1.2 Imaging Assessment of Structural Abnormalities

There are many methods available to multidisciplinary teams investigating possible structural anomalies of the female genital tract. Frequently the age of the patient and the clinical presentation will determine the imaging approach. For example, the approach

Table 2 VCUAM classification (Oppelt et al. 2005)

Vagina (V)	
0	Normal
1a	Partial hymenal atresia
1b	Complete hymenal atresia
2a	Incomplete septate vagina <50%
2b	Complete septate vagina
3	Stenosis of the introitus
4	Hypoplasia
5a	Unilateral atresia
5b	Complete atresia
S1	Sinus urogenitalis (deep confluence)
S2	Sinus urogenitalis (middle confluence)
S3	Sinus urogenitalis (high confluence)
C	Cloacae
+	Other
#	Unknown
Cervix (C)	
0	Normal
1	Duplex cervix
2a	Unilateral atresia/aplasia
2b	Bilateral atresia/aplasia
+	Other
#	Unknown
Uterus (U)	
0	Normal
1a	Arcuate
1b	Septate <50% of the cavity
1c	Septate >50% of the cavity
2	Bicornuate
3	Hypoplastic uterus
4a	Unilateral rudimentary or hypoplastic
4b	Bilateral rudimentary or hypoplastic
+	Other
#	Unknown
Adnexa (A)	
0	Normal
1a	Unilateral tubal malformation, ovaries normal
1b	Bilateral tubal malformation, ovaries normal
2a	Unilateral hypoplasia/gonadal streak
2b	Bilateral hypoplasia/gonadal streak
3a	Unilateral aplasia

(continued)

Table 2 (continued)

3b	Bilateral aplasia
+	Other
#	Unknown
Associated malformation (M)	
0	None
R	Renal system
S	Skeleton
C	Cardiac
N	Neurological
+	Other
#	Unknown

taken for a neonate with pelvic mass would be quite different to that taken for an adolescent with primary amenorrhoea or a young adult patient experiencing difficulty in conceiving.

Broadly speaking the main weapons in our armamentarium are ultrasound, contrast catheter studies, magnetic resonance imaging (MRI), hysterosalpingography (HSG) and laparoscopy. The gold standard for the evaluation of Müllerian abnormalities in adult practice remains HSG and laparoscopy (Deutch and Abuhamad 2008), which obviously have the disadvantage of being invasive in nature, and in the case of HSG, utilising ionising radiation and being inappropriate for paediatric and adolescent patients. There are relatively little data in the literature evaluating the diagnostic accuracy for MRI and ultrasound methods aside from the evaluation of uterine anomalies, and even this data are often based on small number of patients and most studies are not contemporaneous, with the most recent MRI study being from 2006 (Deutch et al. 2006).

1.2.1 Magnetic Resonance Imaging

Magnetic resonance imaging has many advantages to recommend it for the evaluation of structural anomalies of the female reproductive tract, principally its non-invasive nature and the lack of ionising radiation. A combination of T1- and T2-weighted images are typically employed, with T1-weighted images being helpful to assess the presence of blood products and T2-weighted images depicting uterine zonal anatomy with the endometrium returning a bright T2 signal, surrounded by a T2 hypointense junctional zone, which typically measures between 8 and 10 mm in adult configuration uteri. A suggested MRI protocol for the evaluation of structural anomalies is shown in Table 3.

Reported sensitivity and specificity of MRI for the detection and classification of Müllerian duct abnormalities varies widely, with one group showing a sensitivity of 77% and specificity of 33% (Letterie et al. 1995) and several other groups reporting sensitivity and specificity of 100% (Deutch et al. 2006; Carrington et al. 1990). The wide variability observed is likely due to several confounding factors including sample size, type of magnet, the specific sequences used and experience of the reporting radiologist, making an assessment of the true accuracy of MRI for depiction of uterine anomalies difficult. Similarly there are limited data evaluating the accuracy of MRI in depicting vaginal anomalies, with one study (Humphries et al. 2008) reporting a good correlation between MRI and surgical findings, but this study stresses the need for good communication between clinical and radiological teams, as this is a challenging area (see Sect. 1.3.10).

1.2.2 Ultrasound Techniques

Newer ultrasound techniques show great promise for the accurate depiction of Müllerian anomalies, particularly three dimension (3D) transvaginal ultrasound and ultrasound hysterosonography. 3D ultrasound allows a 3D rendering of the uterus generated from 2D images. This allows depiction of the internal cavitary arrangement of the uterus and the external contour, best depicted via a true coronal view of the uterus. This enables accurate differentiation of septate, subseptate, bicornuate and arcuate uteri, with Kupešić et al. (2002) finding an overall accuracy of 99.4% for the differentiation of septate uteri from other types of uterine abnormality. The ability of MRI to perform this differentiation varies widely in the literature, ranging from a sensitivity and specificity of 100% (Pellerito et al. 1992) to a sensitivity as low as 28% (Deutch et al. 2006). In order to maximise diagnostic accuracy of MRI it is imperative to align coronal plane images to the long axis of the uterus, allowing accurate depiction of the external contour (Imaoka et al. 2003; Brown 2006).

Ultrasound hysterosonography utilises either sterile water or saline to 'opacify' the endometrial cavity, with a high sensitivity and specificity for distinguishing septate and bicornuate uteri (Puscheck and Cohen

Table 3 Suggested MRI protocol for the evaluation of structural abnormalities of the female genital tract

Sequence	Slice thickness (mm)	Base resolution	FOV phase	TR	TE	Averages
Upper abdomen						
T2 Tru-Fisp Cor breath hold	5	256	93.8	4.07	2.04	1
T1 2D FLASH axial multi breath hold	6	256	68.8	113	4.91	1
Administer IV buscopan						
Pelvis						
T2 TSE sagittal and axial	6	256	100	4,510	97	3
T2 TSE coronal angled to long axis of the uterus	6	256	100	4,510	97	3
T1 SE axial	5	320	75	500	12	2
Administer IV gadolinium						
T1 SE fat sat. axial and sagittal	5	320	75	595	12	2

2008). Despite the attractiveness of these newer ultrasound techniques used in adult patients, the need for a cavitary transducer with or without cervical catheterisation limits their use in paediatric and adolescent patients. Given these limitations, the most practical means of pre-operative evaluation of structural anomalies of the female genital tract in paediatric and adolescent patients remains a combination of transabdominal ultrasound and MRI (Lang et al. 1999), with catheter studies being utilised in the setting of cloacal or UGS anomalies.

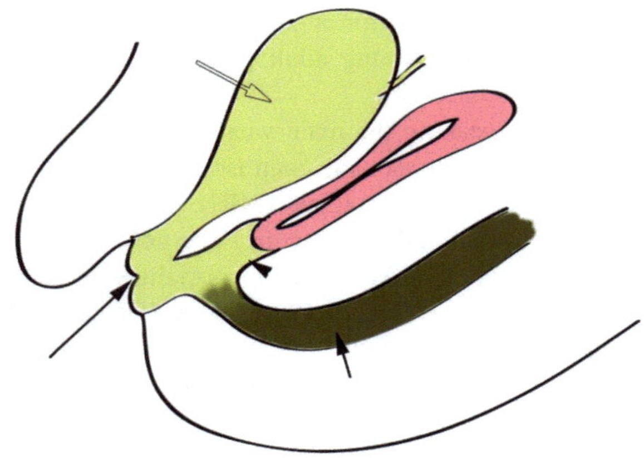

Fig. 2 *Cloacal anomaly:* Line diagram depicting the anatomy of cloacal anomaly. There is a common perineal opening (*long arrow*), which is formed by the confluence of the genital tract (*arrowhead*), hindgut (*short arrow*) and urinary tract (*open arrow*)

1.3 Structural Abnormalities

1.3.1 Cloacal Malformation

Failure of separation of the embryological cloaca by the urorectal septum into rectum and UGS at approximately 5 weeks of gestation results in a persistent common confluence of the urinary tract, genital tract and hindgut (Fig. 2). This uncommon abnormality, with an incidence of approximately 1 in 50,000 births (Warne et al. 2002) affects only patients who are phenotypically female, as opposed to the more severe, less frequent and of different embryological origin, cloacal exstrophy which may affect both males and females. The clinical phenotype is extremely variable.

The prenatal diagnosis of cloacal anomaly can be challenging, with a spectrum of abnormalities described on ultrasound including a bilobed dilated cystic pelvic mass comprising the vagina and bladder (Warne et al. 2002). Possible associated findings include foetal ascites, thought to be secondary to retrograde flow of urine into the peritoneal cavity via the fallopian tubes, and hydronephrosis if there is sufficient bladder outflow obstruction. Maternal MRI may help to identify cloacal anomaly (Hung et al. 2008) antenatally and differentiate simple hydrocolpos from that associated with cloacal anomaly, with lack of normal T1 hyperintense bowel content adjacent to the bladder being reported as being discriminatory (Picone et al. 2007). Alternative diagnoses presenting as cystic pelvic masses in female neonates include rectal duplication cysts, anterior meningocele and sacrococcygeal teratoma, and these should be considered when faced with this clinical scenario (Table 4).

Table 4 Differential diagnosis of pelvic mass in a female neonate

1. Hydrometrocolpos
Cystic
Multiple internal echoes ± layering
May identify uterus superior to the mass
If large may appear as an abdominal mass
2. Rectal duplication cyst
Cystic
Clearly defined wall—may be able to identify bowel wall layers
Tubular ± internal echoes if haemorrhagic
3. Sacrococcygeal teratoma
Mixed solid and cystic ± calcification
May be purely cystic with septations
May be external swelling
4. Anterior meningocele
Cystic
Associate spinal anomalies may need plain film/US/CT/MRI to evaluate
5. Pelvic neuroblastoma
Usually solid
Classically with fine calcifications
"Ill" child
6. Bladder rhabdomyosarcoma
Solid mass ± cystic necrosis
Older child
Abdominal mass ± liver lesions/lymphadenopathy

Postnatally the primary aim of imaging is to define the anatomy for surgical planning and this is usually undertaken via the common perineal channel and/or via the distal limb of a defunctioning colostomy, which is performed to divert the bowel content away from the urogenital tract (Jaramillo et al. 1990). This is usually undertaken using fluoroscopic techniques, with contrast agent introduced via catheters. This procedure can be challenging and may yield ambiguous results. More recently, there have been case reports detailing the use of cross sectional imaging to define the anatomy more accurately. Adams et al. (2006) describe a technique in a single case using multi-detector computed tomography (MDCT) in which contrast material is introduced via catheter to the perineal orifice and delayed scanning is performed after intravenous contrast injection, to produce a combined CT 'cystogram' and CT urogram, to good effect. 3D magnetic resonance (MR) genitography is also feasible, using a 3D spoiled gradient echo technique following instillation of gadolinium via the perineal opening, in combination with contrast injection into either colostomy or vesicostomy if present (Baughman et al. 2007), with the advantage of no radiation burden.

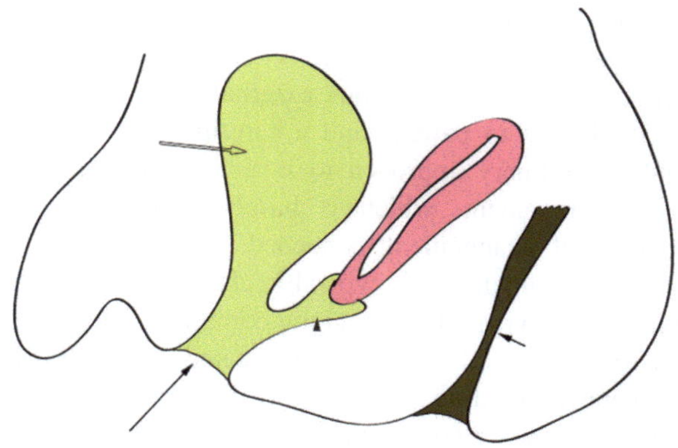

Fig. 3 *Urogenital sinus*: Line diagram depicting the anatomy of the urogenital sinus anomaly. The common perineal opening (*long arrow*) is formed by the confluence of the vagina (*arrowhead*) and urethra (bladder—*open arrow*). The anus (*short arrow*) opens separately, but may not be in the expected normal position

Associated abnormalities are frequently encountered in patients with cloacal anomaly, particularly spinal dysraphism, with an incidence of approximately 50% (Jaramillo et al. 1990; Dick et al. 2001) for which spinal ultrasound has a high sensitivity. Given the high incidence of associated spinal anomalies, care should be taken to also evaluate this if an MRI is performed to define the anatomy, as described above. Double uterus and vagina are also seen in approximately 50% of cases, although this may be difficult to define in a neonate if there is no obstruction present, and should ideally be evaluated after puberty.

1.3.2 Urogenital Sinus

Division of the cloaca by the urorectal septum at approximately 5 weeks of gestation leads to a common urogenital channel (the urogenital sinus) and rectum. Failure of division of the UGS leads to a persistent sinus that can be observed at birth (Fig. 3). The majority of patients with a UGS have ambiguous external genitalia and this condition is most commonly associated with congenital adrenal hyperplasia

(CAH), although UGS anomalies can also occur in the absence of a disorder of sex development. The presence of ambiguous external genitalia is of great distress to parents and a careful and sensitive multidisciplinary approach to investigation and further management, which is based on the precise anatomical arrangement, is needed.

UGS anomalies are typically classified as being either high (where there is a long common channel) or low (where the channel is low, located closer to the perineum) (Hendren and Crawford 1969). Alternative classification systems exist, using the degree of masculinisation of the external genitalia (Prader 1954), or a combination of masculinisation, phallic size and the true location of the vaginal meatus in relation to the bladder neck and perineal meatus (Rink et al. 2005).

Imaging investigation of patients with UGS typically include ultrasound to look for the presence or absence of a uterus, identify the gonads, evaluate the kidneys and to look for associated anomalies. The spine should also be evaluated using either ultrasound or MRI depending on the age of the child. As for cloacal anomalies, catheter studies are usually performed to define the luminal anatomy. It has been reported that this can be performed using ultrasound contrast agent, where local experience allows (Kopac et al. 2009).

1.3.3 Septate Uterus and Bicornuate Uterus

Septate uterus accounts for over 50% of all Müllerian duct abnormalities, owing to a failure in resorption of the uterovaginal septum, and is associated with high incidence of spontaneous abortion and poor obstetric outcome (Heinonen et al. 1982; Maneschi et al. 1993; Propst and Hill 2000). The septum may either be complete, extending to the external os (septate uterus) or partial (subseptate), with a variable length (Fig. 4). Complete septae may extend into the upper vagina in approximately 25% of cases (Propst and Hill 2000) and duplication of the cervix can also be observed.

Bicornuate uterus accounts for approximately 10% of all Müllerian abnormalities. There is failure of fusion of the uterovaginal horns at the level of the fundus, with communication between the two cavities inferiorly. The cleft may extend to the level of the internal os (complete bicornuate uterus) or a variable distance from the fundus (partial bicornuate configuration). There is a degree of variation in the exact manifestation of the bicornuate abnormality (Toaff et al. 1984) and duplicated cervices can be seen, as a longitudinal upper vaginal septum in up to 25% of cases (Fig. 5a–e).

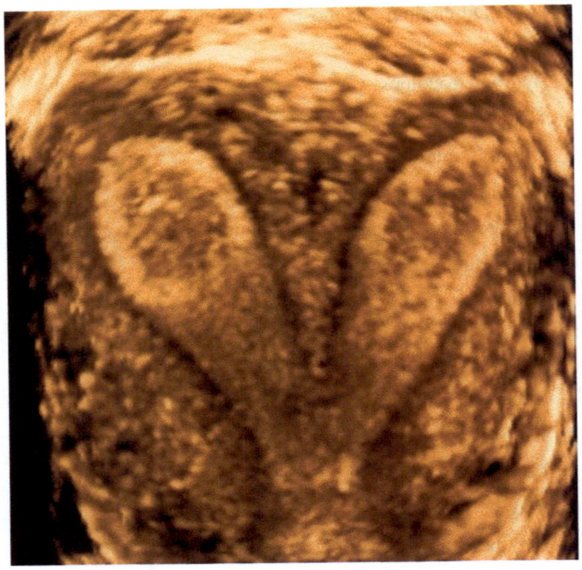

Fig. 4 *Subseptate US*: 3D ultrasound coronal view of the uterus showing a normal external fundal contour and an internal septum, which does not extend to the level of the cervix

Owing to different treatment approaches (hysteroscopic septoplasty for septate uterus, surgical approach for bicornuate uterus) it is important to differentiate the septate uterus from the bicornuate uterus and HSG, ultrasound (US) and MRI can all be used. At HSG an angle of <75° between the uterine horns suggests a septate uterus and an angle of >105° is said to be more consistent with a bicornuate uterus, however, there is overlap in the appearances of the two entities at HSG and the overall accuracy of HSG for differentiating between septate and bicornuate uteri is only 55% (Reuter et al. 1989). Both ultrasound and MRI can depict the internal architecture of the uterus and assess the external uterine contour in an attempt to differentiate between septate and bicornuate uteri. On US a septum appears as an intermediate echogenicity structure separating the cavity, which when complete has a hypoechoic lower portion, thought to be secondary to fibrosis. On MR imaging the septum appears isointense to the adjacent myometrium, with a caudal low-signal intensity segment extending to the os when complete, being the MR correlate of the hypoechoic fibrous portion seen on US. Evaluation of the external

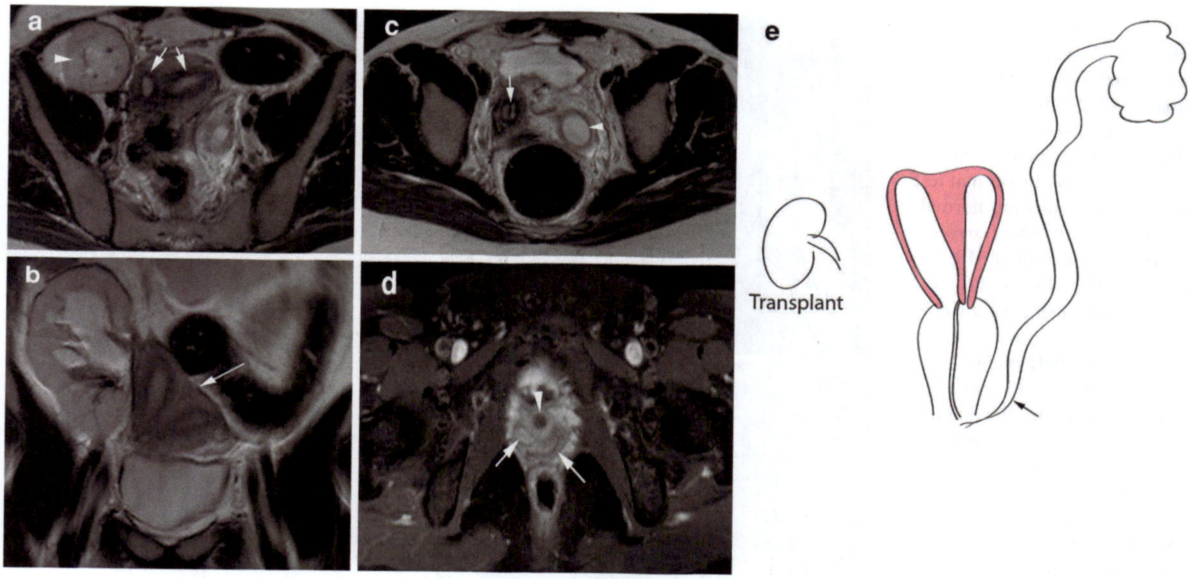

Fig. 5 *Septate uterus and double vagina*: **a** Axial T2-weighted MR image (TR 7560 ms, TE 96 ms), demonstrating a double cavity uterus (*arrows*) and a right iliac fossa renal transplant (*arrowhead*). **b** Coronal T2-weighted MR image demonstrating that there is no significant indentation in the fundal contour (*arrow*). **c** Axial T2-weighted MR image at the level of the cervix, demonstrating double cervix (bicollis) (*short arrow*) and dilated left ureter (*arrowhead*). **d** Axial post-Gadolinium fat-saturated T1-weighted MR image (TR 595 ms, TE 12 ms) showing two distal vaginal lumens (*arrows*), lying adjacent to the urethra (*arrowhead*). **e** Line diagram overview of the anatomy of this case. Note left hydroureter (*arrow*), which could be confused for hydrosalpynx without upper abdominal images

uterine configuration on a true orthogonal long axis view of the uterus is used to differentiate septate from bicornuate uterus. An interostial line is drawn and the degree of fundal indentation assessed. If the indentation is below the interostial line, or <5 mm above it, the uterus is considered to be bicornuate or didelphyic. If the indentation is more than 5 mm above the interostial line the uterus is septate (Homer et al. 2000; Fedele et al. 1988).

1.3.4 Arcuate Uterus

Despite being originally classified as a subset of bicornuate uterus by Buttram and Gibbons (1979), there is some debate as to whether an arcuate uterus should be considered a congenital abnormality or variant of normal. There is a mild indentation of the uterine fundus by myometrium that appears identical to the remainder of myometrium on both US and MRI, with no low reflectivity/low T2 signal fibrous component seen. The external uterine contour is normal and there is no division of the uterine horns (Pellerito et al. 1992) (Fig. 6).

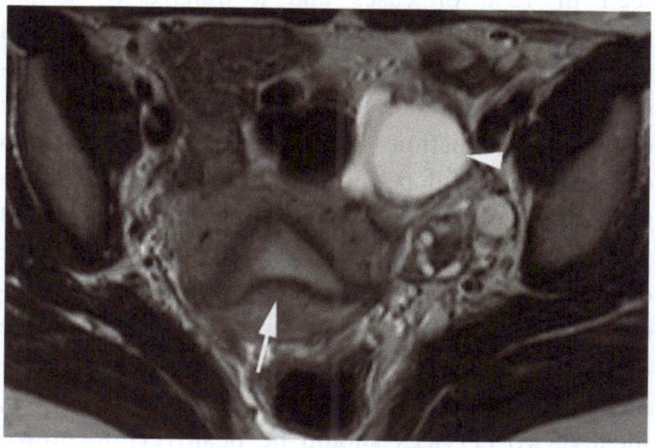

Fig. 6 *Arcuate uterus*: Axial T2-weighted MRI image (TE 7560 ms, TR 96 ms) showing normal external uterine contour, with mild indentation of the endometrium at the uterine fundus (*arrow*). Note is made of left hydrosalpynx (*arrowhead*)

1.3.5 Uterus Didelphys

Uterus didelphys results from almost total failure of fusion of the two Müllerian ducts, resulting in non-communicating hemiuteri and cervices, each with its own fallopian tube. A longitudinal vaginal septum is

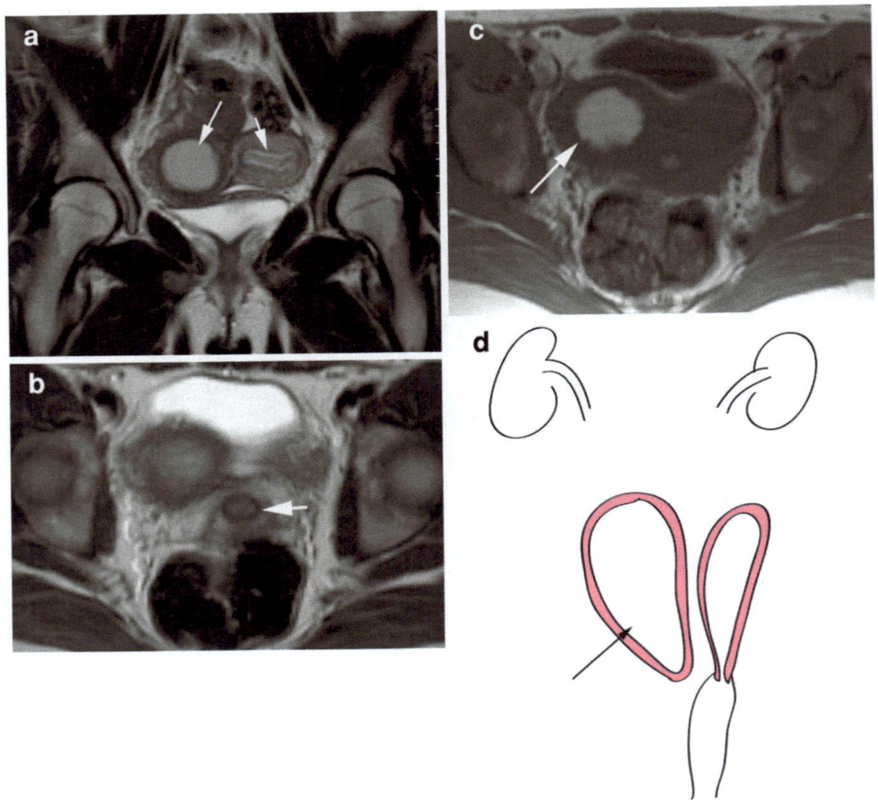

Fig. 7 *Uterus didelphys with obstructed right hemi-uterus*: **a** Coronal T2-weighted MR image (TR 5940 ms, TE 74 ms) demonstrating a distended right hemi-uterus (*long arrow*) and a normal left hemi-uterus, showing normal zonal anatomy (*short arrow*). **b** Axial T2-weighted MR image (TR 5940 ms, TE 74 ms) demonstrating a single cervix (*short arrow*). **c** Axial T1-weighted MR image (TR 578 ms, TE 13 ms) demonstrating haemorrhagic content of the right hemi-uterus (*arrow*). **d** Line diagram depicting the anatomy of this case. Didelphic uterus with an obstructed right hemi-uterus (*arrow*). The left hemi-uterus and vagina are normal

seen in 75% of cases and a transverse vaginal septum may also be seen. This can manifest as unilateral haematocolpos, usually becoming symptomatic at menarche. Retrograde menstruation may occur if obstruction is present and can lead to endometriosis and pelvic adhesions. Imaging investigations demonstrate two separate uterine cavities with a large cleft seen between them. The uterine cavities are of expected size, have normal endometrial–myometrial zonal anatomy and maintain the normal endometrial–myometrial ratio. No communication exists between the two cavities (Fig. 7a–d). Ideally two cervices should be positively identified in order to make the diagnosis (Carrington et al. 1990).

1.3.6 Unicornuate Uterus

Failure of development of one Müllerian duct results in ipsilateral maldevelopment of the uterus and vagina, with contralateral unicornuate uterus accounting for approximately 20% of all Müllerian abnormalities. In one-third of cases there is complete agenesis of the uterus ipsilateral to the abnormal Müllerian duct, manifesting as an isolated contralateral unicornuate uterus (Fig. 8). In approximately two-thirds of cases there is a rudimentary uterine horn ipsilateral to the Müllerian duct abnormality, which may either have a cavity (33%) or be non-cavitary (33%). Cavitary rudimentary horns may communicate with the unicornuate uterus in approximately 10% of all cases. The abnormality is usually asymptomatic but may manifest with cyclical pain if there is a non-communicating cavitary rudimentary horn, and resection of this is advised both for symptomatic relief and to avoid complication of ectopic pregnancy, which can occur via transperitoneal sperm migration (Rolen et al. 1966).

1.3.7 DES-Exposed Uterus

The synthetic oestrogen diethylstibisterol (DES) was used during 1950–1970s to treat recurrent spontaneous abortions and premature delivery. Although exposure is associated with structural abnormalities in female children exposed in utero (AFS group VII) (chiefly a T-shaped uterine cavity), this group will not be considered here as DES was discontinued in 1971

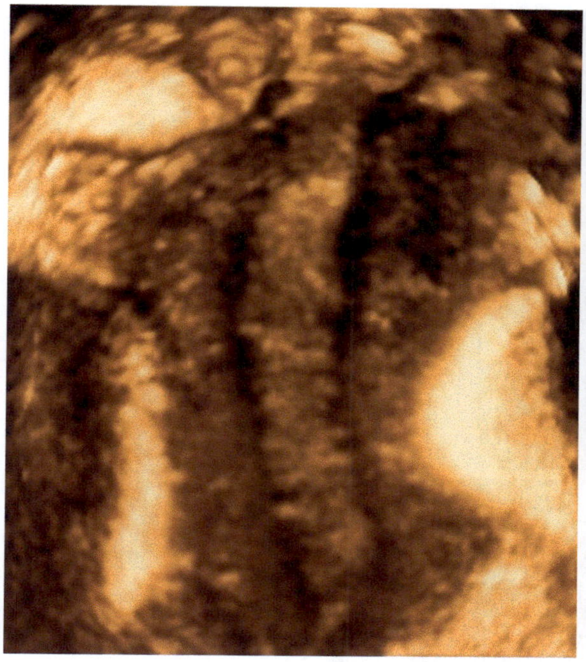

Fig. 8 *Unicornuate uterus*: 3D ultrasound coronal view of the uterus showing a 'finger' like appearance, typical of a unicornuate uterus

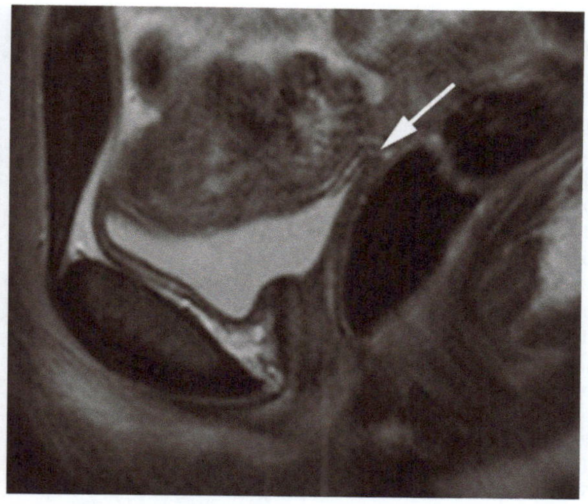

Fig. 9 *Rokitansky syndrome*: Sagital T2-weigted MR image (TR 4510 ms, TE 97 ms) demonstrating absence of the uterus. Note the 'pointed' configuration of the bladder (*arrow*) posteriorly, which is frequently observed in the absence of uterine tissue

and thus current paediatric and adolescent patients do not fall into the cohort of those exposed.

1.3.8 Mayer–Rokitansky–Kuster–Hauser Syndrome

Mayer–Rokitansky–Kuster–Hauser (MRKH) syndrome is a disorder of Müllerian duct formation in patients who are genotypically female, typically presenting with primary amenorrhoea (Oppelt et al. 2006). The exact cause for the failure of Müllerian development is unclear but is thought to occur between 4th and 12th week of gestation.

The syndrome was originally believed to be sporadic, but familial clusters have more recently led a search for a genetic cause. One of the most widely investigated group of genes investigated are the WNT genes, in particular the WNT4 gene that acts as a suppressor of male sexual differentiation (Jordan et al. 2001). WNT4 deficiency has been described in small series of patients with Müllerian duct failure, but crucially these patients also have androgen excess (Biason-Lauber et al. 2004, 2007) and it has been suggested that this defines WNT4 deficiency as a separate clinical entity to MRKH syndrome (Biason-Lauber et al. 2007). More recently a genetic study of 11 members of the same family with MRKH syndrome failed to observe causal mutations in several WNT genes, suggesting that mutations in the coding sequence of these genes are not responsible for MRKH (Ravel et al. 2009).

MRKH typically consists of a solid rudimentary bipartite uterus and a solid vagina without a lumen (vaginal 'agenesis') (Fig. 9). The ovaries, fallopian tubes and kidneys are normal in typical MRKH, resulting in normal female secondary sexual characteristics. MRKH has a variable expression, for example vaginal anomalies vary from complete agenesis, through short distal vagina and absent proximal 2/3, to an almost normal appearance. Similarly the uterus can contain functioning endometrial tissue and this can lead to cyclical pain and endometriosis if there is vaginal agenesis.

In addition to the typical cluster of findings described above, there are some patients who have atypical features with associated anomalies of the renal tract or ovaries being observed. Furthermore, Duncan et al. (1979) described a combination of Müllerian duct aplasia (MU), renal aplasia (R) and cervical somite dysplasia (CS) as a second atypical form of MRKH syndrome, the so-called MURCS association. It has been further suggested that the

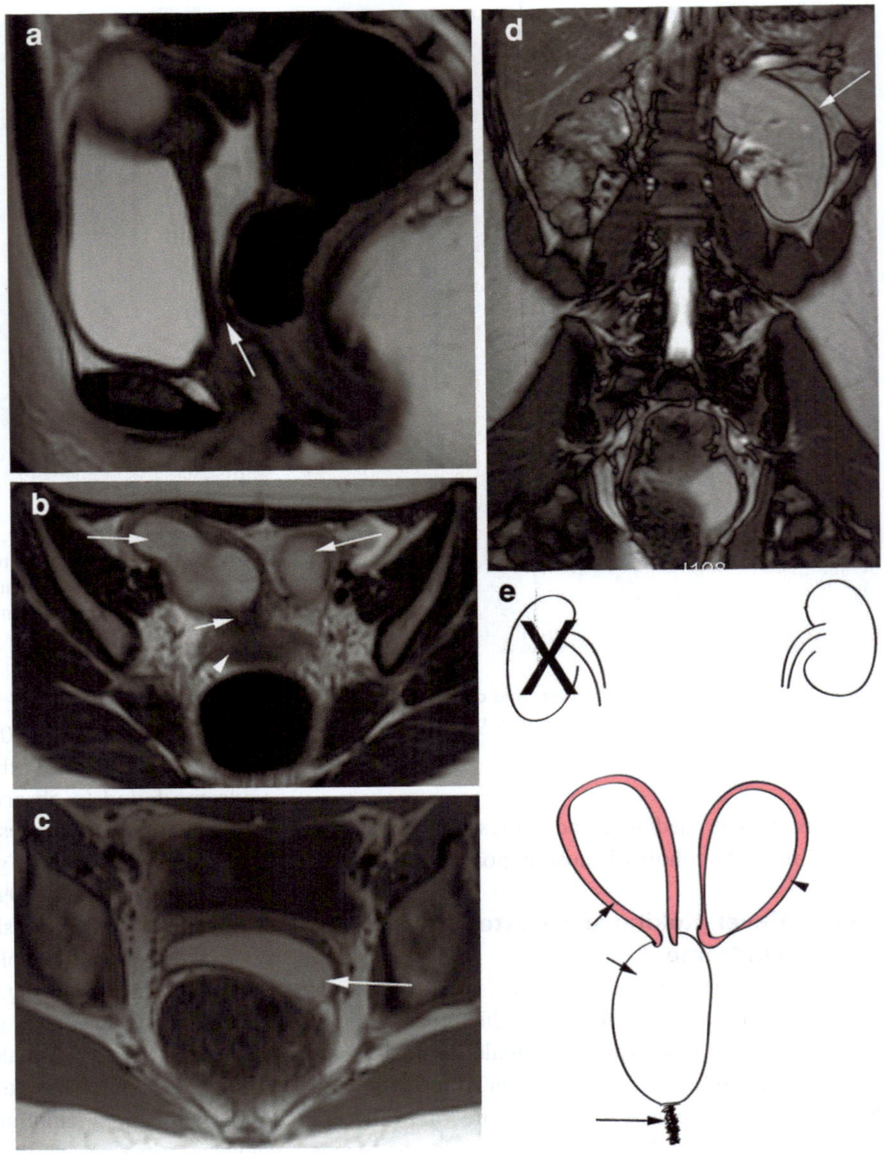

Fig. 10 *Obstructed uterus didelphys, distal vaginal atresia and renal agenesis (Variant of HWWS)*: **a** Sagital T2-weighted MR image (TR 6150 ms, TE 71 ms) demonstrating a fluid-filled proximal vagina, with no discernable distal vaginal tissue (*arrow*). **b** Axial T2-weighted MR image (TR 6150 ms, TE 71 ms) demonstrating two hemi-uteri (*long arrows*). The right uterus has a cervix (*short arrow*) connecting to the sole vagina (*arrowhead*). **c** Axial T1-weighted MR image (TR 578 ms, TE 13 ms) demonstrating haemorrhagic content within the distended proximal vagina (*arrow*). **d** Coronal Tru-Fisp MR image (TR 4.3 ms, TE 2.15 ms) of the upper abdomen, demonstrating a solitary left kidney (*arrow*). **e** Line diagram depicting the anatomy of this case. Distal vaginal agenesis (*arrow*) causing obstruction of the right hemi-uterus and vagina (*short arrows*), with a non-communicating left hemi-uterus (*arrowhead*). Note right renal agenesis

atypical and MURCS groups be described as a GRES syndrome (Genital Renal Ear and Skeletal syndrome) (Strubbe et al. 1994). A review of 53 patients with MRKH syndrome, found typical features in approximately 50%, MURCS association in 30% and atypical features in 20%, with renal anomalies being the most frequent associated abnormality (Oppelt et al. 2006). MRI clearly defines the abnormality, with sagittal images being the most useful for identifying the rudimentary uterus.

1.3.9 Herlyn–Werner–Wunderlich Syndrome

Herlyn–Werner–Wunderlich syndrome (HWWS) is a rare abnormality consisting of uterus didelphys, renal agenesis and a vaginal septum on the side ipsilateral to the renal absence, usually resulting in vaginal obstruction. The exact incidence of HWWS is difficult to determine, with little data available in the literature. A single centre study (Gholoum et al. 2006) of all patients evaluated with uterine or vaginal anomalies over a 22-year period found that 15% had

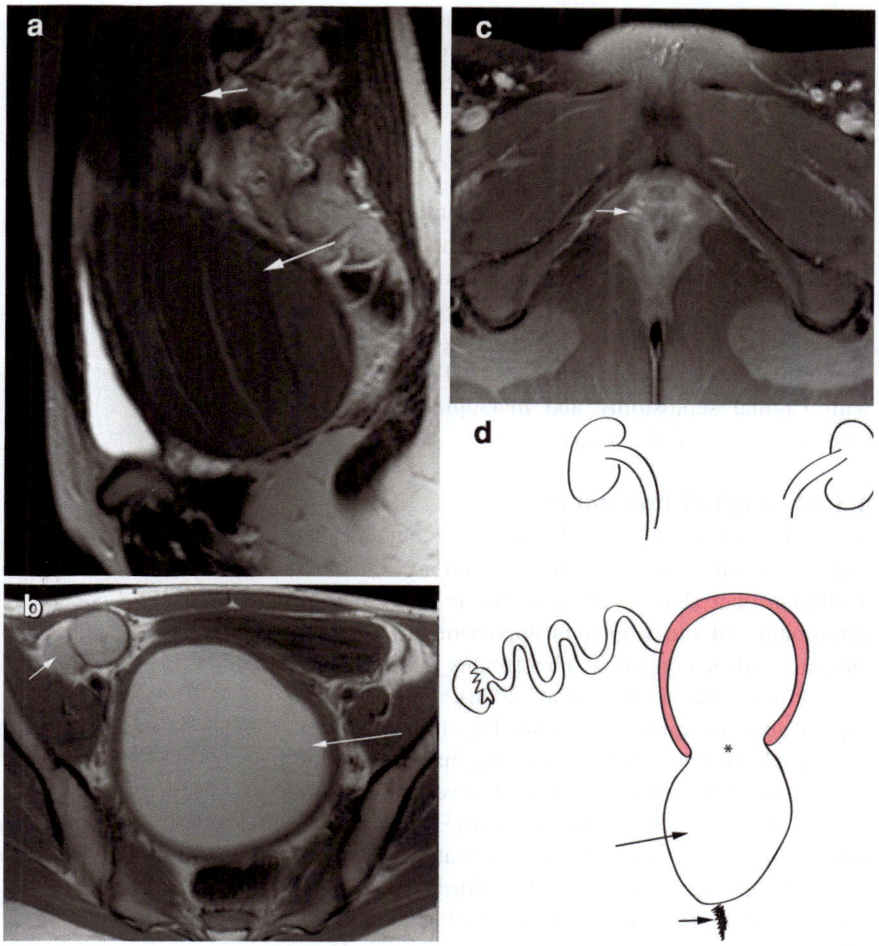

Fig. 11 *Distal vaginal agenesis*: **a** Sagital T2-weighted MR image (TR 8490 ms, TE 132 ms) demonstrating a bilobed dilated structure with low T2 signal contents (*arrows*), displacing the urinary bladder. **b** Axial T1-weighted MR image (TR 595 ms, TE 12 ms) demonstrating T1 shortening of the contents of the dilated structure, consistent with blood products (*long arrow*). There is also right haematosalpynx (*short arrow*). **c** Axial post-Gadolinium fat-saturated T1-weighted MR image (TR 595 ms, TE 12 ms) demonstrating an absence of the expected vaginal tissue posterior to the urethra, with only venous plexus present (*short arrow*). **d** Line diagram depicting the anatomy of this case. Combination of distended uterus and vagina (*long arrow*), with a widely open internal os (*asterisk*), appreciated as bilobed structure on MR imaging. The distal vagina was not present (*short arrow*). Note right haematosalpynx

HWWS. Patients usually present with abdominal pain or a pelvic/abdominopelvic mass (Gholoum et al. 2006) and the cause for the pain may remain occult for some time after initial presentation as menstruation occurs via the non-obstructed contralateral vagina. It may be only when the cyclical nature of the pain is recognised that a Müllerian duct abnormality is sought out. Interestingly the abnormality is overwhelmingly more common on the right (Gholoum et al. 2006); the cause for this is not known.

In addition to the classical abnormality, it is well recognised that there is a degree of variability. Communication between the two uteri or two vaginas is observed occasionally (Acien et al. 1987) and a degree of obstruction of the contralateral vagina has also been described (Gholoum et al. 2006) (Fig. 10a–e).

Ultrasound is an excellent means of recognising the anomaly, with didelphic uterus, haematocolpos secondary to the obstructed vagina and absent ipsilateral kidney readily seen. MRI is useful to clarify the anatomy and to confirm the haemorrhagic nature of the contents (Orazi et al. 2007). Although the most uncommon of all Müllerian duct abnormalities, awareness of the condition is vital in order to make the diagnosis. It has been suggested that all female infants with multicystic dysplastic kidneys or unilateral renal agenesis be carefully evaluated for the presence of uterus didelphys and an obstructed hemivagina (Orazi et al. 2007). As stated earlier, uterovaginal anomalies in the neonatal period can be very difficult to identify, even with the residual presence of maternal hormones making the uterus more prominent than later in infancy. Such an approach to identifying HWWS as advocated by Orazi et al. would therefore require long-term follow-up, at least until the onset of puberty.

Accurate identification of patients with HWWS is important, as if left untreated there is a risk for endometriosis, pelvic adhesions and infection (Zurawin et al. 2004; Olive and Henderson 1987; Haddad et al. 1999). Surgical treatment of these patients has been reported to have a good outcome, with Gholoum et al. (2006) reporting cessation of symptoms in 11 of 12 patients with HWWS treated with vaginal septostomy and marsupialisation at a median follow-up of 3 years.

1.3.10 Vaginal Anomalies

There are a variety of vaginal structural anomalies that may be encountered, often in association with other Müllerian duct abnormalities, with one study finding abnormality of the vagina in approximately 68% of patients with a congenital abnormality of the upper genital tract (Humphries et al. 2008). The principal vaginal abnormalities are agenesis (Fig. 11a, b), as seen in MRKH syndrome, a transverse vaginal septum and duplication of the vagina secondary to a vertical septum.

A transverse vaginal septum may occur at any point, but is most often encountered at the junction between the upper and the middle third (Blask et al. 1991). A complete septum leads to haematocolpos where there is functioning endometrial tissue. 'Double vagina' is most often seen in the setting of uterine duplication anomalies.

It is important to accurately define vaginal anatomy in the setting of an obstructive congenital anomaly as the capacity and length of the distal vaginal segment is an important factor in determining the surgical approach. Proximal segments with good length and capacity can be treated via a perineal rather than abdominal incision and may not require a graft or intestinal bridge to facilitate anastomosis.

Various techniques are available for assessing the vagina in this group of patients with the use of a cotton bud to determine the length of the distal segment being a bedside test that is readily performed. Trans-abdominal ultrasound has limited utility and cavitary ultrasound is poorly tolerated and is often inappropriate for many adolescent and paediatric patients. Although some authors advocate the use of jelly or other means of distending the vagina to improve its depiction (Olpin and Heilbrun 2009), it has been shown that using small field of view T2-weighted and post-contrast fat-saturated T1-weighted images is a reliable method for evaluating the vagina (Fig. 12a, b) (Humphries et al. 2008). The added advantage of MRI over clinical 'cotton bud method' or ultrasound methods is that the proximal vagina can be defined accurately and easily assessed.

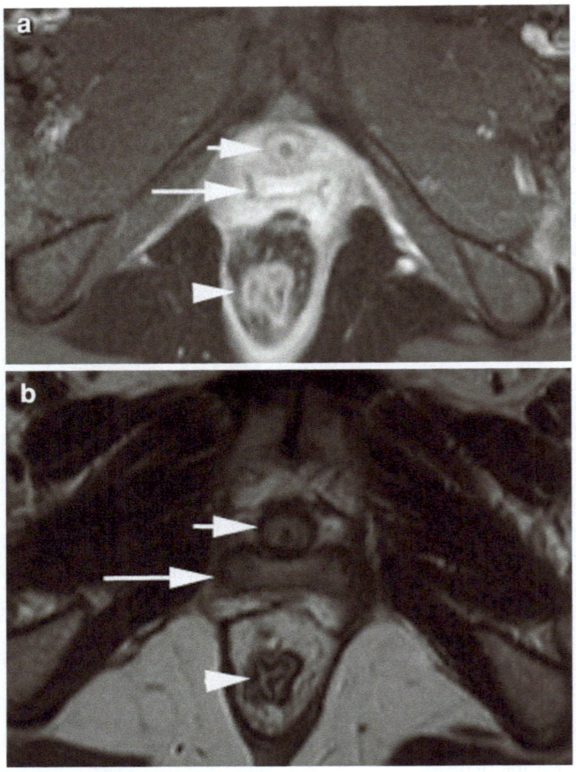

Fig. 12 *Normal vagina MRI*: Axial post-Gadolinium fat-saturated T1-weighted (TR 595 ms, TE 12 ms) (**a**) and T2-weighted (TR 7560 ms, TE 96 ms) MRI images (**b**), showing normal H-shaped configuration of the vagina (*arrow*), interposed between the urethra (*short arrow*) and rectum (*arrowhead*)

2 Conclusion

Structural abnormalities of the paediatric and adolescent female genital tract are a complex, heterogeneous group of disorders with a variety of clinical and radiological manifestations. There are a number of imaging investigations available that may be used to evaluate patients with suspected structural anomalies.

Imaging should be tailored to the clinical presentation and age of the patient, with ultrasound and MRI being the mainstays in the paediatric and adolescent age groups. Close interaction between clinical and radiological teams is vital to ensure that both groups understand and can communicate effectively with one another in order to avoid ambiguity when describing abnormalities. This in turn allows high quality, accurate examinations, facilitating appropriate management decisions.

3 Acknowledgment

Many thanks to Mr. Davor Jurkovic (University College London Hospital) for providing the 3D ultrasound images used in this chapter.

References

Acien P (1992) Embryological observations on the female genital tract. Hum Reprod 7:437–445

Acien P, Arminana E, Garcia-Ontiveros E (1987) Unilateral renal agenesis associated with ipsilateral blind vagina. Arch Gynecol 240:1–8

Acien P, Acien M, Sanchez-Ferrer M (2004) Complex malformations of the female genital tract. New types and revision of classification. Hum Reprod 19:2377–2384

Adams ME, Hiorns MP, Wilcox DT (2006) Combining MDCT, micturating cystography, and excretory urography for 3D imaging of cloacal malformation. AJR Am J Roentgenol 187:1034–1035

Baughman SM, Richardson RR, Podberesky DJ et al (2007) 3-Dimensional magnetic resonance genitography: a different look at cloacal malformations. J Urol 178:1675–1678; discussion 1678–1679

Biason-Lauber A, Konrad D, Navratil F et al (2004) A WNT4 mutation associated with Mullerian-duct regression and virilization in a 46, XX woman. N Engl J Med 351:792–798

Biason-Lauber A, De Filippo G, Konrad D et al (2007) WNT4 deficiency—a clinical phenotype distinct from the classic Mayer-Rokitansky-Kuster-Hauser syndrome: a case report. Hum Reprod 22:224–229

Blask AR, Sanders RC, Rock JA (1991) Obstructed uterovaginal anomalies: demonstration with sonography. Part II. Teenagers. Radiology 179:84–88

Brown MA (2006) MR imaging of benign uterine disease. Magn Reson Imaging Clin N Am 14:439–453

Buttram VC, Gibbons WE (1979) Müllerian anomalies: a proposed classification (an analysis of 144 cases). Fertil Steril 32:40–46

Byrne J, Nussbaum-Blask A, Taylor WS et al (2000) Prevalence of Müllerian duct anomalies detected at ultrasound. Am J Med Genet 94:9–12

Carrington BM, Hricak H, Nuruddin RN et al (1990) Müllerian duct anomalies: MR imaging evaluation. Radiology 176:715–720

Deutch TD, Abuhamad AZ (2008) The role of 3-dimensional ultrasonography and magnetic resonance imaging in the diagnosis of Mullerian duct anomalies: a review of the literature. J Ultrasound Med 27:413–423

Deutch T, Bocca S, Oehninger S et al (2006) Magnetic resonance imaging versus three-dimensional transvaginal ultrasound for the diagnosis of Müllerian anomalies. Fertil Steril 86:S308

Dick EA, de Bruyn R, Patel K et al (2001) Spinal ultrasound in cloacal exstrophy. Clin Radiol 56:289–294

Duncan PA, Shapiro LR, Stangel JJ et al (1979) The MURCS association: Mullerian duct aplasia, renal aplasia, and cervicothoracic somite dysplasia. J Pediatr 95:399–402

Fedele L, Ferrazzi E, Dorta M et al (1988) Ultrasonography in the differential diagnosis of "double" uteri. Fertil Steril 50:361–364

Gholoum S, Puligandla PS, Hui T et al (2006) Management and outcome of patients with combined vaginal septum, bifid uterus, and ipsilateral renal agenesis (Herlyn-Werner-Wunderlich syndrome). J Pediatr Surg 41:987–992

Haddad B, Barranger E, Paniel BJ (1999) Blind hemivagina: long-term follow-up and reproductive performance in 42 cases. Hum Reprod 14:1962–1964

Heinonen PK, Saarikoski S, Pystynen P (1982) Reproductive performance of women with uterine anomalies. An evaluation of 182 cases. Acta Obstet Gynecol Scand 61:157–162

Hendren WH, Crawford JD (1969) Adrenogenital syndrome: the anatomy of the anomaly and its repair. Some new concepts. J Pediatr Surg 4:49–58

Homer HA, Li TC, Cooke ID (2000) The septate uterus: a review of management and reproductive outcome. Fertil Steril 73:1–14

Humphries PD, Simpson JC, Creighton SM et al (2008) MRI in the assessment of congenital vaginal anomalies. Clin Radiol 63:442–448

Hung YH, Tsai C, Ou C et al (2008) Late prenatal diagnosis of hydrometrocolpos secondary to a cloacal anomaly by abdominal ultrasonography with complementary magnetic resonance imaging. Taiwan J Obstet Gynecol 47:79–83

Imaoka I, Wada A, Matsuo M et al (2003) MR imaging of disorders associated with female infertility: use in diagnosis, treatment, and management. Radiographics 23:1401–1421

Jaramillo D, Lebowitz RL, Hendren WH (1990) The cloacal malformation: radiologic findings and imaging recommendations. Radiology 177:441–448

Jordan BK, Mohammed M, Ching ST et al (2001) Up-regulation of WNT-4 signaling and dosage-sensitive sex reversal in humans. Am J Hum Genet 68:1102–1109

Kopac M, Riccabona M, Haim M (2009) Contrast-enhanced voiding urosonography and genitography in a baby with ambiguous genitalia and urogenital sinus. Ultraschall Med 30:299–300

Kupešić S, Kurjak A, Skenderovic S et al (2002) Screening for uterine abnormalities by three-dimensional ultrasound improves perinatal outcome. J Perinat Med 30:9–17

Lang IM, Babyn PS, Oliver GD (1999) MR imaging of paediatric uterovaginal anomalies. Pediatr Radiol 29:163–170

Letterie GS, Haggerty M, Lindee G (1995) A comparison of pelvic ultrasound and magnetic resonance imaging as diagnostic studies for Müllerian tract abnormalities. Int J Fertil Menopausal Stud 40:34–38

Maneschi F, Marana R, Muzii L et al (1993) Reproductive performance in women with bicornuate uterus. Acta Eur Fertil 24:117–120

Marten K, Vosshenrich R, Funke M et al (2003) MRI in the evaluation of Mullerian duct anomalies. Clin Imaging 27:346–350

Nahum GG (1998) Uterine anomalies. How common are they, and what is their distribution among subtypes? J Reprod Med 43:877–887

Nazir Z, Rizvi RM, Qureshi RN et al (2006) Congenital vaginal obstructions: varied presentation and outcome. Pediatr Surg Int 22:749–753

Olive DL, Henderson DY (1987) Endometriosis and Mullerian anomalies. Obstet Gynecol 69:412–415

Olpin JD, Heilbrun M (2009) Imaging of Müllerian duct anomalies. Clin Obstet Gynecol 52:40–56

Oppelt P, Renner SP, Brucker S et al (2005) The VCUAM (Vagina Cervix Uterus Adnex-associated Malformation) classification: a new classification for genital malformations. Fertil Steril 84:1493–1497

Oppelt P, Renner SP, Kellerman A et al (2006) Clinical aspects of Mayer-Rokitansky-Kuester-Hauser syndrome: recommendations for clinical diagnosis and staging. Hum Reprod 21:792–797

Oppelt P, von Have M, Paulsen M et al (2007) Female genital malformations and their associated abnormalities. Fertil Steril 87:335–342

Orazi C, Lucchetti MC, Schingo PMS et al (2007) Herlyn-Werner-Wunderlich syndrome: uterus didelphys, blind hemivagina and ipsilateral renal agenesis. Sonographic and MR findings in 11 cases. Pediatr Radiol 37:657–665

Pellerito JS, McCarthy SM, Doyle MB et al (1992) Diagnosis of uterine anomalies: relative accuracy of MR imaging, endovaginal sonography, and hysterosalpingography. Radiology 183:795–800

Picone O, Laperelle J O, Sonigo P et al (2007) Fetal magnetic resonance imaging in the antenatal diagnosis and management of hydrocolpos. Ultrasound Obstet Gynecol 30:105–109

Prader A (1954) Genital findings in the female pseudohermaphroditism of the congenital adrenogenital syndrome; morphology, frequency, development and heredity of the different genital forms. Helv Paediatr Acta 9:231–248

Propst AM, Hill JA 3rd (2000) Anatomic factors associated with recurrent pregnancy loss. Semin Reprod Med 18:341–350

Puscheck EE, Cohen L (2008) Congenital malformations of the uterus: the role of ultrasound. Semin Reprod Med 26:223–231

Raga F, Bauset C, Remohi J et al (1997) Reproductive impact of congenital Müllerian anomalies. Hum Reprod 12:2277–2281

Ravel C, Lorenço D, Dessolle L et al (2009) Mutational analysis of the WNT gene family in women with Mayer-Rokitansky-Kuster-Hauser syndrome. Fertil Steril 91:1604–1607

Reuter KL, Daly DC, Cohen SM (1989) Septate versus bicornuate uteri: errors in imaging diagnosis. Radiology 172:749–752

Rink RC, Adams MC, Misseri R (2005) A new classification for genital ambiguity and urogenital sinus anomalies. BJU Int 95:638–642

Rolen AC, Choquette AJ, Semmens JP (1966) Rudimentary uterine horn: obstetric and gynecologic implications. Obstet Gynecol 27:806–813

Salim R, Woelfer B, Backos M et al (2003) Reproducibility of three-dimensional ultrasound diagnosis of congenital uterine anomalies. Ultrasound Obstet Gynecol 21:578–582

Strubbe EH, Cremers CW, Willemsen WN et al (1994) The Mayer-Rokitansky-Kuster-Hauser (MRKH) syndrome without and with associated features: two separate entities? Clin Dysmorphol 3:192–199

Subramanian S, Sharma R, Gamanagatti S et al (2006) Antenatal MR diagnosis of urinary hydrometrocolpos due to urogenital sinus. Pediatr Radiol 36:1086–1089

The American Society of Reproductive Medicine (ASRM) (1988) The American Fertility Society classifications of adnexal adhesions, distal tubal occlusion, tubal occlusion secondary to tubal ligation, tubal pregnancies, Mullerian anomalies and intrauterine adhesions. Fertil Steril 49:944–955

Toaff ME, Lev-Toaff AS, Toaff R (1984) Communicating uteri: review and classification with introduction of two previously unreported types. Fertil Steril 41:661–679

Warne S, Chitty LS, Wilcox DT (2002) Prenatal diagnosis of cloacal anomalies. BJU Int 89:78–81

Zurawin RK, Dietrich JE, Heard MJ et al (2004) Didelphic uterus and obstructed hemivagina with renal agenesis: case report and review of the literature. J Pediatr Adolesc Gynecol 17:137–141

Normal Growth and Puberty

Caren J. Landes and Joanne C. Blair

Contents

1 **Introduction** 82

2 **Endocrinology of the Female Reproductive Tract** 82
2.1 Infancy 82
2.2 Childhood 83
2.3 Puberty 83

3 **Normal Anatomy and Imaging Appearances of the Female Reproductive Tract** 85
3.1 Vagina 85
3.2 Uterus 86
3.3 Rectouterine Pouch 91
3.4 The Adnexa 92

4 **Menstrual Cycle** 97
4.1 Endocrinology of the Normal Menstrual Cycle 97
4.2 Ultrasound Imaging of the Endometrium During the Menstrual Cycle 97
4.3 Zonal MR Anatomy of the Uterus During the Menstrual Cycle 101
4.4 Zonal MR Anatomy of the Ovary During the Menstrual Cycle 102

5 **Adrenal Gland** 103

6 **Pituitary** 103

7 **Assessment of Skeletal Maturity and Bone Age** 105

8 **Bone Mineralization** 107
8.1 Evaluation of Bone Mass 108

References 111

C. J. Landes (✉)
Department of Radiology,
Alder Hey Children's Hospital NHS Foundation Trust,
Liverpool, L12 2AP, UK
e-mail: caren.landes@alderhey.nhs.uk

J. C. Blair
Department of Endocrinology,
Alder Hey Children's Hospital NHS Foundation Trust,
Liverpool, L12 2AP, UK

Abstract

The appearances of the female reproductive tract during infancy, childhood and adolescence are regulated by the hypothalamic-pituitary-ovarian axis. During neonatal life and early infancy the development of the reproductive tract is stimulated by high levels of gonadotropins and oestrogen. During childhood, production of these hormones falls to rise again in late childhood and pubertal years. This chapter describes normal development, anatomy and diagnostic imaging appearances of the female reproductive tract in the context of the changes in hormone production that regulate development. Normal growth and bone maturation including the acquisition of bone mass is also discussed.

Abbreviations

IVC	Inferior vena cava
DHEA	Dehydroepiandrosterone
DHEAS	Dehydroepiandrosterone sulphate
VCUG	Voiding cystourethrogram
DWI	Diffusion weighted-imaging
GnRH	Gonadotropin-Releasing Hormone
hCG	human chorionic gonadotropin
h	Hours
H	Height
W	Width
D	Depth
MHz	Megahertz
ml	Millilitre

G. Mann et al. (eds.), *Imaging of Gynecological Disorders in Infants and Children*, Medical Radiology. Diagnostic Imaging, DOI: 10.1007/174_2011_309, © Springer-Verlag Berlin Heidelberg 2012

cm	centimetre
mm	Millimetre
cm^3	Cubic centimetre
s	Seconds
m	metre
SPAIR	Spectral Adiabatic Inversion Recovery
MFO	Multifollicular ovary
TSE	Turbospin Echo
T1W	T1-weighted
T2W	T2-weighted
AP	Anteroposterior
US	Ultrasound
CT	Computed Tomography
MRI	Magnetic Resonance Imaging
MR	Magnetic Resonance
SD	Standard deviation
LH	Luteinising hormone
FSH	Follicle stimulating hormone
DXA	Dual-emission X-ray absorptiometry
ADH	Anti-diuretic hormone (ADH)
FCR	Fundocervical ratio
G&P	Greulich & Pyle
IV	Intravenous
SMS	Skeletal maturity score
TW	Tanner-Whitehouse
TW2	Tanner-Whitehouse 2
TW3	Tanner-Whitehouse 3
BMD	Bone mineral density
g/cm^2	Grams per square centimetre
ROI	Region of interest
BMC	Bone mineral content
QCT	Quantitative computed tomography
QUS	Quantitative ultrasound
SOS	Speed of sound
BUA	Broadband ultrasound attenuation
dB	Decibel

1 Introduction

The appearances of the female reproductive tract during infancy, childhood and adolescence reflect the hormonal milieu at each stage of development. During neonatal life and early infancy hormones of maternal, placental, fetal and neonatal origin stimulate the development of the reproductive tract. In late infancy gonadotropin and oestrogen levels fall, rising again in the late childhood and pubertal years as the hypothalamic-pituitary–gonadal axis once again becomes active and an ovulatory cycle is established in late adolescence.

This chapter describes the normal development, anatomy and diagnostic imaging appearances of the female reproductive tract during each of these phases of life. A brief description of the normal appearances of the pituitary and adrenal glands is included. Normal growth and bone maturation including the acquisition of bone mass is also discussed. These developmental changes are set in the context of normal hormonal changes that are described briefly.

2 Endocrinology of the Female Reproductive Tract

2.1 Infancy

The hypothalamic-pituitary-ovarian pathway is well developed at the time of birth. Gonadotropin and ovarian sex steroid secretion are important for the stimulation of germ cell division and follicular development. By 5–6 months gestation the ovary has approximately 6–7 million primordial follicles. This number falls to 2–4 million in the neonate and by puberty only 400,000 remain (Baker 1963).

At delivery the infant is exposed to an abrupt withdrawal of maternal and placental hormones and the hypothalamic-pituitary-ovarian axis escapes the inhibitory effect of maternal oestrogen. At the time of delivery serum oestrogen levels are high and gonadotropins are low, but as the inhibitory effect of maternal oestrogen wanes during the first week of life gonadotropin concentrations rise. In female infants follicle stimulating hormone (FSH) is the dominant hormone of the postnatal gonadotropin surge (Winter et al. 1975), stimulating a rapid increase in ovarian follicular maturation during the first 4 months of life (Polhemus 1953). Serum FSH peaks around 3–6 months of age and declines from the age of 12 months, becoming unmeasurable by the age of 2 years. The more modest postnatal rise in luteinizing hormone (LH) stimulates the secretion of oestrogen from ovarian follicles during the first 2–4 months of age (Winter et al. 1976).

Serum prolactin increases threefold in the last trimester of pregnancy and falls rapidly in the first eight weeks of life in the term infant. In contrast, prolactin levels rise steadily during the first few weeks of life in the preterm infant (Mckiernan and Hull 1981).

2.2 Childhood

During early childhood the activity of the hypothalamic-pituitary-ovarian axis is downregulated under the influence of the central nervous system pathways. Reactivation of the hypothalamic-pituitary–gonadal axis is seen in girls from the age of 5–6 years.

Between the ages of 6 and 8 years the activity of the microsomal enzyme p450c17 in the zona reticularis of the adrenal cortex increases. This increase in enzyme activity induces the synthesis and secretion of the adrenal androgens dehydroepiandrosterone (DHEA), its sulphate (DHEAS) and androstendione.

2.3 Puberty

2.3.1 Regulation of the Onset of Puberty

Pubertal and skeletal maturation seem to be regulated by similar mechanisms. Girls generally enter puberty when they achieve a pubertal bone age and pubertal development correlates better with bone age than chronological age, height or weight particularly approaching menarche.

The first signs of pubertal development are seen in 99% of girls between the ages of 8 and 13 years. Pubertal development in girls below this age is traditionally considered to be 'precocious' and the absence of any signs of pubertal development in girls aged more than 13 years is considered 'delayed'. However, data from a North American cross sectional study of more than 17,000 girls report that 27% of African American girls and 7% of white girls had breast development or pubic hair growth below the age of 7 years (Herman-Giddens et al. 1997). In response to these data the definition of precocious puberty has been revised, with puberty being considered precocious in African American girls aged less than 6 years and white girls aged less than 7 years (Kaplowitz et al. 1999).

The mechanisms by which the onset of puberty is initiated are obscure however, epidemiological studies have identified a number of factors that influence the timing of puberty. The age of menarche in mothers is related to the timing of puberty in daughters and recent genetic studies have identified a number of genes that may, in part, explain this observation (Kadlubar et al. 2003; Stavrou et al. 2002; Xita et al. 2005). The age at onset of puberty is also influenced strongly by environmental factors of which nutrition may be the most important. Early severe protein malnutrition presenting as marasmus delays the timing of puberty (Galler et al. 1987) and chronic malnutrition delays menarche by approximately 2 years (Kulin et al. 1982). Conversely, an inverse relationship exists between body mass index, fat mass and age at the onset of puberty (Kaplowitz et al. 2001). Leptin (a hormone secreted by fat cells) appears to play a significant role. Leptin signals that caloric intake and fat stores are adequate, inhibits appetite and stimulates gonadotropin secretion. An adequate level of leptin is critical for the attainment of puberty, and leptin deficient subjects have been observed to have delayed puberty, with the onset of gonadotropin secretion once leptin is administered (Farooqi et al. 1999). These data have led to speculation that the secular trend towards an earlier age at the start of puberty and menarche (Euling et al. 2008) may be related to the increasing prevalence of childhood obesity.

The effect of in utero nutrition on the timing of puberty is controversial. In some studies girls born small for gestational age are reported to have an earlier onset of puberty than those born appropriate for gestational age (Lazar et al. 2003; Ibáñez et al. 2000; Veening et al. 2004) while others report no effect of birth weight on the timing of puberty (Powls et al. 1996). Studies that include early childhood growth suggest that the relationship between birth weight and puberty is mediated through early growth in childhood, with those growing most rapidly experiencing the onset of puberty at an earlier age (dos Santos Silva et al. 2002).

2.3.2 Endocrine Changes During Puberty

During the late prepubertal years pulses of gonadotropin-releasing hormone (GnRH) are secreted with increased frequency, initially during sleep (Landy et al. 1990). Serum concentrations of FSH rise to levels in excess of LH at the earliest stages of development but as the amplitude of GnRH pulses increases LH secretion becomes dominant as puberty progresses.

The gonadotropins act in concert to stimulate ovarian oestrogen synthesis and secretion. Pulses of

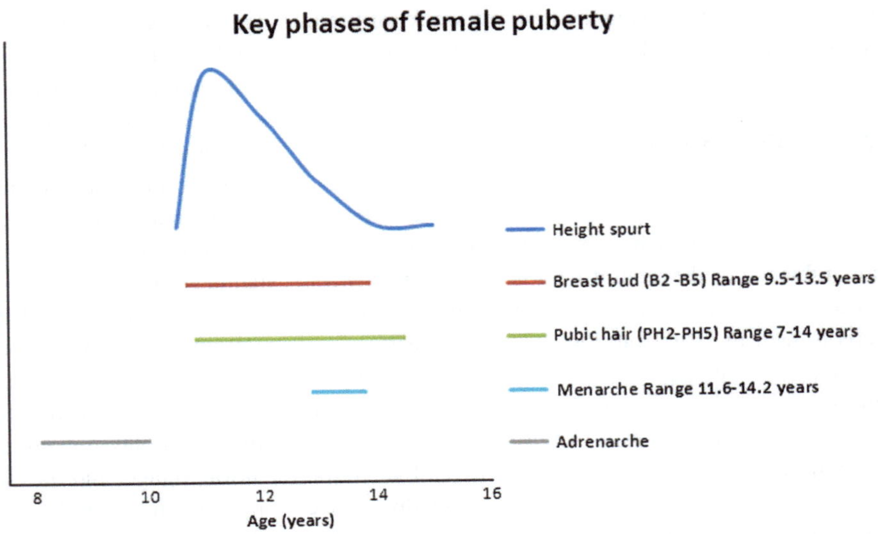

Fig. 1 Line diagram summarising the typical sequence of events during pubertal maturation in girls. Menarche occurs after attainment of Tanner stage 4 (B4) breast development (Tanner 1975)

gonadotropins are observed only during the sleeping hours during early puberty, and levels of oestrogen rise in the morning (Norjavaara et al. 1996). By mid puberty the diurnal pattern of oestrogen secretion is most marked with highest levels being observed in the late night and early morning hours. As girls near completion of puberty this diurnal pattern of sex steroid secretion wanes and a year following menarche differences in day time and night time sex steroid secretion are no longer evident.

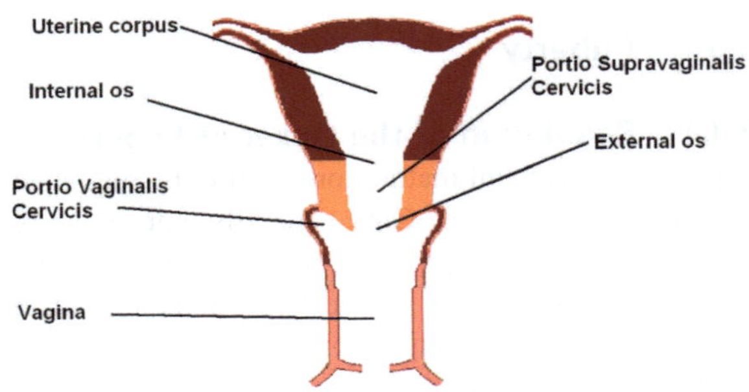

Fig. 2 Schematic diagram of the vagina and cervix in coronal cross-section

2.3.3 Physical Changes During Puberty

Breast development or 'thelarche' is the earliest sign of puberty in around 90% of Caucasian girls and it generally coincides with the onset of the pubertal growth spurt. Circulating oestrogens initiate stromal and ductal tissue growth and promote adipose tissue deposition. Ductal growth is mediated by oestrogens, prolactin and growth hormone but is independent of progesterone. Progesterones enable lobular growth and alveolar budding. The pubertal development of the female breast—described in accordance with the Tanner staging system (Marshall and Tanner 1969) is discussed further in chapter—Breast disorders. The development of pubic and axillary hair usually occurs after breast development but this may be the first sign of puberty, particularly in girls of African descent. The key events of female pubertal maturation are summarised in Fig. 1.

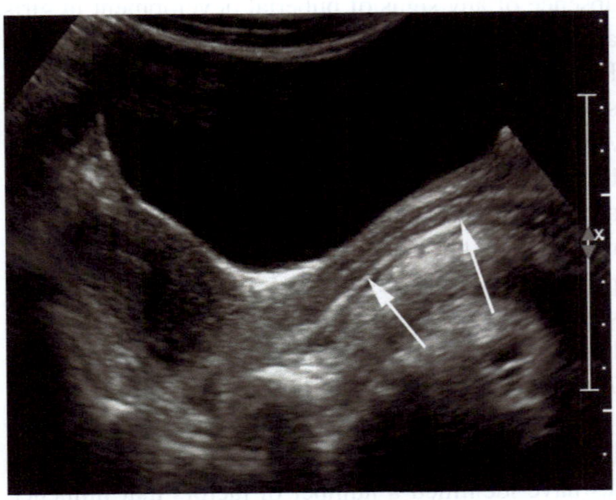

Fig. 3 US of the vagina. Longitudinal US scan showing the typical multi-layered appearance of the vagina (*arrows*)

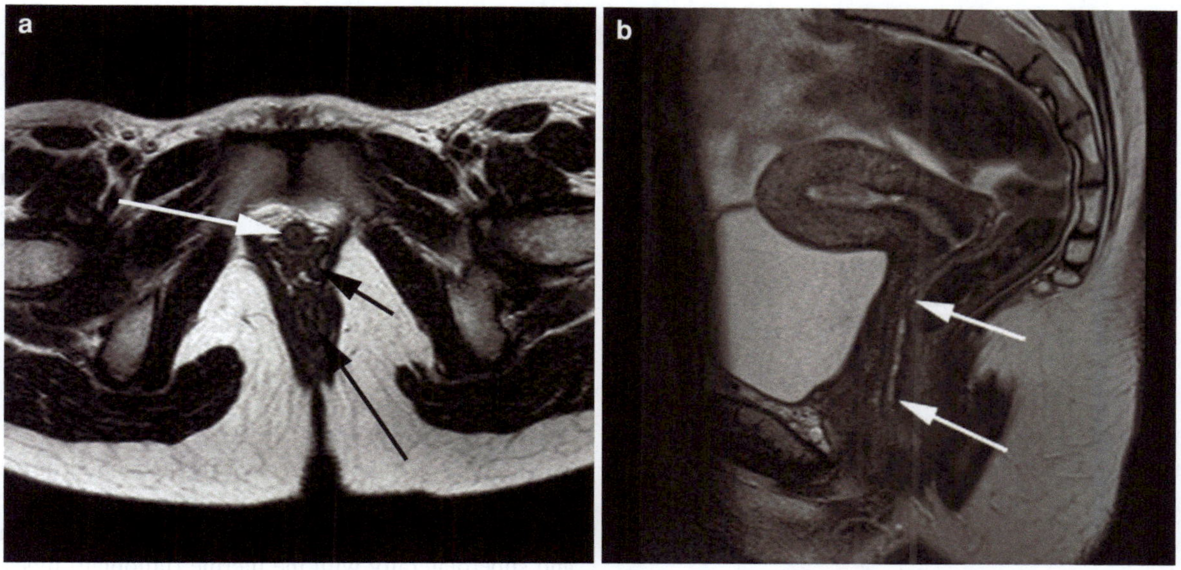

Fig. 4 MRI of the vagina. **a** Axial T2 TSE image. The vagina is often H-shaped in cross-section (*short black arrow*), the urethra lies anteriorly (*white arrow*), the rectum lies posteriorly (*black arrow*). **b** Sagittal T2 TSE image of the vagina (*arrows*) showing the multilayered appearance of the vagina. The innermost layer (vaginal mucosa), is of high signal intensity; the middle layer (muscularis), is of low signal intensity; and the outer layer (paravaginal tissues and venous plexuses), is of high signal intensity

Girls experience a growth spurt early in puberty. The timing of menarche is closely related to a bone age of 13 years and once menarche has been attained girls grow a further 5.0–7.5 cm in height. As puberty nears completion high concentrations of oestrogen induce epiphyseal fusion and the cessation of growth.

3 Normal Anatomy and Imaging Appearances of the Female Reproductive Tract

3.1 Vagina

3.1.1 Anatomy

The vagina is a flattened fibromuscular conduit which connects to the external genitalia to the uterine cervix extending upwards from the urethral insertion at the introitus to the level of lateral vaginal fornices (Fig. 2). The urinary bladder lies anterior to the vagina and the rectum lies posterior to it. Overdistension of the urinary bladder may distort the position of the vagina and uterus.

3.1.2 Imaging

3.1.2.1 Ultrasound Morphology

Visualisation of the lower vagina by transabdominal ultrasound can be limited by an unfavourable acoustic window. The upper and middle thirds of the vagina should be readily seen. The sonographic appearances of the vagina scanned transabdominally depend on the angle of insonation and can range from a hypoechoic to a hyperechoic structure (Beuscher-Willems 2006). With careful scanning it should be possible to resolve the multi-layered structure of the vagina; with a hyperechoic outer circumference representing the serosa, inner hypoechoic muscularis and typically a hyperechoic luminal echo (Fig. 3). The presence of fluid within the lumen may result in a central echo of variable echotexture. Fluid may fill the vagina due to retrograde reflux of urine from the bladder and should not be confused with hydrocolpos. The presence of an echogenic intraluminal foreign body in the vagina which demonstrates multiple reverberation artefacts or posterior acoustic shadowing is usually accounted for by a tampon in a postmenarchal girl.

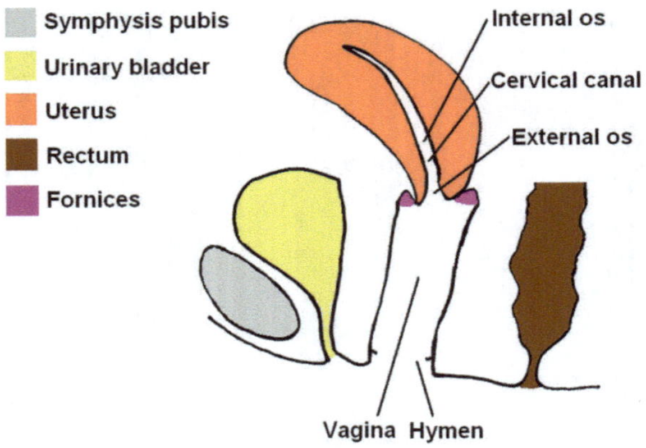

Fig. 5 Schematic diagram of the female internal genitalia and gynaecological tract in sagittal cross-section

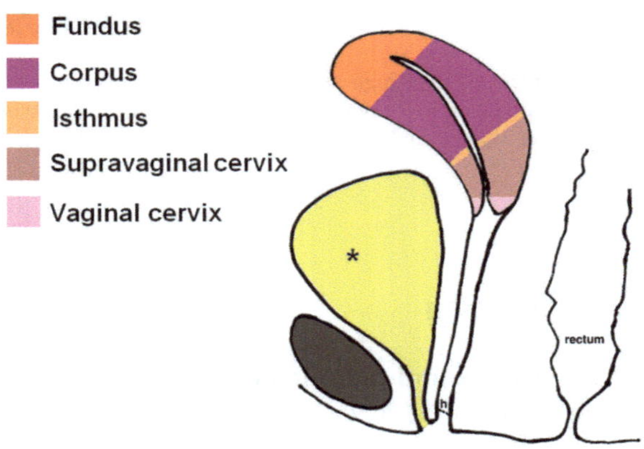

Fig. 6 Schematic diagram of the uterine segments in sagittal cross-section. Urinary bladder (*)

Transperineal US is useful to visualise the lower vagina. Transvaginal and transrectal ultrasound can be used to document the appearances of the vagina but have very limited application in children and should only be considered after exhausting all other available imaging strategies, particularly MRI.

3.1.2.2 MRI Morphology

On T2-weighted (T2W) images the vagina comprises of three distinct layers, typically appearing 'H-shaped' in cross-section. The inner mucosal layer and luminal secretions within the vaginal canal are seen together as a high signal intensity stripe on T2W images and low signal on T1-weighted (T1W) images. The middle submucosal/muscular layer is of low signal on both T1W and T2W images (Fig. 4). The outer adventitial layer is of high signal on T2W imaging due to slow flowing blood in the vaginal venous plexus (López et al. 2005). On T2W fat-saturated images the vagina is of low to intermediate signal intensity. The mucosa or muscularis cannot be differentiated as distinct layers on T1W sequences. Following intravenous gadolinium contrast medium administration the most conspicuous enhancement is seen in the muscularis and outer venous plexuses.

3.2 Uterus

3.2.1 Anatomy

The uterus is a hollow muscular organ centred in the lower pelvis between the rectum and urinary bladder (Fig. 5). Inferiorly, it is contiguous with the vagina and superolaterally with the uterine (fallopian) tubes.

Anatomically the uterus consists of three layers; the endometrium (mucosa), myometrium (muscularis) and perimetrium (serosa).

The uterus consists of three distinct segments; the cervix, isthmus (lower uterine segment) and corpus (body) (Fig. 6).

The uterine cervix comprises the portio supravaginalis cervicalis, the portion of the cervix which does not protrude into the vaginal lumen (endocervix) and the intravaginal portio vaginalis cervicalis (Fig. 2). The cervix is separated from the uterine corpus by the impression of the internal os and demarcates the level of the uterine arteries. The external cervical os demarcates the lower margin of the uterine cavity.

The uterine isthmus is a small structure, which from an imaging standpoint, is only important in the gravid uterus and will not be considered further here.

The long axis of the corpus may flex forward onto the urinary bladder (anterversion) and flex backwards with increasing bladder volume (retroversion) (Fig. 7). The angle between the long axis of the corpus relative to the long axis of the cervix and isthmus is referred to as anteflexion if acute and retroflection if obtuse (Fig. 7).

The uterus is supported by adjacent soft tissues (parametrium and paracolpium), and ligamentous attachments to the pelvic floor and sidewall (see adnexal structures). The uterus is covered by peritoneum which forms peritoneal recesses (Fig. 8) (see rectouterine pouch).

Arterial blood supply to the uterus is via the uterine and ovarian arteries (Fig. 9). The uterine

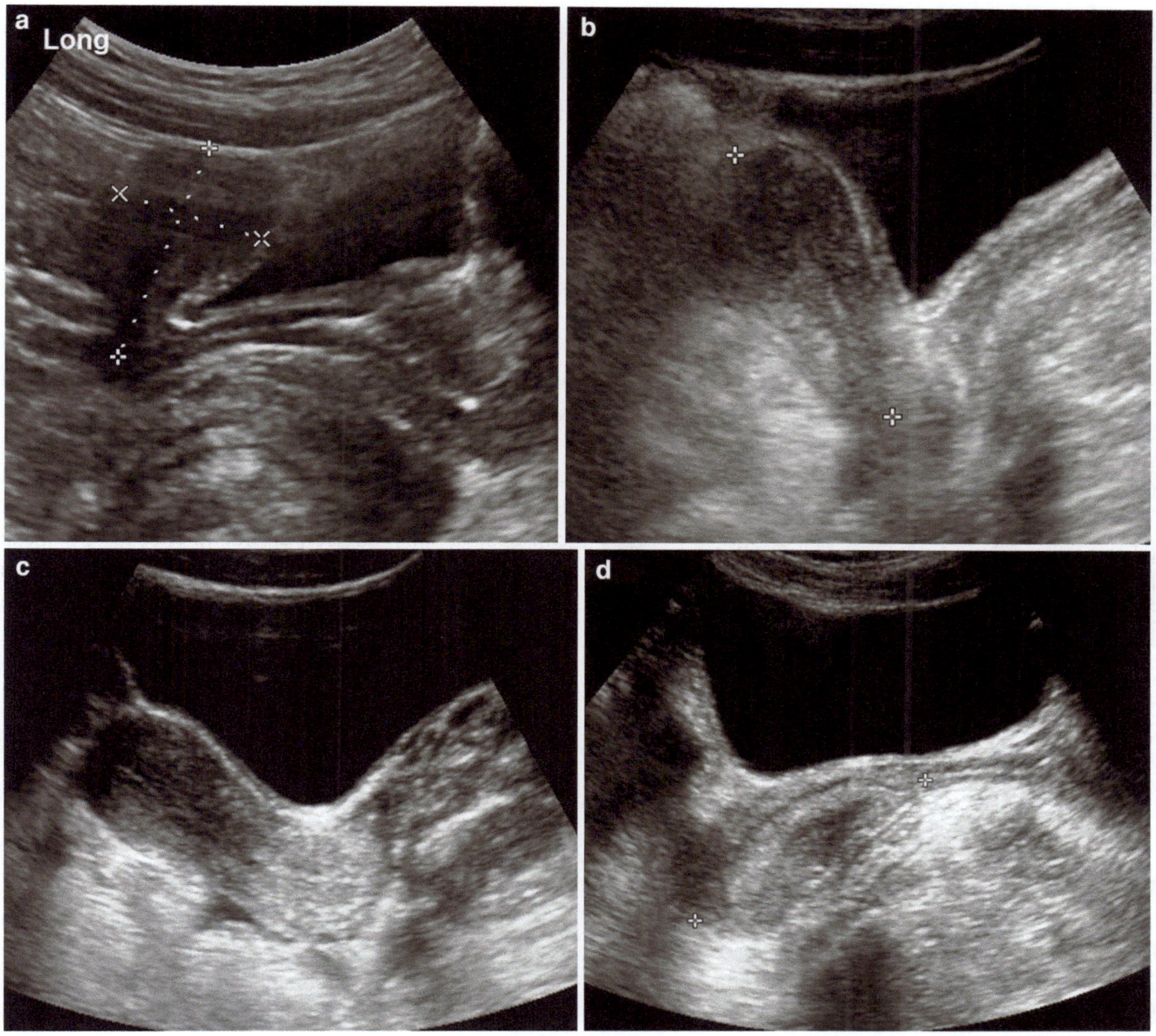

Fig. 7 Uterine position and the effect of bladder filling on uterine shape. **a** Longitudinal US scan shows an underfilled bladder resulting in pronounced anteflexion of the uterus (between callipers). **b** The same child with a more distended urinary bladder and 'normal' anteverted uterus (between callipers). The posterior wall of the uterus is not well seen due to adjacent bowel gas. **c** A further delay in scanning has achieved an optimal bladder volume sufficient to displace bowel in order to fully visualise the uterus. Over-distension of the bladder compresses the uterus, making the fundal prominence less apparent. **d** Longitudinal US scan showing a retroverted uterus (between callipers)

arteries enter the uterus at the isthmus via the cardinal ligaments with ascending and descending branches which along with the ovarian artery supply the fallopian tubes.

Lymphatic drainage of the cervix is via parametrial and iliac lymph nodes; drainage of the corpus is through the broad ligaments into para-aortic lymph nodes.

The cavity of the uterus can be demonstrated to good effect with water soluble contrast medium, appearing slit-like in parasagittal planes and cone shaped in the coronal plane. In practice, such imaging is of little diagnostic value in children but remains integral to the work-up of infertility (Fig. 10).

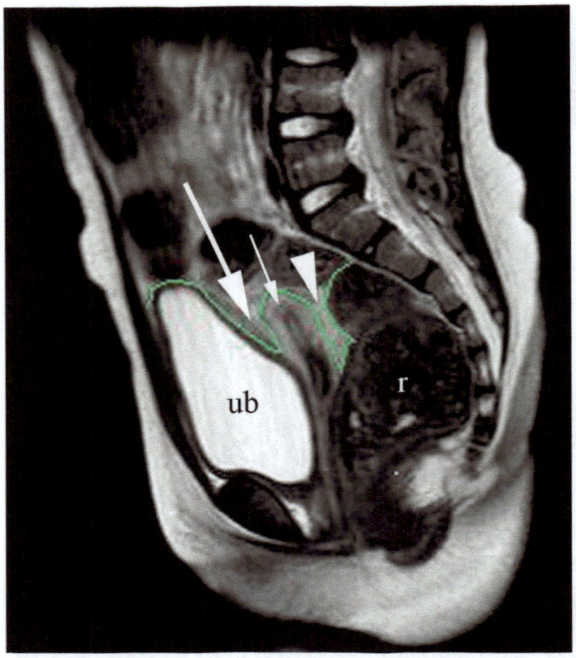

Fig. 8 The abdominopelvic peritoneal reflections. Sagittal T2W scan in a 2-year-old showing the location of the peritoneum (*green line*) draped over the urinary bladder (UB), uterus (*small arrow*) and rectum (R). The vesicouterine (*large arrow*) and rectouterine pouch (*arrowhead*)

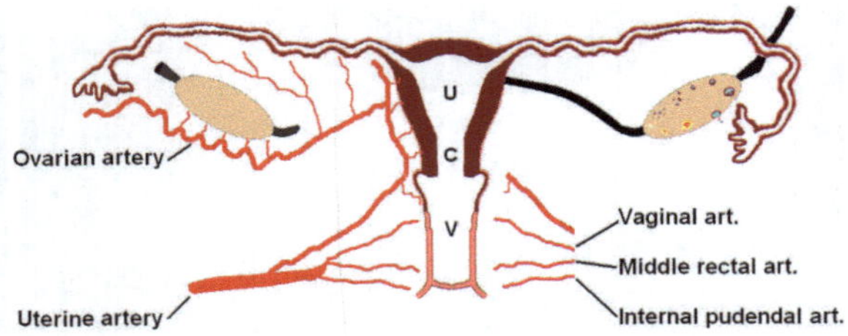

Fig. 9 Line diagram showing the arterial blood supply of the female genital tract. Uterus (U), cervix (C) and vagina (V)

3.2.2 Imaging

3.2.2.1 Uterine Cervix

On MRI the cervix uteri consists of three distinct layers on T2W imaging. The MR appearances of the cervix show much less variation when compared with the uterine corpus for any given age or phase of the menstrual cycle. The zonal anatomy of the cervix comprises: an inner high signal intensity central zone (endocervical glands and mucous) which is of variable width and related to the physiologic changes of menstruation, an intermediate layer called the 'junctional zone' or 'endometrio-myometrial interface' which is hypointense on all spin-echo pulse sequences (fibrous stroma) and an outer layer isointense to myometrium (Fig. 11). Following intravenous gadolinium administration the junctional zone shows less marked enhancement compared to the mucosa, submucosal and myometrium.

At genitography the presence of a cervical impression on the vaginal vault is an important indirect marker of the presence of intact Müllerian structures (Fig. 12).

Nabothian cysts are retention cysts of the uterine cervix related to healing cervicitis and are a common incidental finding in women of child bearing age but can occasionally be seen earlier in life. At US these are typically small, thin-walled hypoechoic cysts measuring a few mm in size (Fig. 13). On MRI the cyst(s) may be slightly high or intermediate signal-intensity on T1W imaging and of high signal intensity on T2W images (Okamoto et al. 2003). No solid component should be evident.

3.2.2.2 Uterine Corpus

Infantile Uterus

During the last trimester of fetal life, growth of the uterus is stimulated by maternal and placental hormones. The myometrium and endometrium hypertrophy in response to oestrogenisation. The appearances of the neonatal uterus reflect waning post-partum maternal hormonal influence. With a full urinary bladder the neonatal uterus should be visible on US (Fig. 14). Tissue harmonic imaging and use of high resolution imaging is helpful in cases where the uterus is not readily visualised. The absence of a uterus in a child with external female genitalia should alert to the possibility of a disorder of sexual differentiation ("Disorders of Sex Development").

The uterine cervix is longer than the uterine corpus. The cervix may initially be up to twice the length of the fundus. In around 60% of infants the uterus is tubular, where the anteroposterior (AP) cervix is equal to the AP fundus (Nussbaum et al. 1986). In 40% of infants the uterus has a characteristic 'spade-shaped', 'heart-shaped' or 'inverted pear-shaped' appearance on longitudinal US (AP cervix is larger than AP fundus). The mean length of the neonatal uterus is 3.4 cm

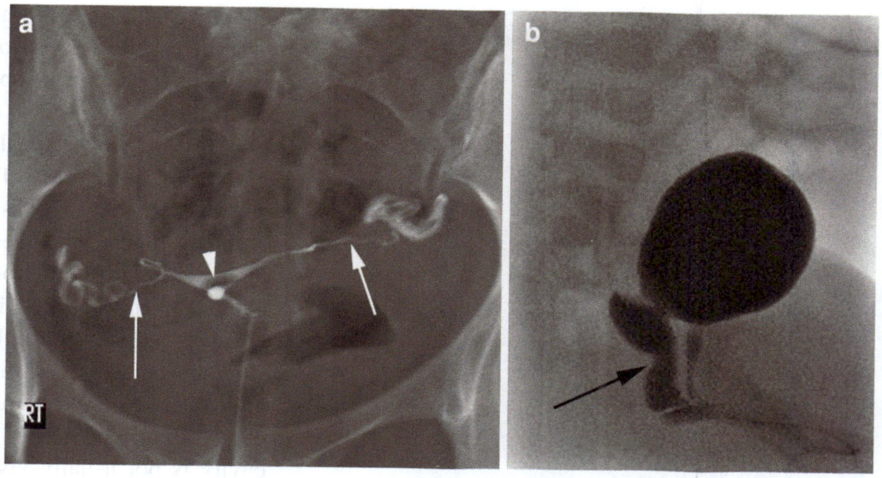

Fig. 10 Contrast studies of the female internal genitalia. **a** Hysterosalpingogram showing normal anatomy and peritoneal spill performed on a 21-year-old nulliparous female investigated for subfertility. The uterine cavity is catheterised *(arrowhead)* and of a normal small volume. The fallopian tubes show normal calibre *(arrows)*. **b** Inadvertent reflux of urine into the vagina *(arrow)* during a voiding cystourethrogram (VCUG) study on a neonate, reflux of urine can also be readily demonstrated on US

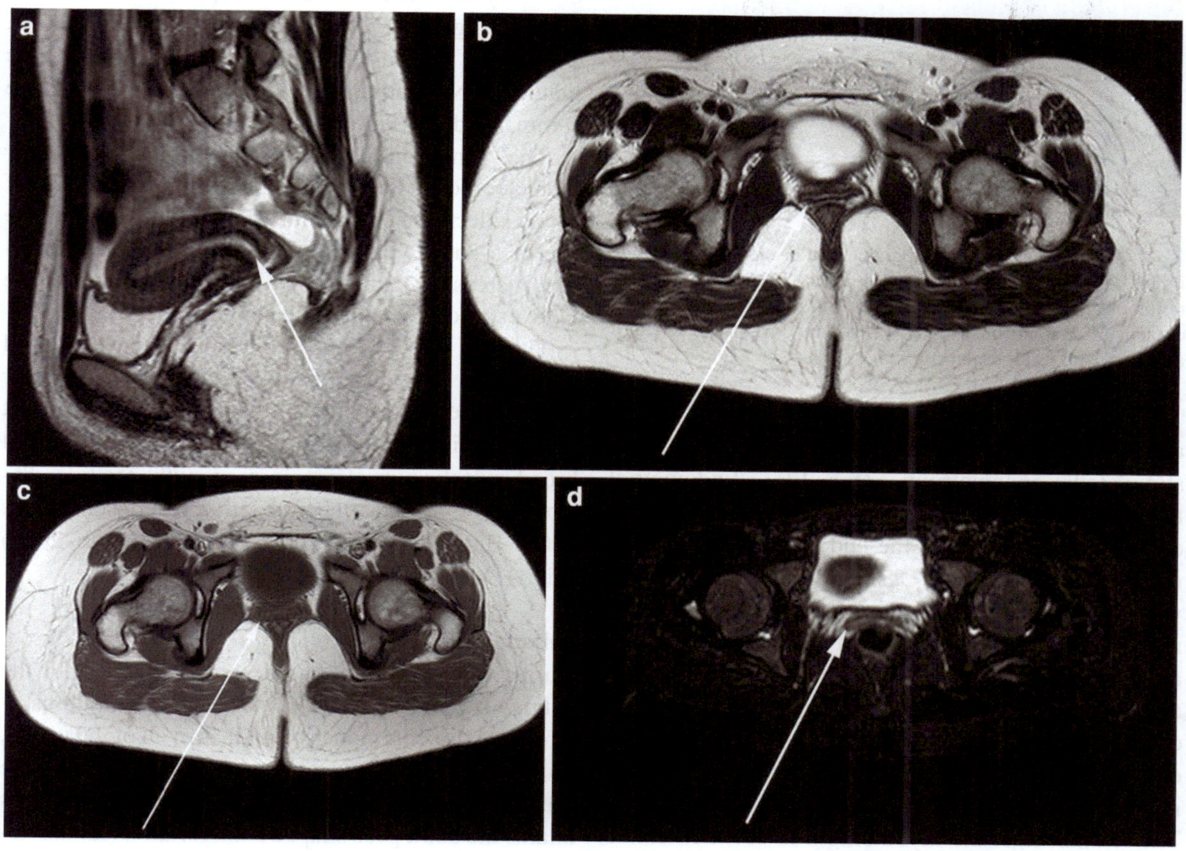

Fig. 11 MRI of the normal cervix. **a** Sagittal T2-weighted TSE image shows a central high signal corresponding to endocervical glands outlined by a peripheral low signal intensity rim *(arrow)*, **b** Axial T2-weighted TSE, **c** Axial T1-weighted TSE and **d** Axial T2-weighted SPAIR images of the cervix *(arrow)*

(2 SD = ± 1.3 cm) with a range of 2.3–4.6 cm (Nussbaum et al. 1986) (Fig. 14). The maximum AP diameter of the uterus is 1.4 cm. The volume range of the neonatal uterus is 2.6–4 ml (Stranzinger and Strouse 2008). Uterine volume and morphology for a given age are summarised in Table 1.

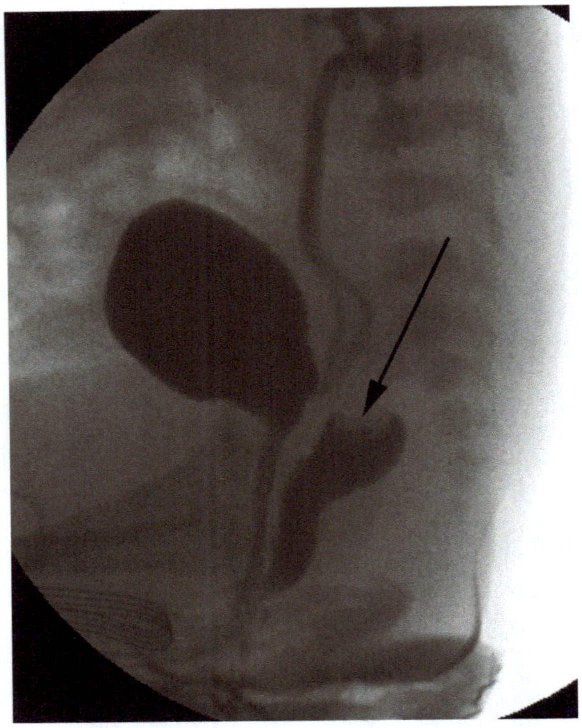

Fig. 12 Voiding cystourethrogram in a 6-month-old female infant with bilateral vesicouereteric reflux. There is inadvertent reflux of urine into the vagina. A cervical impression (*arrow*) is demonstrated upon the vaginal vault implying the presence of an intact Müllerian organ (uterus)

The endometrial cavity is visible on ultrasound as a uniform bright echogenic stripe representing the stimulated endometrium (Fig. 14). Endometrial thickness is measured from echogenic border to echogenic border across the endometrial cavity on a midline sagittal image. Oestrogenisation of the cervical and vaginal mucoid glands results in physiologic mucoid secretions and vaginal discharge. A small amount of fluid in the uterine cavity is present in around a quarter of neonatal uteri. The endometrial echo may be surrounded by a thin uniform hypoechoic myometrial halo. The halo may represent neonatal myometrial vascular engorgement and haemorrhage. The remainder of the myometrium is of intermediate homogeneous echotexture. As maternal oestrogen is withdrawn the endometrial lining may be shed and the vaginal discharge may become blood stained.

Prepubertal Uterus

Between the first and fourth months of life, postnatal regression of the uterus is observed. The endometrial stripe is no longer visible (Fig. 15). The uterus decreases to 2.6–3.0 cm in length and becomes tubular in shape. Up until the second year of life the uterus is quiescent and shows little growth. Stanhope et al. (1985) found no uterine growth until 10 years of age but used uterine cross-sectional area data. It is generally accepted that the uterine fundus and cervix grows in length and diameter during childhood remaining approximately equal in proportion in the prepubertal period (Bridges et al. 1996). Using uterine volume measurements, the uterus shows slow growth between 2 and 8 years and retains its tubular shape (Orsini et al. 1984; Salardi et al. 1985). The endometrial cavity is not usually visualised until around the age of 7-8 years. There is a weak positive correlation between age and uterine length (Badouraki et al. 2008), but uterine length is a key marker of pelvic maturity. Normative ranges for uterine length are summarised in (Fig. 16).

The fundocervical ratio (FCR—anteroposterior diameter of fundus/anteroposterior diameter of cervix) decreases to a minimum value between the age of 5 and 6 years (Nussbaum et al. 1986), gradually increasing thereafter so that by 12 years of age FCR exceeds 1 in all subjects (Griffin et al. 1995).

Uterine artery Doppler ultrasound may be used to confirm the onset of puberty. Pulsed Doppler demonstrates a narrow systolic waveform without positive diastolic flow in prepubertal girls and broad systolic waveform is seen with positive diastolic flow in postpubertal girls (Ziereisen et al. 2001; Battaglia et al. 2002; Battaglia et al. 2003) (Fig. 17).

Pubertal Uterus

During puberty the uterus descends further into the pelvis. The influence of increasing concentrations of circulating sex hormones result in growth of the uterus, this may precede ovarian growth by 2 years. The fundal diameter exceeds that of the cervix. The uterus attains the adult pear-shaped configuration (fundus-to-cervix ratio 2/1 to 3/1) and measures 5–8 cm in length, with an AP diameter of 1.6–3.5 cm (Haber and Mayer 1994; Holm et al. 1995; Griffin et al.1995; Bridges et al. 1996; Buzi et al. 1998) (Fig. 18).

The endometrium, initially seen as a thin echogenic interface, increases in thickness and is a key marker of pubertal progression. Following the establishment of

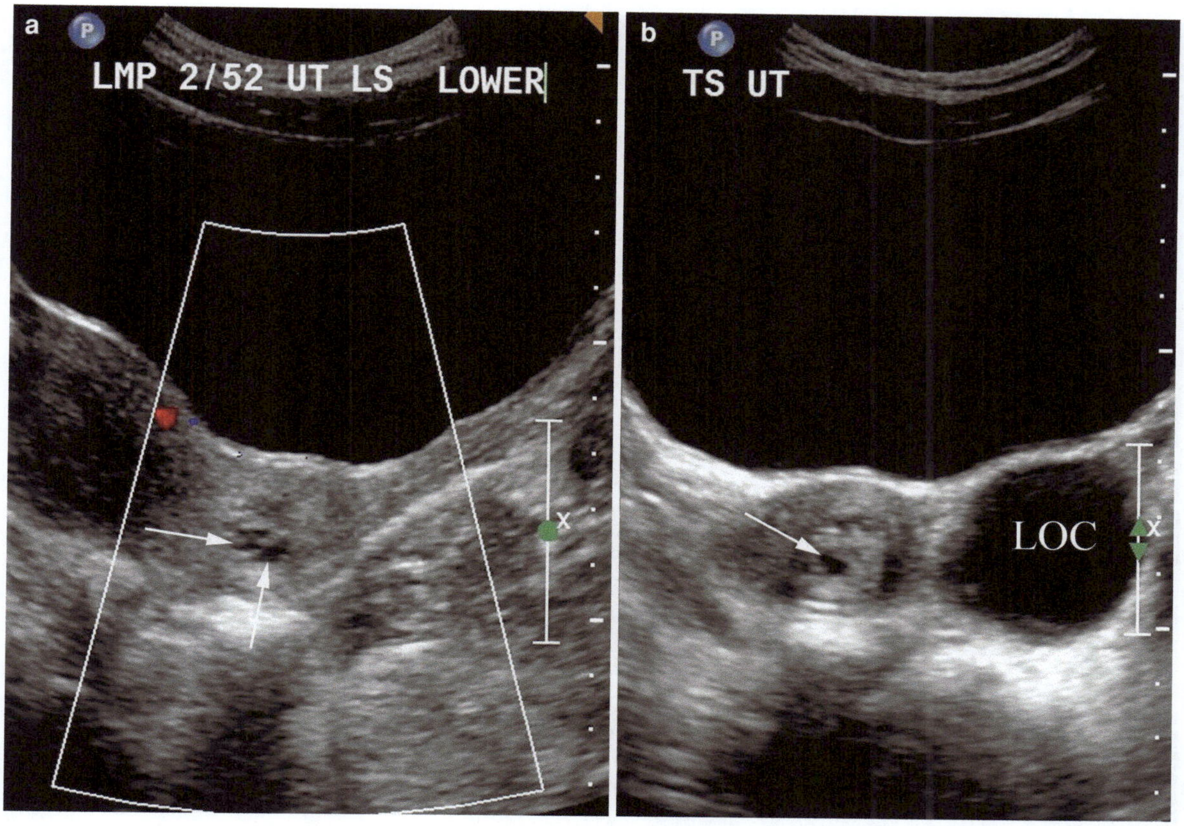

Fig. 13 Nabothian cyst (Nabothian follicle). **a** Longitudinal colour Doppler US, **b** Transverse US images showing small anechoic cervical cysts (*arrows*). These mucoid inclusion cysts are of no clinical significance. An incidental simple left ovarian cyst (LOC) was noted which resolved on a 6 week follow-up scan

menstrual cycles the endometrium undergoes cyclical changes in sonographic appearances described further (see menstrual cycle).

The suggested cut-off value for defining a pubertal uterus is a uterine length of 4 cm (Herter et al. 2002; Badouraki et al. 2008). An endometrial thickness of 6-8 mm implies imminent menarche (Stranzinger and Strouse 2008).

3.3 Rectouterine Pouch

3.3.1 Anatomy

The rectouterine pouch also referred to as the pelvic cul-de-sac or pouch of Douglas is the intraperitoneal recess between the anterior aspect of the rectum and posterior margin of the uterus (Fig. 8).

3.3.2 Imaging

Free fluid may accumulate in this potential anatomic space and its volume can be estimated by ultrasound using the formula $(H \times W \times D) \times 0.53$. Bowel lying in the pouch can be distinguished from other structures by virtue of its content and presence of peristalsis.

Physiologic free fluid can be observed in the recto-uterine pouch during all phases of the menstrual cycle and peaks in the secretory phase (Fig. 19). The volume of fluid accumulated in the pouch varies according to hormonal status and phase of the menstrual cycle (Davis and Gosink 1986). Physiologic pelvic free fluid is typically most abundant in the secretory phase of the menstrual cycle. Haemorrhagic ascites may be seen during periovulation. Minimal physiological pelvic free fluid has been demonstrated in premenarchal children, but the presence of pelvic fluid was significantly greater

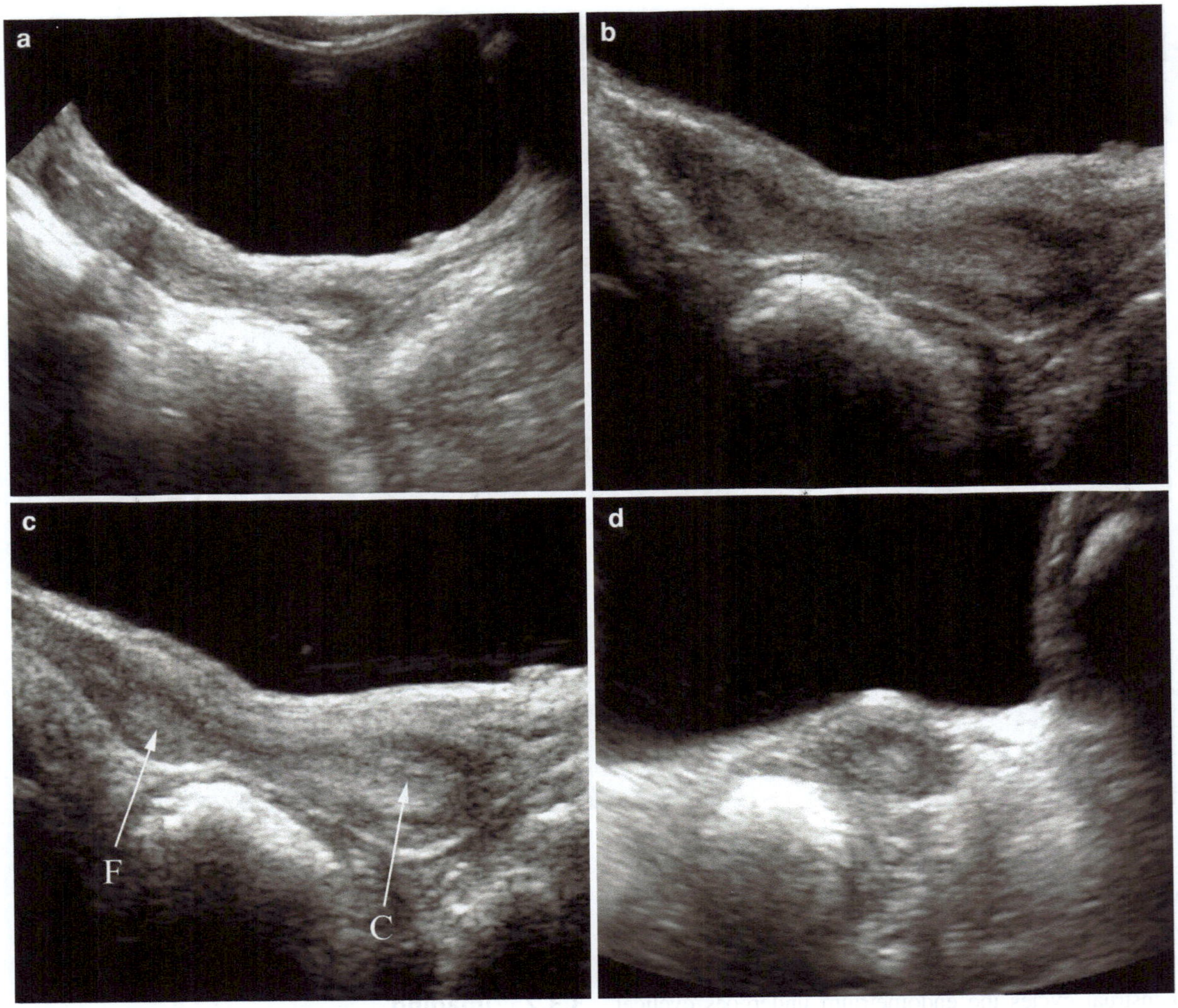

Fig. 14 Neonatal uterus. Maternal and placental hormones stimulate the uterus, the endometrial stripe is visible as a thin central echogenic band. The neonatal uterus is spade-shaped (inverted pear-shape) as in this example imaged using **a** 8.5 MHz curvilinear, **b** 12.5 MHz linear, and **c** 17.5 MHz curvilinear probes—the cervix (C) can be more prominent than the fundus (F) in the neonate. Tubular uterine morphology which is characteristic of a prepubertal uterus is also a common configuration of the uterus in neonates (see Fig. 15). **d** Transverse image of the uterine cervix in a neonate using a 17.5 MHz probe

in the symptomatic group than in the asymptomatic group (Rathaus et al. 2003).

3.4 The Adnexa

The female adnexa or extrauterine appendages are located in the lower pelvis and consist of the ovaries, fallopian tubes, suspensory ligaments and supporting soft tissues.

3.4.1 Fallopian Tubes

The fallopian tube extends from the lumen of the superolateral margin of the uterus to the ipsilateral ovary. The segmental anatomy of the fallopian tube is summarised in (Fig. 20). The medial or intramural portion of the fallopian tube is intrauterine (uterine and interstitial). The extrauterine fallopian tube comprises of three segments and lies in the peritoneal fold (mesosalpinx) in the superior margin of the broad ligament. The isthmus lies adjacent to the uterine wall and is the

Table 1 Uterine dimensions and morphology during childhood and adolescence After Haber and Mayer (1994); Cohen et al. (1990)

Age	Uterine volume (ml) [uterine length × anteroposterior depth]	Fundocervical ratio [anteroposterior diameter of fundus/anteroposterior diameter of cervix]	Uterine shape	Endometrial stripe
Neonate	2.6–4	1:2	Spade shape	Echogenic
3 months–1 year	0.8–1.3	1:1	Tubular shape	Hypoechoic
1–2 years	0.8–1.3	1:1	Tubular shape	Hypoechoic
2–8 years	0.8–1.6		Tubular shape	Hypoechoic
8–16 years	0.8–25	3:1	Pear shape after puberty	Cyclical changes after puberty

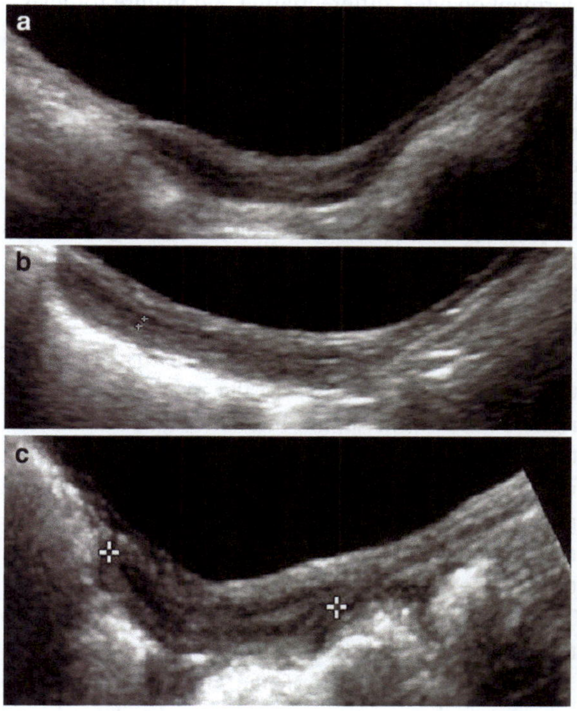

Fig. 15 Longitudinal ultrasound appearances of prepubertal uterus at different ages. **a** Imaging obtained in a 1-year-old girl shows a 'near' tubular uterus with marginal prominence of the cervix. **b** Imaging obtained in a 4-year-old girl shows a tubular uterus with no differentiation between the cervix and fundus (AP depth of cervix is equal to that of the fundus) and a barely perceptible endometrial lining seen as a thin echogenic line (between callipers). **c** Imaging of a an 8-year-old girl, the uterus undergoes growth during adrenarche but retains prepubertal tubular morphology

narrowest segment. The majority of the length is comprised by the ampulla which is more capacious. The infundibulum is in direct continuity with the peritoneal cavity and comprises multiple projections or fimbriae. The fimbriae ovarica lie in contact with the ovary. In the reproductively mature adolescent, the fallopian tubes can measure approximately 9–15 cm in length with a luminal diameter of 2–4 mm.

The fallopian tubes are tortuous, lack defined interfaces and are poor acoustic reflectors (Timor-Tritsch 2006). Non-dilated healthy fallopian tubes are rarely demonstrated by ultrasound or MRI unless outlined by adjacent pelvic fluid. (Brown and Ascher 2006).

3.4.2 Suspensory Ligaments and Parametrium

Peritoneal reflections from the ventral and dorsal surface of the uterus form a double fold of peritoneum giving rise to the broad ligament which extends laterally to the pelvic sidewalls and caudally condenses into the paired cardinal ligaments. The cardinal ligaments separate the paravaginal soft tissues from the parametrium. The free margin of the broad ligament is formed laterally by the ovarian ligament and medially by the fallopian tubes (Fig. 21). The ovarian ligaments extend from the uterine cornu to the ovary and are remnants of the gubernaculum.

The parametrial tissues lie between the portio supravaginalis cervicalis and urinary bladder, extending laterally to invest between the layers of the broad ligaments. The parametrium contains the

Fig. 16 Uterine length versus age (Griffin et al. 1995)

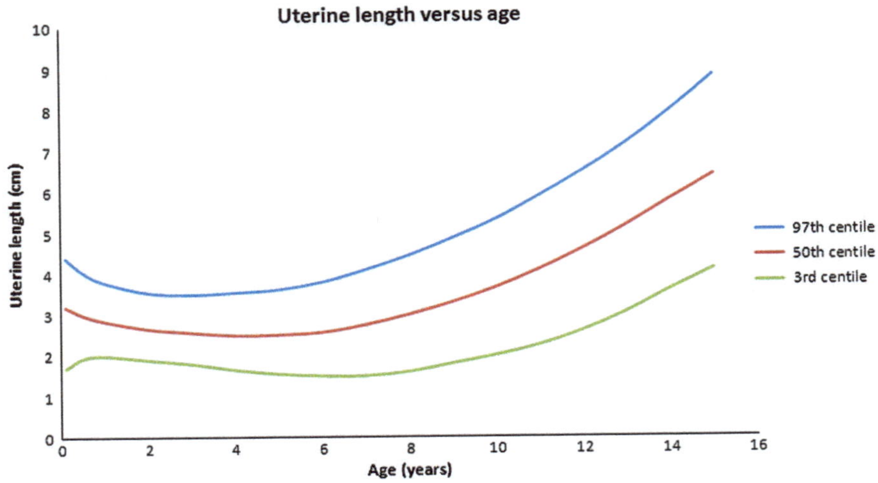

fallopian tubes, uterine and ovarian vasculature, ovarian ligament, round and uterosacral ligaments, lymphatics, ureters and Wolffian vestiges. The round ligaments form from the remnant of the gubernaculum between the uterus and labium majorum. The parametrium normally enhances following intravenous gadolinium.

The paired uterosacral ligaments extend from the cervix or vagina to insert into the sacrospinous ligament/coccygeus muscle complex in most females, or occasionally insert into the pyriformis muscle or sacrum (Umek et al. 2004). The vesicouterine ligament extends from the posterior wall of the urinary bladder to the cervix.

3.4.3 The Ovary

3.4.3.1 Anatomy

Each ovary is anchored within the peritoneal cavity by the mesovarium to the posterior margin of the broad ligament, suspensory (infundibulopelvic) ligament in the superolateral wall of the broad ligament to the pelvic sidewall, and ovarian (utero-ovarian) ligament to the uterine cornu (Clement 2002).

Neonatal ovaries are typically spherical in shape and located in the superior margin of the broad ligaments. The neonatal ovary comprises anatomical and functional components similar to those of pubertal and postmenarchal ovaries. The ovaries consist of an inner central medulla and outer cortex (Fig. 22). The medulla contains loose connective tissue, blood vessels, lymphatics and nerves. The peripheral cortex consists of an outer surface germinal epithelium, underlying tunica albuginea and deeper functional layer containing dormant oocytes, differentiating and mature follicles.

The paired retroperitoneal ovarian arteries arise directly from the abdominal aorta and along with the ovarian veins course along the ventral aspect of the psoas muscles, crossing the common iliac vessels and ureter at or near the pelvic brim, before entering the suspensory ligament of each ovary. The ovarian vascular pedicle along with communicating branches from the uterine vessels enter the ovarian medulla at the hilum in the peritoneal fold of the mesovarium (Fig. 9) via the ovarian ligament.

The venous drainage of the ovaries is by way of the pampiniform plexuses to the ovarian veins. The right ovarian vein drains into the IVC and the left typically into the left renal vein. On cross-sectional imaging, particularly CT (computed tomography), the position of an ovary may be inferred by following the retroperitoneal course of the ovarian vein which leads to the suspensory ovarian ligament (Lee et al. 2003). The ovarian veins are typically larger and lie lateral to the accompanying artery.

Lymphatic drainage of the ovaries follows the course of the ovarian arteries to the lateral and pre-aortic lumbar nodes.

3.4.3.2 Imaging Appearances

Neonatal Ovary

The sonographic appearances of the ovaries in neonates and infants typically include heterogeneous stroma with peripherally distributed microcystic follicles which are anechoic, thin walled and measure less than 9 mm in diameter (Fig. 23). The mean

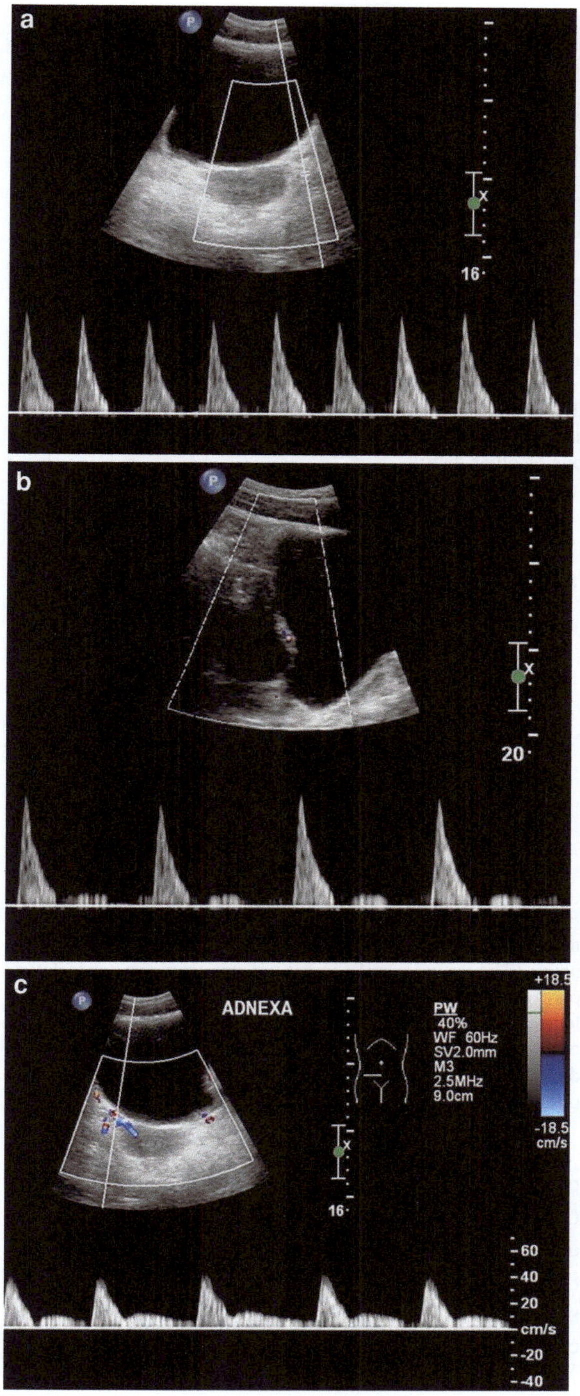

Fig. 17 Assessment of pubertal development using Pulsed-Wave Doppler interrogation of the uterine artery. **a** Typical prepubertal waveform with narrow systolic envelopes and absent diastolic flow. **b** Typical pubertal waveform with systolic flow and interrupted diastolic flow. **c** Typical waveform at the end of puberty with a broad systolic phase and continuous diastolic flow

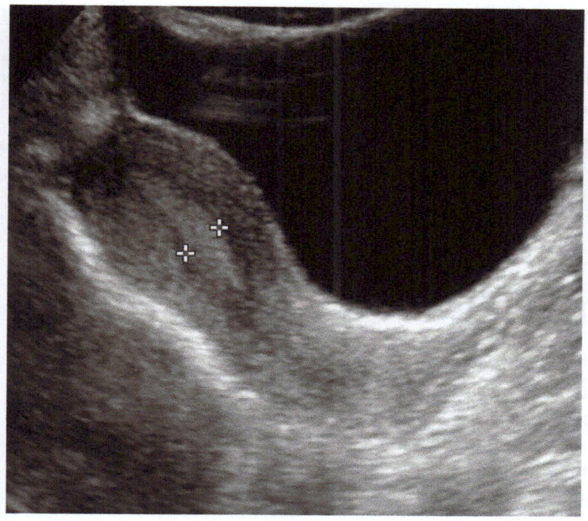

Fig. 18 Normal pubertal uterus. Longitudinal US shows a pear-shaped configuration of the uterus. The anteroposterior diameter of the fundus is larger than the cervix. The echogenic endometrial lining (between callipers) is well seen

neonatal follicular diameter is 7 mm. Using the formula for a prolate ellipsoid (0.523 × length, height × width) mean ovarian volume in infants and neonates is 1.06 cm^3 (Cohen et al. 1993).

Neonatal ovarian cysts develop from ovarian follicles. In utero, follicular development is mediated predominately by fetal pituitary FSH secretion, but also maternal human chorionic gonadotropin (hCG) and oestrogens. In the neonate and premenarchal child low-level pulsatile GnRH secretion promotes continual follicular development. A neonatal physiological ovarian cyst should not exceed 3 cm in diameter (Seigel 2010).

Prepubertal and Premenarchal Ovary

The ovaries are quiescent in early childhood appearing relatively homogeneous with few follicles (Fig. 24). Ovarian volume increases throughout childhood, reflecting an increase in the size and number of antral follicles and amount of stroma derived from follicular atresia (Porcu 2004). Under the age of 6 years mean ovarian volumes are stable and do not exceed 1 cm^3 (Table 2). Normative values for ovarian volume for a given age are summarised in Fig. 25.

Mean ovarian volumes in prepubertal girls (6–10 years old), range from 1.2 to 2.3 cm^3, increasing

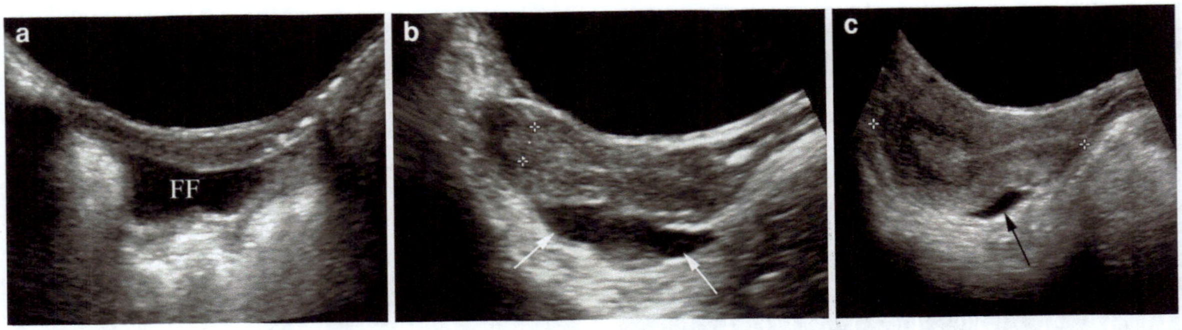

Fig. 19 Pelvic free fluid. Intraperitoneal free fluid preferentially pools in the recto-uterine pouch in the supine or erect positions. **a** Trace free fluid (FF) thought to relate to rapid rehydration in this young child scanned for suspected renal tract infection. **b** Anechoic free fluid in pelvis (*arrows*) is a non-specific finding but should alert the operator to look for ascites and an underlying pathologic cause. Anechoic free fluid is a normal finding in the late menstrual cycle. **c** Echogenic free fluid (*black arrow*) deep into the uterus in this teenager with suspected appendicitis. Echogenic free fluid may relate blood, pus or other debris

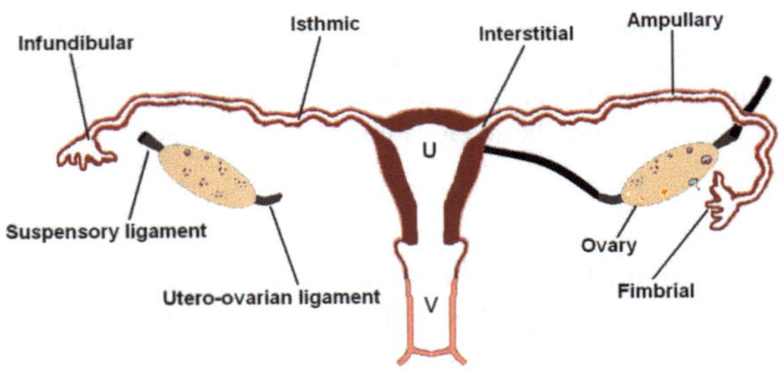

Fig. 20 Line diagram showing the segmental anatomy of the normal fallopian tube. There are four segments, from the medial to lateral aspect: the intramural interstitial portion which is contiguous with the uterine fundus, the isthmus, the ampulla, and the infundibulum at the fimbriated portion. Uterus (U) and vagina (V)

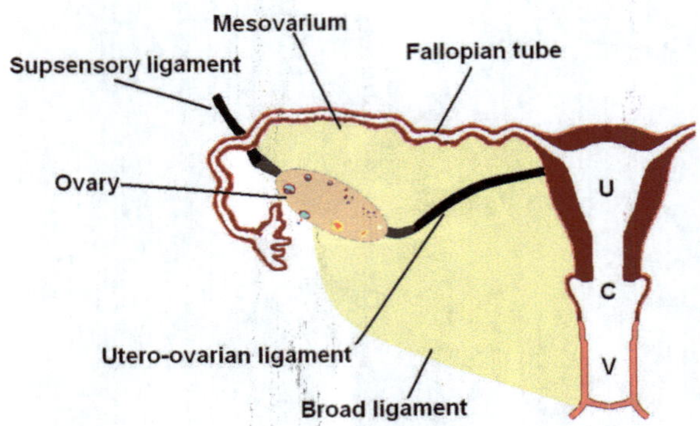

Fig. 21 Line diagram (*anterior view*) showing the broad ligament and ovarian attachments in relation to the fallopian tube and uterus. The suspensory ligament extends from the superolateral part of the broad ligament to the pelvic sidewall. The medially located utero-ovarian ligament is enclosed between the two peritoneal layers of the broad ligament. The pelvic ligaments are difficult to visualise on cross-sectional imaging in children unless outlined by fluid. Uterus (U), cervix (C) and vagina (V)

around the time of the growth spurt (7–9 years old) which also coincides with nocturnal pulsatile LH secretion. In the years immediately prior to menarche, enhanced gonadotropin secretion is sufficient to drive follicular growth and oestrogen production. At this time the ovaries attain multifollicular morphology (Fig. 26) comprising more than six anechoic follicles each of which are at least 4 mm in diameter (Adams et al. 1985). These appearances coupled with fibrosis of the cortex and partial luteinisation of the theca interna often make the ovaries indistinguishable from adolescent ovaries. In premenarchal girls (11–12 years old), mean ovarian volumes range from 2 to 4 cm^3 (Cohen et al. 1993). Ovarian follicles are seen in around 70% of girls aged 2 to 12 years.

Non-visualisation of one or both ovaries by transabdominal ultrasound scanning is occasionally encountered. At least one ovary was identified in 82% of patients aged between 2 and 12 years and in 87% of patients over 5 years, while both ovaries were demonstrated in 65 and 80% of cases respectively (Orsini et al. 1984). With modern US equipment, it should be possible to visualise both ovaries in most children with transabdominal scanning.

Pubertal Ovaries

At puberty the ovaries grow further in size and descend deeper into the pelvis. The ovaries contain both stimulated and unstimulated cortical follicles (Fig. 27). Large stimulated follicles may distort ovarian shape and tend to make ovarian calculation

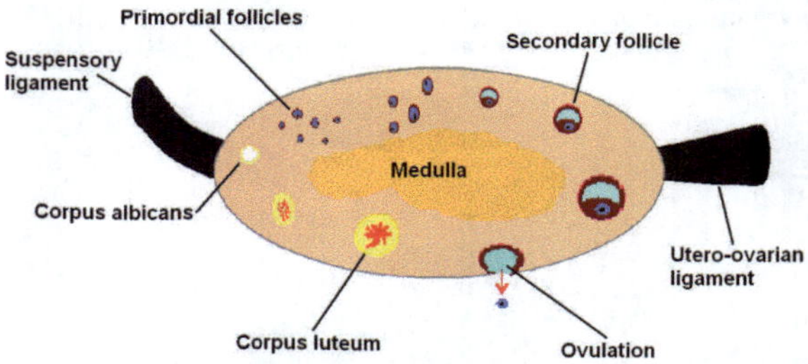

Fig. 22 Schematic diagram of the human ovary showing the central medulla and cyclical development of ovarian follicles within the cortex

less reproducible. Mean ovarian volume is typically quoted as 9.8 cm^3 (Table 2) but volumes are highly variable depending on the stage of the menstrual cycle (see Sect. 4). Ranges for ovarian dimensions include: length 2.5–5.0 cm, width 1.5–3.0 cm and depth 0.6–1.5 cm (Orsini et al. 1984).

4 Menstrual Cycle

4.1 Endocrinology of the Normal Menstrual Cycle

The establishment of regular ovulatory menstrual cycles heralds full reproductive maturity. Menstrual cycles are often irregular in adolescence and initially characterised by anovulatory cycles. Earlier onset of menarche, before 12 years, is associated with a higher proportion of ovulatory cycles in the first gynaecologic year (year following menarche) (Diaz et al. 2006). The ovulatory menstrual cycle is divided into three phases: follicular, ovulatory and luteal. These phases are characterised by changes in the morphology of the uterus and ovary and are summarised in Fig. 28.

4.1.1 Follicular Phase

Ovarian follicles are sensitive to oestrogen. Most ovarian follicles are non-ovulatory appearing as simple anechoic structures with imperceptible walls and a diameter of less than 10 mm. During the early follicular phase FSH and LH levels rise as the pituitary escapes from the negative feedback effect of progesterone, oestradiol and inhibin secreted towards the end of the luteal phase (Fig. 29). The rise in FSH stimulates a pool of secondary antral follicles in the ovary to enter the final stages of follicular development. Each follicle demonstrates a different sensitivity to FSH and only one will respond maximally to become the dominant (Graafian) follicle (Fig. 30) with a diameter of 18–30 mm (some authors may use a cut-off value of 25 mm for the definition of a follicle). By day seven of the menstrual cycle, the dominant follicle is usually evident. As FSH levels fall towards the end of the follicular phase the other follicles become atretic.

4.1.2 Ovulation

During the ovulatory phase, a positive feedback loop between the pituitary and ovary sees the pituitary secrete increasing amounts of LH in response to oestradiol that in turn stimulates further LH secretion. This leads to the mid-cycle LH surge that stimulates a proteolytic cascade resulting in the protrusion of the follicle on the ovarian surface and follicular rupture with conversion of the dominant follicle into the corpus luteum. The fimbriae ovarica of the fallopian tube pick up the oocyte, surrounded by its cumulus and antral fluid. Oestradiol levels fall approximately 12 h following follicular rupture.

4.1.3 Luteal Phase

Progesterone secretion rises steadily to peak seven days following ovulation, to coincide with the time of blastocyst implantation. If fertilisation and implantation take place the trophoblast secretes hCG ensuring the production of progesterone until the placenta is fully formed by 12 weeks gestation. If fertilisation does not take place, oestradiol and progesterone levels fall in the mid-luteal phase and luteal regression begins. A scar is left on the ovary that gradually becomes avascular over subsequent cycles (corpus albicans).

4.2 Ultrasound Imaging of the Endometrium During the Menstrual Cycle

The endometrium undergoes morphological and functional changes during the menstrual cycle which can be divided into three phases: menstrual, proliferative (follicular) and secretory (luteal). The cyclical ovarian changes described parallel the endometrial changes in the follicular and luteal phases.

4.2.1 Menstruation

During menstruation (days 0–5), the endometrium appears as a thin echogenic 'stripe' measuring 1–4 mm

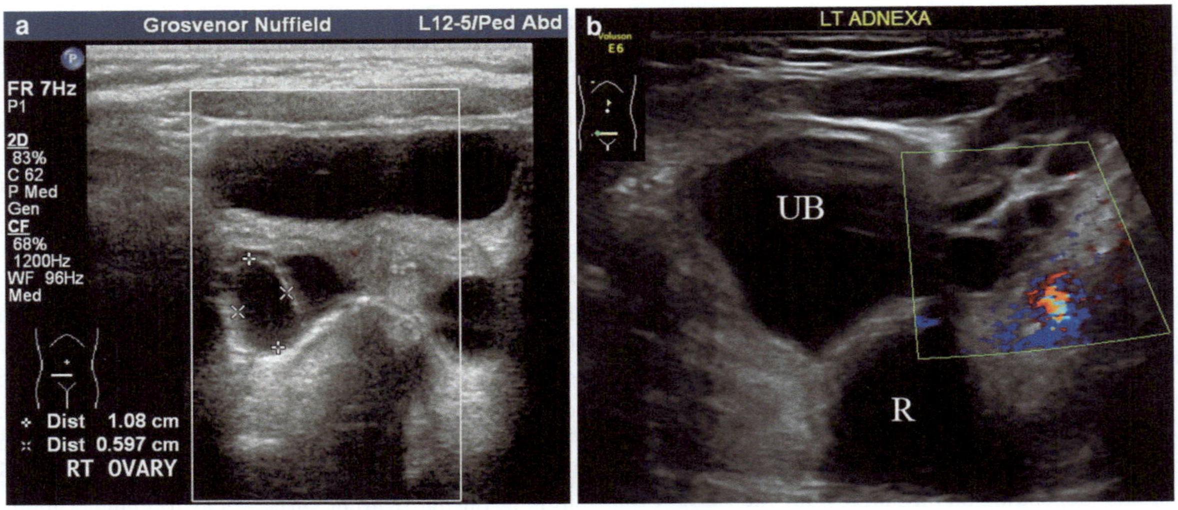

Fig. 23 Neonatal ovary. **a** Transverse colour Doppler linear transducer sonogram shows macrocystic anechoic follicles in both ovaries, the largest measuring just over 1 cm (between callipers) in diameter in the right ovary. Neonatal follicles exceeding 1 cm in diameter are functional cysts and are a very common finding reflecting transient maternal hormonal influence. **b** Transverse colour Doppler linear transducer sonogram showing a normal left ovary containing several follicles with a diameter smaller than 1 cm

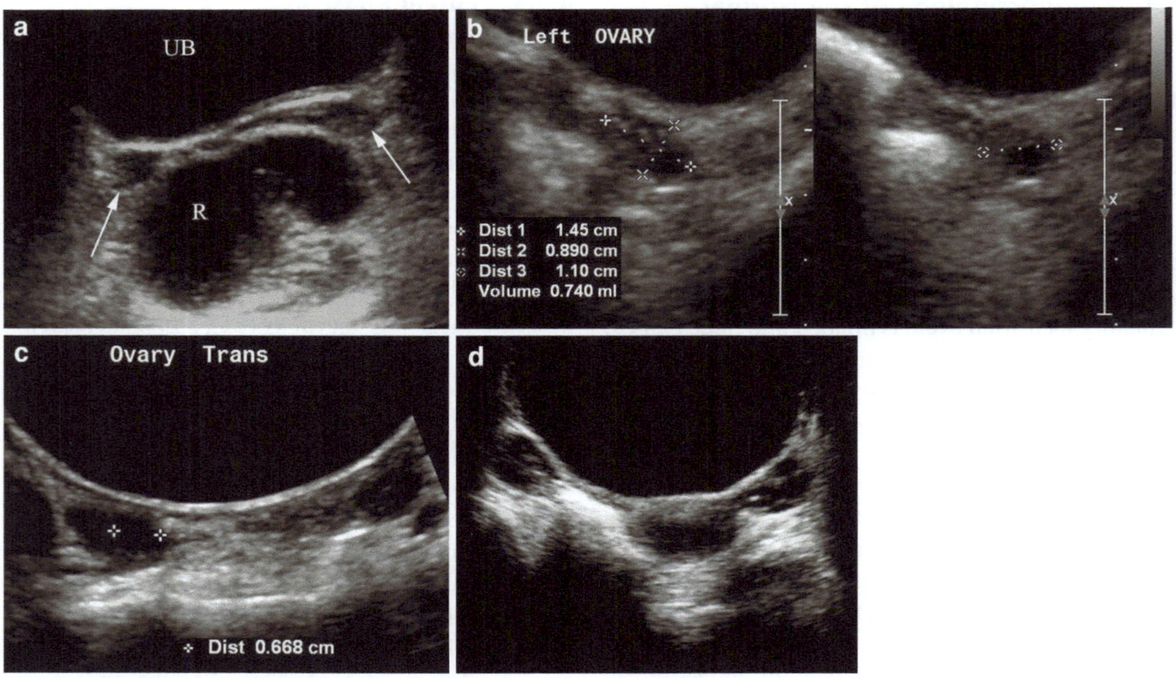

Fig. 24 Prepubertal ovary. **a** Transverse US scan obtained in a 1-year-old girl showing normal ovaries (*arrows*) with scant visible follicles, urinary bladder (UB), rectum (R). **b** Composite focused oblique views provide a calculated ovarian volume of just under 1 cm^3. **c** Transverse US scan obtained in a 5-year-old girl shows normal ovaries with visible follicles (largest between callipers). The ovarian volume is 2 cm^3. **d** Transverse sonograms in an 8-year-old girl showing both ovaries contain small cystic follicles. Ovarian morphology is of limited value in assessing pubertal status as follicles are visible at all ages. Ovarian volume is a good discriminator but should be interpreted in the context of the uterine length

Table 2 Normal ovarian volumes in neonates, infants and throughout childhood

Chronological age	Mean volume (cm^3)	Standard deviation (cm^3)
Birth to 3 months	1.1	1.0
4–12 months	1.1	0.7
13–24 months	0.7	0.4
2 years	0.8	0.4
3 years	0.7	0.2
4 years	0.8	0.4
5 years	0.9	0.02
6 years	1.2	0.4
7 years	1.3	0.6
8 years	1.1	0.5
9 years	2.0	0.8
10 years	2.2	0.7
11 years	2.5	1.3
12 years	3.8	1.4
13 years	4.0.2	2.3
Postpubertal	9.8	0.6

Data (birth to 24 months) summarised from Cohen et al. (1993)
Data (2–13 years) summarised from Orsini et al. (1984)

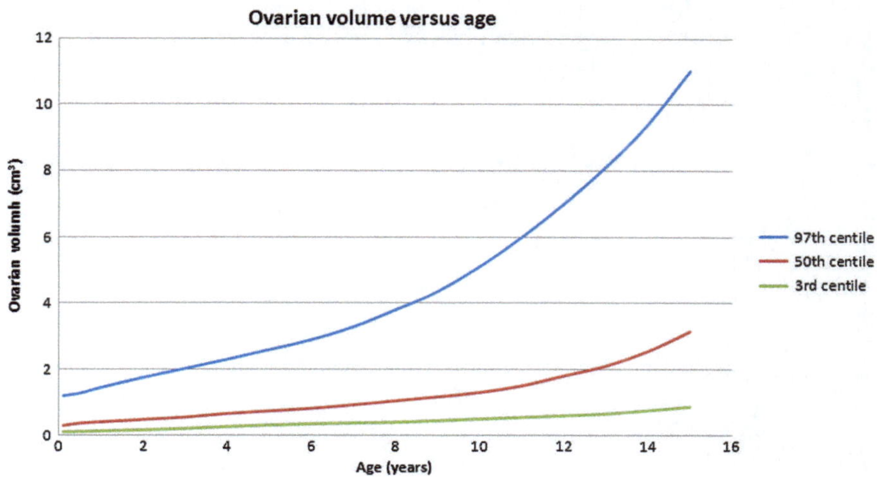

Fig. 25 Ovarian volume versus age (Griffin et al. 1995). Once the effects of maternal hormonal influence have subsided during infancy the ovaries are quiescent and show relatively stable volumes with slow growth in childhood. Ovarian growth is accelerated during adrenarche and pubarche

thickness. Heterogeneity of the endometrial echoes during menstruation results from sloughed endometrial tissues (stratum functionalis) and blood break down products. The endometrium may enter a transient period of repair called the 'resting period' for 1–2 days.

4.2.2 Proliferative Phase

The proliferative phase of the menstrual cycle (variable duration of between days 6 and 14) lasts until ovulation and represents the preparation of the endometrium for implantation of a fertilised ovum. The proliferative phase heralds the onset of endometrial hypertrophy under the influence of oestrogens secreted by Graafian follicle in the ovary. Endometrial thickness ranges from 5–7 mm (Fig. 31). The endometrial echogenicity relative to the myometrium becomes more pronounced reflecting glandular, stromal and capillary development (Fleischer 1999). In the late proliferative phase, the endometrium develops a transitory multilayered appearance and can measure up to 11 mm in

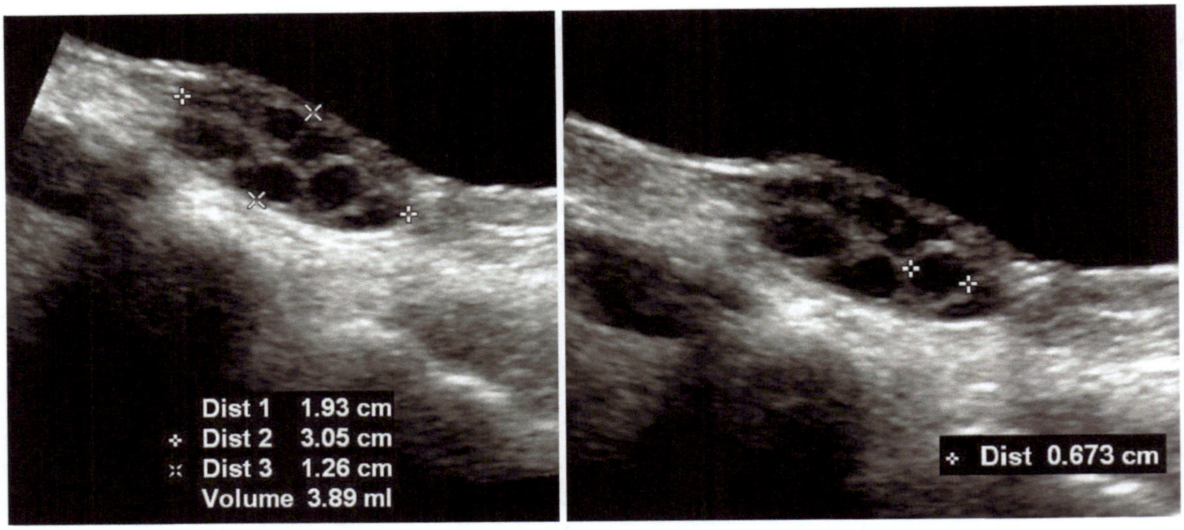

Fig. 26 Multifollicular ovary (MFO). Composite oblique US images of a MFO. MFO refers to an ovary with normal stromal content containing at least six anechoic small follicles (2–9 mm in diameter) visible in a single image plane

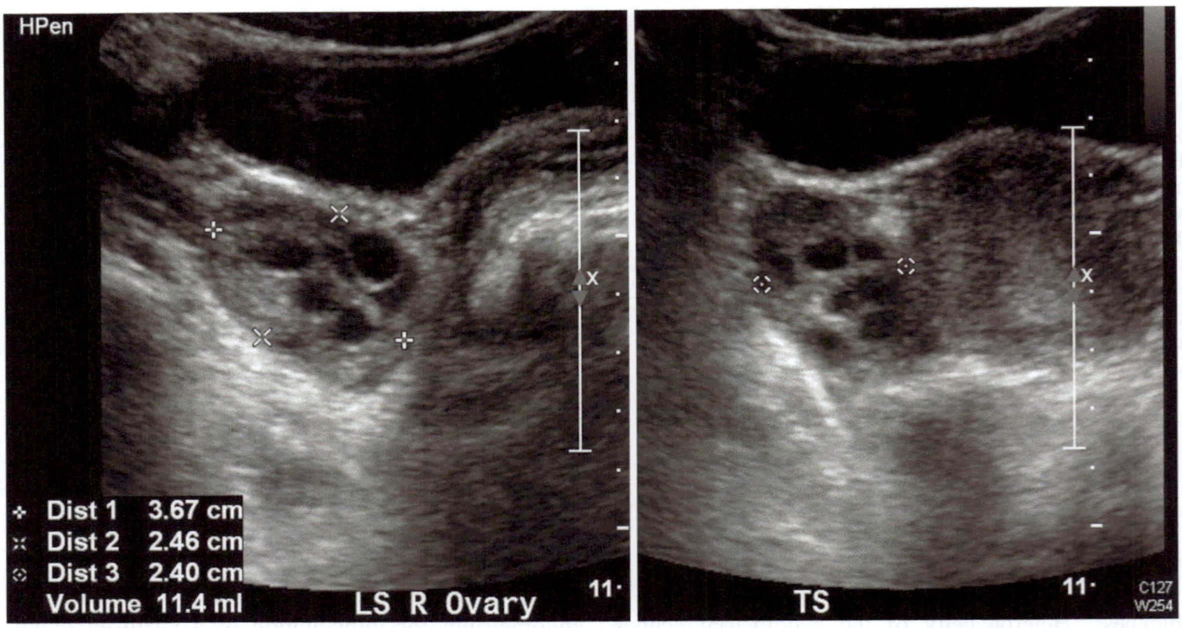

Fig. 27 Postmenarchal ovary. Composite oblique US images of the left ovary of a 14-year-old girl demonstrating multiple follicles with a volume of 11.4 cm^3

thickness. The basal layer is echogenic. A thin echogenic median layer forms a central interface with the hypoechoic inner functional layer (Nalaboff et al. 2006). The multi-layered appearance usually disappears 48 h after ovulation.

4.2.3 Secretory Phase

The secretory phase lasts 14 days. Endometrial thickness and echogenicity increases further during the secretory phase under the influence of progesterone produced by the corpus luteum in the ovary.

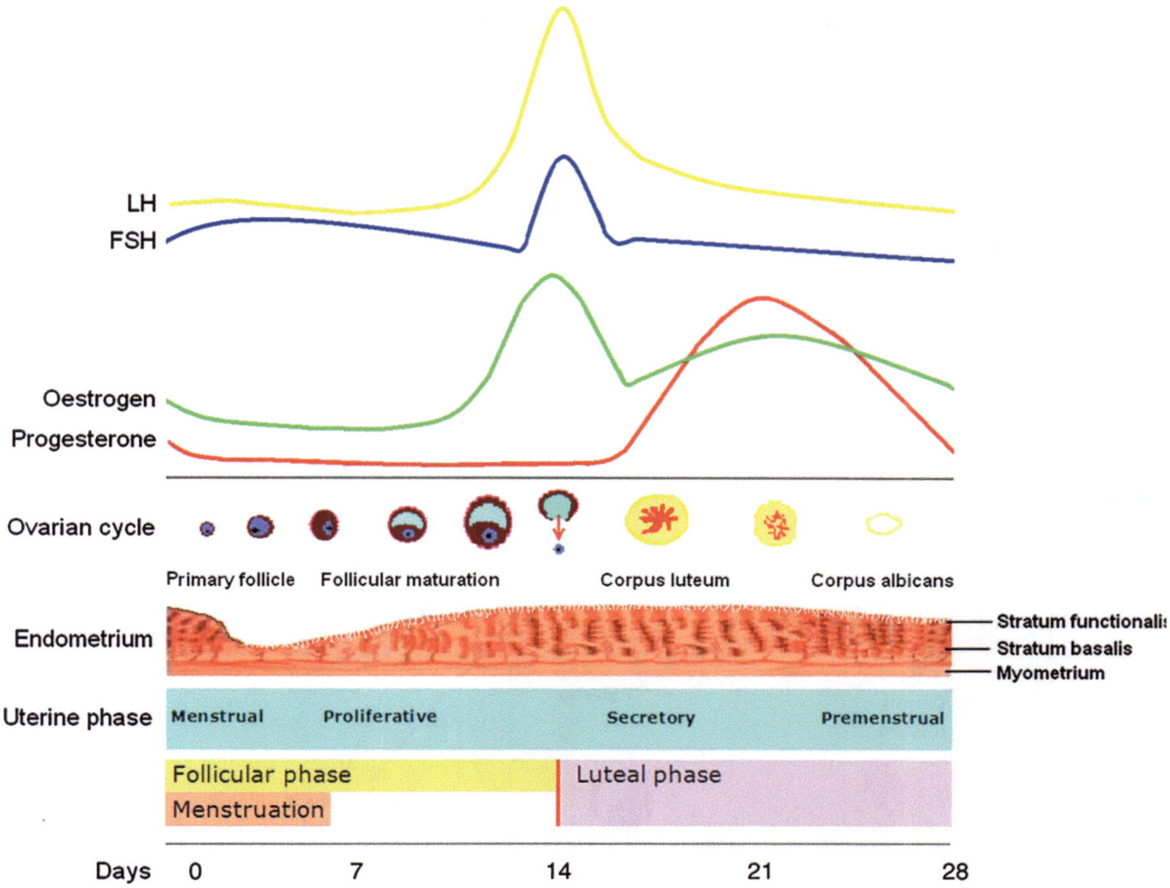

Fig. 28 Schematic overview of the menstrual cycle (cycle length typically 28 days duration). Menstruation lasts around 3–5 days and results in shedding of the endometrial lining. The secretory phase lasts for 14 days. Average hormonal values and the duration of a menstrual cycle may vary from cycle to cycle in the same individual

The endometrial thickness may range from 7–16 mm and reaches maximal depth in the mid-secretory phase. Increased endometrial echogenicity reflects mucoid glandular distension with nutrients and stromal oedema, the latter may result in increased posterior acoustic enhancement. The nutrients (glucose, fructose and glycogen) are secreted into the endometrial canal to nourish any implanted ovum. In the absence of a fertilised ovum the corpus luteum involutes and the functional endometrial layer undergoes involution and necrosis resulting in the onset of menstruation.

4.3 Zonal MR Anatomy of the Uterus During the Menstrual Cycle

On MR imaging the normal endometrium is best demonstrated on T2W images. On T2-weighted imaging the normal zonal anatomy of the uterus includes the endometrium, which is of uniformly high signal intensity and varies in thickness with menstrual phase, the inner myometrium (junctional zone) which is of uniformly low signal intensity (Nalaboff et al. 2006) (Fig. 32), and the intermediate signal intensity outer myometrium.

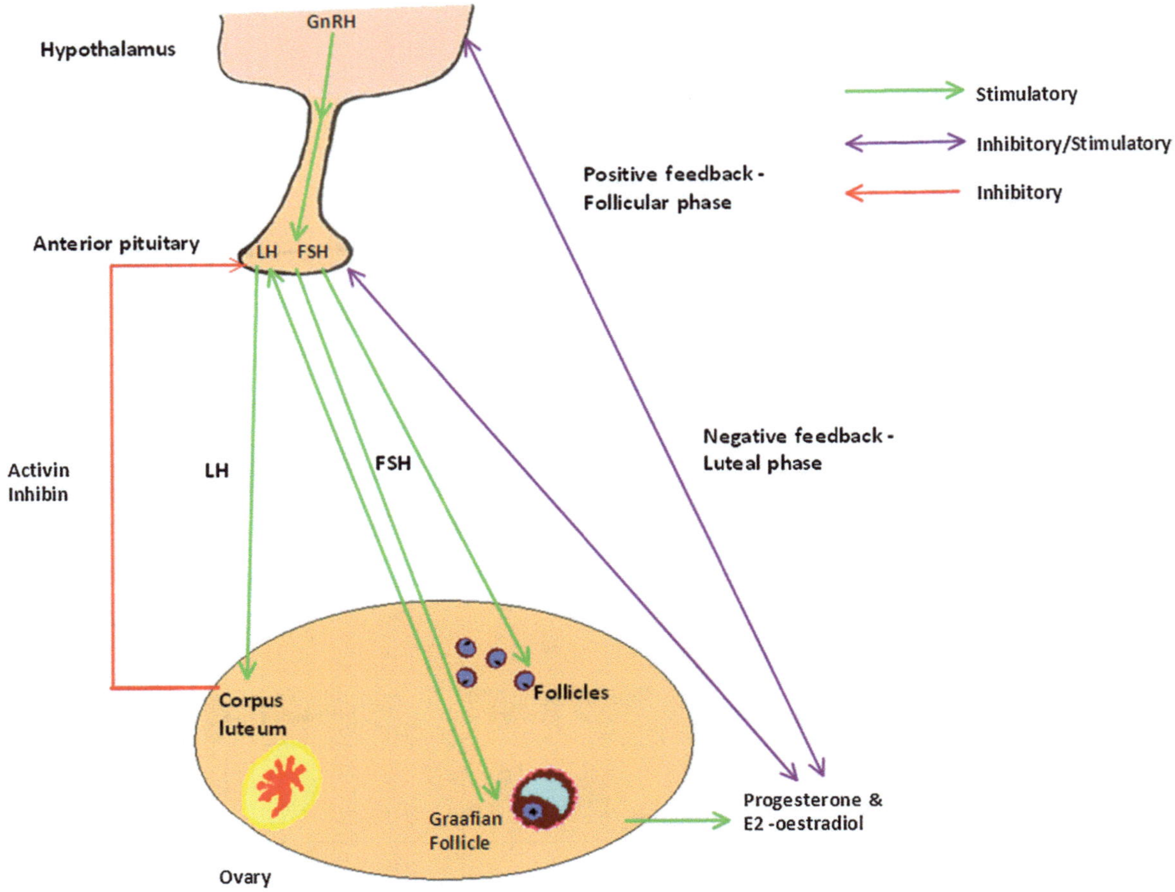

Fig. 29 Schematic overview of the key constituent hormonal pathways and feedback mechanisms of the hypothalamic-pituitary-ovarian axis

The endometrium varies in thickness between 3 mm (proliferative phase) and 7 mm in the secretory phase). During menstruation, myometrial thickness and signal intensity decreases on T2W images. Consequently, the junctional zone may become indistinct or show apparent thickening which mimics adenomyosis (Takeuchi et al. 2010). Myometrial T2W signal intensity is also slightly decreased during the early proliferative phase. The outer myometrium signal on T2W imaging increases slightly during the secretory phase. Both ultrasound and MRI depict zonal architecture of the uterus but the thickness of the endometrium, junctional zone and outer myometrium differ between the two modalities.

Like CT, T1W images are poor at demonstrating zonal anatomy with the uterine corpus appearing homogeneously isointense to skeletal muscle. There is strong enhancement of the endometrium and outer myometrium on T1W images following gadolinium. Zonal enhancement of the uterus may also be seen in arterial phase contrast-enhanced imaging with CT (Fig. 33).

4.4 Zonal MR Anatomy of the Ovary During the Menstrual Cycle

The postmenarchal ovaries show distinct zonal anatomy on T2W imaging. The cortex is of low-signal intensity and contains high-intensity follicles which usually make the ovaries easy to locate on T2W sequences (Fig. 34). The medulla is of intermediate signal-intensity. During menstruation ovarian volumes decrease, follicular size decreases and medullary signal-intensity decreases. The ovaries are of low-to

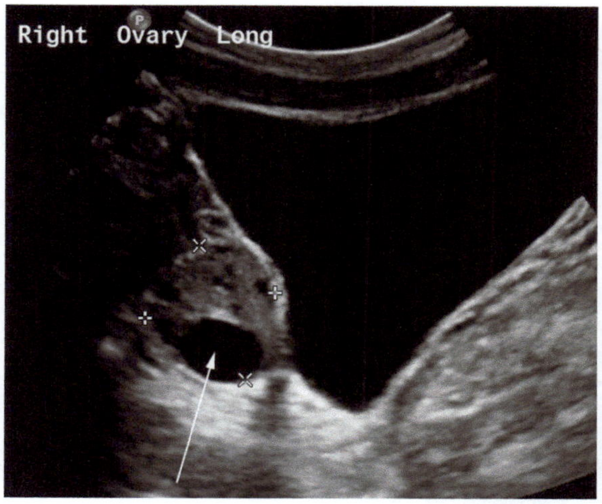

Fig. 30 Dominant follicle. Normal appearances of ovary (between callipers) on day 13 post-menstruation of a 28-day menstrual cycle. An anechoic dominant follicle (*arrow*) is depicted with several subordinate follicles

intermediate-signal intensity on T1W imaging with follicles typically isointense to fluid and are more difficult to visualise.

The ovaries gradually enlarge during the proliferative phase. Maximal ovarian size is attained during periovulation with the presence of a dominant follicle. The medulla has high signal intensity due to stromal oedema and neovascularisition. On diffusion weighted-imaging (DWI), the ovarian stroma has low signal intensity during menstruation, and higher signal intensity during periovulation (Takeuchi et al. 2010).

5 Adrenal Gland

Imaging of the adrenal glands is important in children with "Disorders of Sex Development" and "Delayed and Precocious Puberty".

Ultrasound is the first line imaging strategy for the evaluation of the adrenals in children, particularly the young. MR is the preferred cross-sectional modality for suspected mass lesions. CT is still used as part of the work up of neuroblastoma.

The sonographic appearance of the normal adrenal gland in children varies with age. The fetal adrenal gland is enlarged by virtue of its thickened cortex. In newborns, the cortex is large and hypoechoic, whereas the medulla is relatively small and hyperechoic (Fig. 35). At birth the fetal adrenal cortex rapidly involutes. With increasing age, the cortex becomes smaller and the medulla relatively larger. The cortex remains hypoechoic and the medulla hyperechoic until age 5–6 months, by which time the gland has become hyperechoic and smaller, with poor or absent sonographic differentiation between cortex and medulla. After 1 year of age, the appearance of the gland is similar to that of the adult gland, with straight or concave borders and a hypoechoic character (Kangarloo et al. 1986). The age-related appearances and size of the adrenals is summarised in Tables 3 and 4. The morphology of the adrenals is variable with the inverted 'V' or 'Y' shapes being the most common.

6 Pituitary

The MR characteristics of the normal pituitary gland in childhood and adolescence are well established. In childhood the pituitary height, signal characteristics and contrast-enhancement pattern follow a predictable pattern of development. The anterior pituitary usually appears hyperintense on T1-weighted MR imaging up until a postnatal corrected age of 2 months and thereafter is isointense to the pons (Kitamura et al. 2008; Argyropoulou et al. 2004). Anterior pituitary signal increases during pregnancy and postpartum. The posterior pituitary signal is bright on T1-weighted imaging at all ages. This is related to the concentration of neurosecretory granules containing antidiuretic hormone (ADH) bound to neurophysin. Plasma ADH concentrations are high in neonates and decrease during the first year of life, this is mirrored by a gradual reduction in posterior pituitary signal from birth until age 1 year after which appearances follow those of an adult. The signal intensity also decreases with dehydration and increases following rehydration (Lee et al. 2001).

Anterior pituitary height varies with age (Fig. 36). In the first year of life there is a weak negative linear correlation with age (Kiortsis et al. 2004). Positive linear correlation is seen thereafter up until puberty at which time a plateau is reached. The upper border of the anterior pituitary is typically convex in the first 2 months of life. The pituitary throughout childhood shows a flat upper surface with a height of 2–6 mm. At

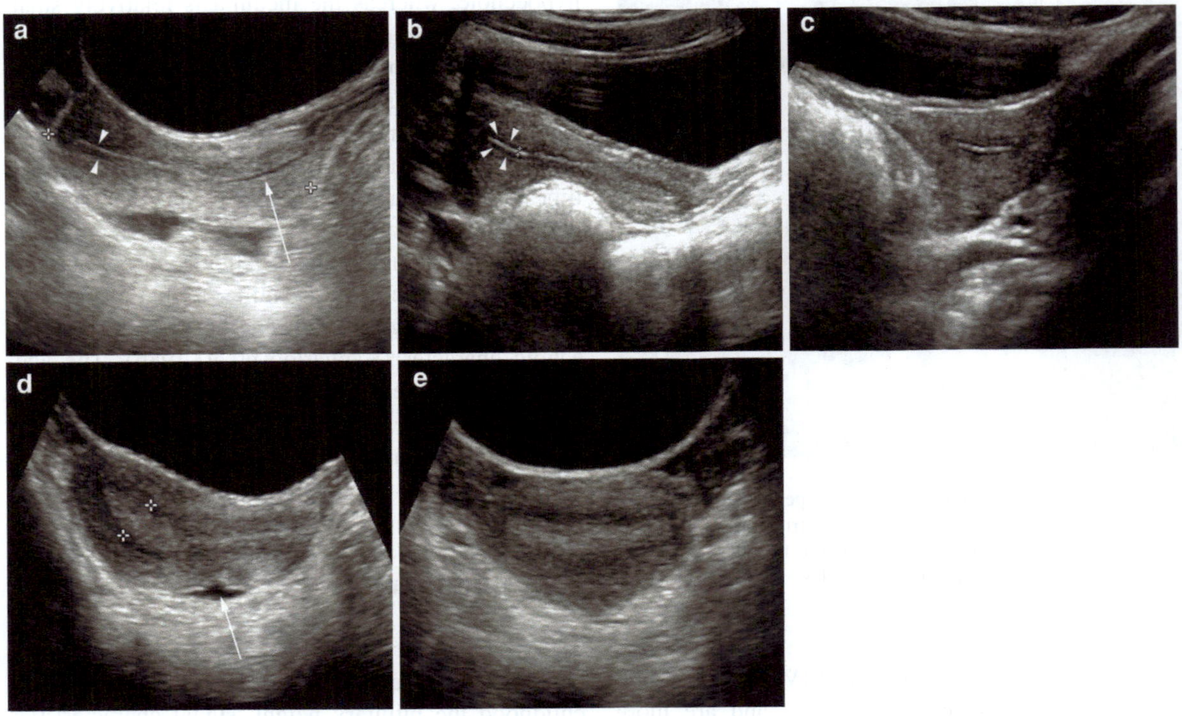

Fig. 31 US of the uterus obtained during various phases of the menstrual cycle. **a** Longitudinal imaging during menstruation shows a thin endometrial lining (*arrowheads*) with a trace of intracavitary fluid (*arrow*). Pelvic free fluid is demonstrated. **b** Longitudinal image during the late proliferative phase of the menstrual cycle showing a multilayered appearance to the endometrium (*arrowheads*). **c** Corresponding transverse image. **d** Longitudinal image during the secretory phase of the menstrual cycle shows a thickened, uniformly echogenic endometrium (between callipers), trace pelvic free fluid is demonstrated (*arrow*). **e** Corresponding transverse image of the uterine corpus

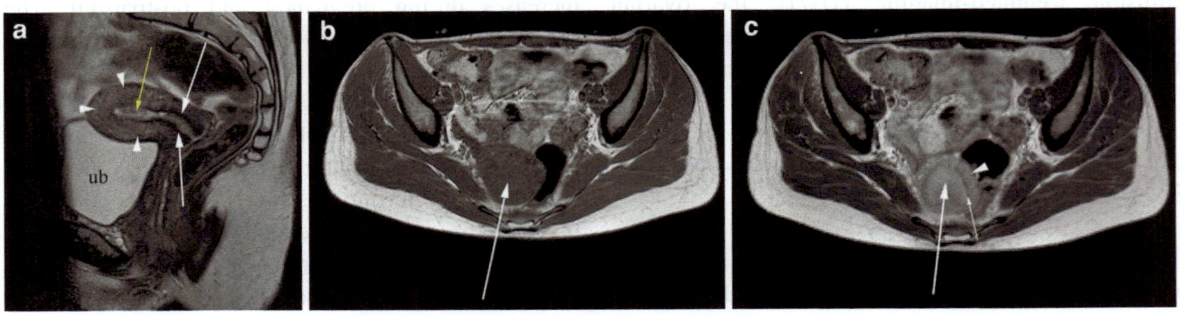

Fig. 32 **a** Normal uterine MRI zonal anatomy. Sagittal T2W MR image depicting the normal endometrium (*yellow arrow*) , junctional zone (*arrows*) and myometrium (*arrowheads*). Urinary bladder. **b** Axial T1W image before IV gadolinium and **c** corresponding axial T1W image post-IV gadolinium, showing enhancing uterine endometrium (*large arrow*) and myometrium (*arrowhead*), the junctional zone (*short arrow*) is much better appreciated on contrast-enhanced imaging

puberty, pituitary enlargement results from physiologic hypertrophy, with normal height values up to 8 mm in boys and 10 mm in girls. The pituitary gland enlarges throughout pregnancy reaching a maximal height of up to 12 mm in the first postpartum week (Elster 1993). Postpubertal females typically have flat or mildly convex glands with a maximal height of 10 mm.

Contrast enhancement of the pituitary fossa follows a predictable pattern. The posterior pituitary and stalk enhance at the same time as the straight sinus

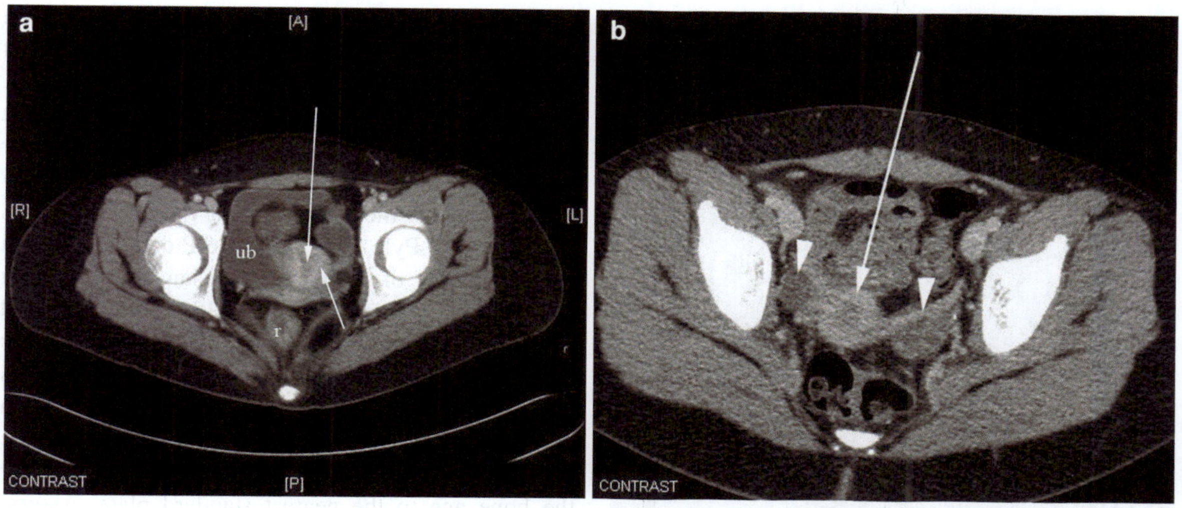

Fig. 33 Axial contrast-enhanced CT uterus and ovaries. **a** The uterus enhances in a predictable fashion with less marked enhancement of the endometrium (*arrow*) relative to the myometrium (*short arrow*), urinary bladder (UB), rectum (R). **b** Normal ovaries (*arrowheads*) with enhancing cortex containing discrete follicles imaged at the level of the uterus (*arrow*). The ovaries can be difficult to visualise in children particularly when there is a paucity of intra-abdominal fat or as is often the case, when the ovaries lie adjacent to the bowel. Contrast-enhanced images are essential but still provide much less information than non-contrasted US or MRI

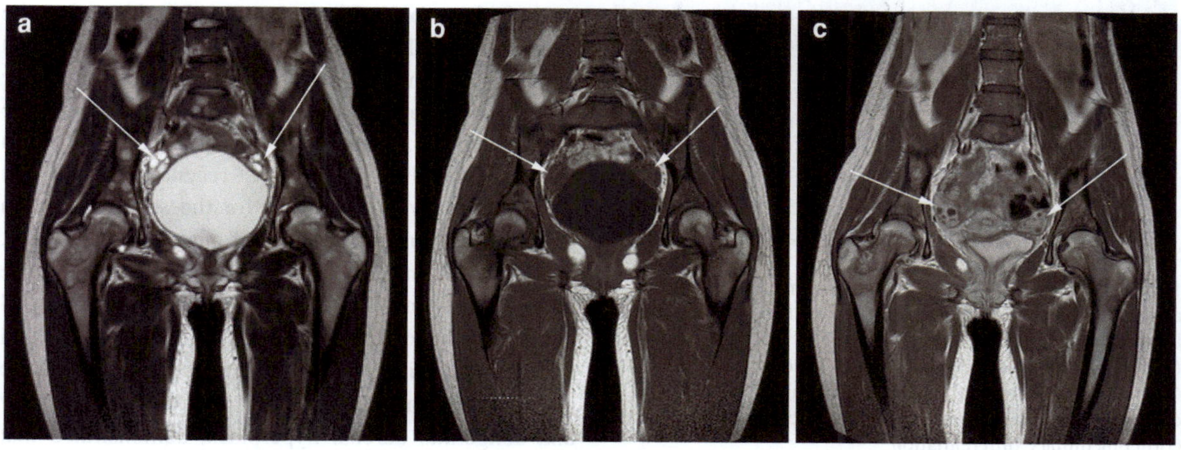

Fig. 34 MRI appearances of normal ovaries. **a** Coronal T2-TSE image of the ovaries in a child with metastatic sarcoma. On T2W-imaging the ovarian cortex is of intermediate signal intensity. The ovarian medulla is isointense to the uterine myometrium. The ovaries contain small hyperintense subcortically located follicles (*arrows*). **b** Coronal T1-TSE and **c** Post IV-gadolinium images. On T1W imaging the ovarian zonal anatomy is difficult to appreciate, the fluid-filled follicles are seen as discrete hypointense areas. The ovarian stroma (*arrows*) shows uniform enhancement following contrast accentuating the non-enhancing follicles

between 9.2 and 18.5 s following injection and the anterior pituitary shortly thereafter by 30 s following injection (Maghnie et al. 1994) (Fig. 37). Abnormalities in this temporal relationship may indicate pathology and have been exploited using dynamic gradient-echo and spin-echo contrast-enhanced pituitary imaging.

7 Assessment of Skeletal Maturity and Bone Age

A reliable method of measuring skeletal maturity (bone age) is important for the analysis of potential disorders of growth and pubertal maturation. Accurate

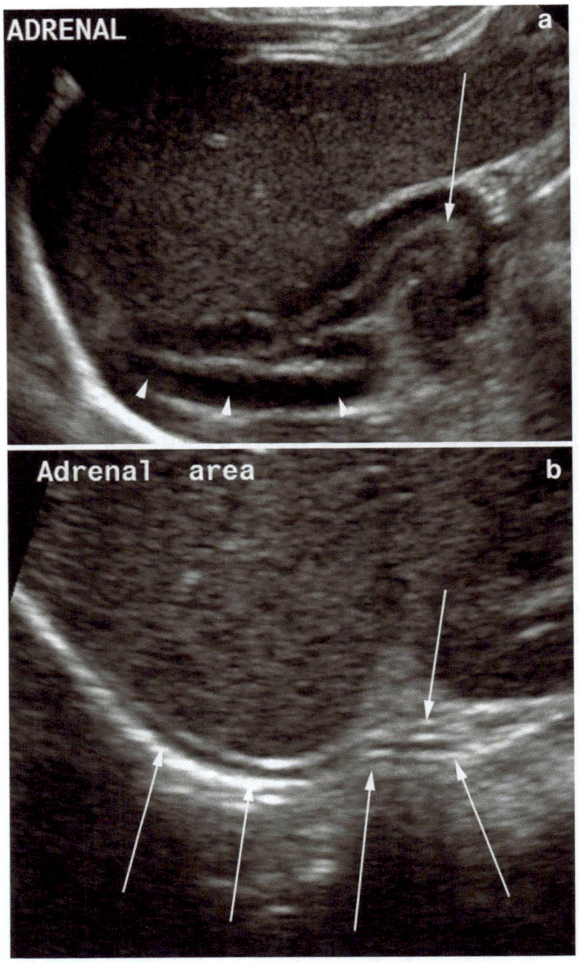

Fig. 35 The normal adrenal gland. **a** Transverse sonogram of a normal relatively large neonatal adrenal gland showing the hypoechoic cortex (*arrowheads*) and echogenic medulla (*arrow*). **b** Longitudinal sonogram of a normal adrenal gland (*arrows*) in a 1-year-old girl. The adrenal gland shows adult characteristics and is uniformly hypoechoic with no appreciable corticomedullary differentiation

knowledge of bone age is also required for bone mass estimation. Pubertal delay and precocious puberty are indicated when the estimated bone age lies two standard deviations below or above the chronological age respectively. In chlidren, bone mass measurements are usually assessed relative to bone age rather than chronological age (see Sect. 8.1.1).

By far the most commonly employed imaging technique involves obtaining a dorsopalmar radiograph of the non-dominant wrist and hand for assessment of skeletal maturity indicators. Carpal bone maturation varies greatly. Bone age estimation based on metacarpal and phalangeal assessment more closely approximates chronological age than wrist and carpal bone readings (Carpenter and Lester 1993).

Several methods are available for the assessment of skeletal age; these may be performed manually or involve automated processing. The most commonly used method is the Greulich and Pyle (G&P) Atlas (Greulich and Pyle 1959). The G&P data are derived from a cohort of affluent Caucasian children from Ohio, USA, examined between 1931 and 1942 and comprises standard radiographic plates for both sexes at a particular chronological age. Each of the images in the G&P atlas represents the median standard for a particular chronological age. The technique is holistic and requires the reader to approximate a best fit for the bone age to the nearest standard plate. Assessments made using the G&P atlas are often very inaccurate. Observer variability and bias related to the prior knowledge of the patient's chronological age influence the derived bone age (Berst et al. 2001).

The Tanner-Whitehouse (TW) method favoured by many centres is more time-consuming and employs an analytical approach (Tanner et al. 1975). It requires the summation of the maturity indicators of 20 individual bones of the hand and wrist to derive a skeletal maturity score (SMS) which correlates with a tabulated bone age for a given sex. Three editions of this scoring system have been published. The most recent edition (TW3) updated the SMS to account for the secular trend in towards earlier maturation (Tanner et al. 2001). The descriptions and manual ratings are the same between versions; however the centile charts for SMS against age have changed. Comparison of the TW2 and TW3 standards in a group of 142 children with idiopathic short stature, constitutional delay of growth and puberty and congenital adrenal hyperplasia demonstrated that TW3 estimates of SMS were younger than TW2, and that this difference increased with age (Ahmed and Warner 2007). The FELS method (Roche et al. 1988) is also an analytical method but less widely used. Currently, TW remains the method of choice and has been shown to be more reliable and reproducible in clinical practice (Bull et al. 1999).

More recently, automated G&P analysis of bone age has been validated in children (Thodberg and Sävendahl 2010). A review of data from 719 patients with various diagnoses reported that 99% of images could be analyzed with an accuracy of 0.7 years (Thodberg 2009) (Fig. 38).

Table 3 Normal adrenal gland size (Oppenheimer et al. 1983)

Age	Gland length (cm)	Limb thickness (cm)	Width (cm)
Neonate	0.9–3.6 (mean 1.5)	0.2–0.5 (mean 0.3)	–
Adult	4–6	0.2–0.6	2–3

Table 4 Age-related sonographic features of normal adrenal glands (Kangarloo et al. 1986)

Age	Borders	Shape and size	Echogenicity
Newborn	Convex	Cortex ≫ Medulla thickness	Cortex hypoechoic
			Medulla hyperechoic
6 weeks–2 months	Convex	Gradual change to medulla > cortex thickness	Cortex hypoechoic
			Medulla hyperechoic
5–6 months	Straight	Decreasing size	Loss of corticomedullary differentiation
			Overall hyperechoic
>1 year	Concave or straight margins	Adult morphology	Loss of corticomedullary
			differentiation
			Hypoechoic

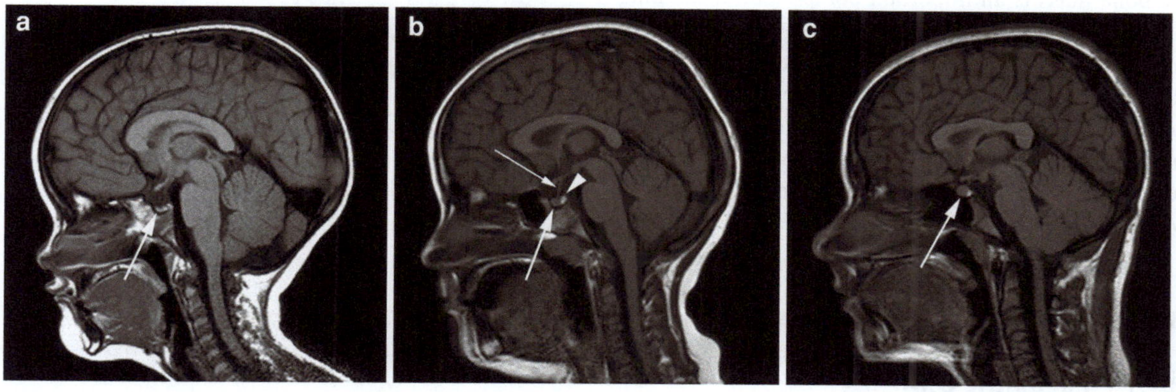

Fig. 36 Appearance of the normal pituitary gland in females on T1W-imaging as a function of age. The posterior pituitary is hyperintense and does not change in appearance with age. **a** During childhood the anterior pituitary may show a concave superior border (*arrow*), but typically **b** has a flat superior border (*arrow*) and measures 2–6 mm in maximal craniocaudal dimension. Posterior pituitary (*arrowhead*), infundibulum (*thin arrow*). **c** During puberty the anterior pituitary (arrow) undergoes physiologic hypertrophy and may attain a height of 10 mm with a convex superior border

8 Bone Mineralization

There are two periods of maximal bone mineralization, the first during infancy and second during pubertal development. Peak accrual of bone mineral occurs during early puberty (typically occurring between 14 and 16 years of age or within 2 years of menarche) with bone mass maximised in young adulthood. By the age of 17 years most girls will have accrued 90% of the total body mineral content.

A number of modifiable factors influence peak bone mass including exercise, nutritional status, body weight and oestrogen profile. Childhood disease and medications may predispose to reduced peak bone mass acquisition, thereby increasing the

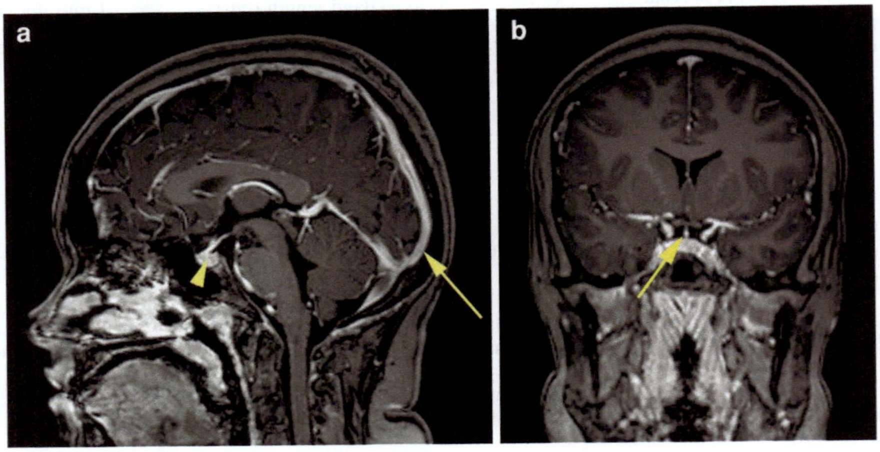

Fig. 37 T1 W-gadolinium enhanced images of the pituitary. **a** Sagittal scan showing enhancement of the anterior pituitary (*arrowhead*) which is similar to that of the dural venous sinuses. **b** Coronal image showing normal enhancement of the pituitary infundibulum (*arrow*)

risk of developing osteoporosis and the long-term fracture rate. These include disorders in girls presenting with delayed puberty ("Delayed and Precocious Puberty") and amenorrhoea ("Menstrual Disorders and Vaginal Discharge"). Accurate evaluation of paediatric bone mass is an important component of the diagnostic work-up of these children. As such there is an increasing desire by clinicians to quantify bone mineral density (BMD) and attempt to improve it. It is generally accepted that the first line of investigation should be a measurement of the Vitamin D levels, since it is recognised that a significant proportion of children are Vitamin D deficient (Ginde et al. 2009).

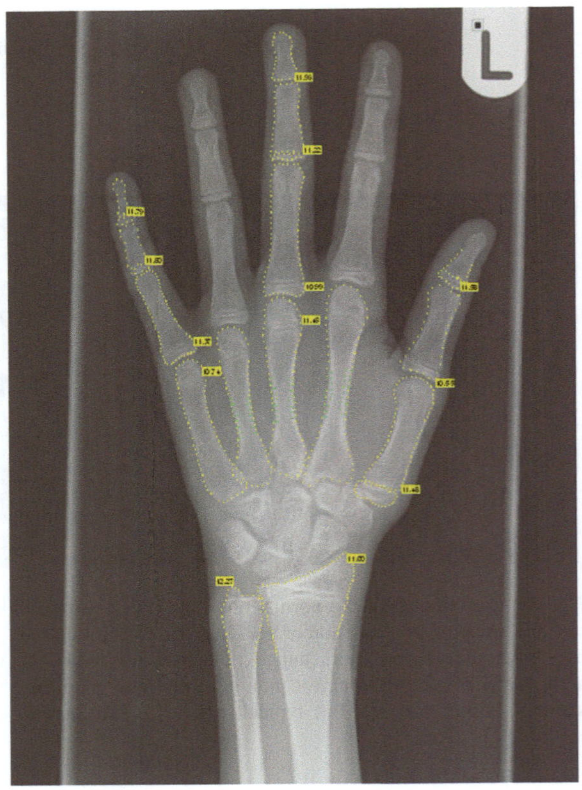

Fig. 38 Automated analysis of bone age using 'BoneXpert' software (Visiana, Holte, Denmark) analysis of a non-dominant wrist and hand radiograph. Results from a teenager with Crohn's disease and delayed pubertal maturation are presented showing delayed bone age. The chronological age is 16 years and 11 months, the Greulich and Pyle age is 11.4 years and TW2 age 13.1 years

8.1 Evaluation of Bone Mass

8.1.1 Paediatric DXA

Dual-energy X-ray absorptiometry (DXA) is used in many paediatric centres as a tool to assess bone density. DXA scans are acquired over a few minutes using a very low ionising radiation dose technique. The principle of DXA imaging relies on the differences in the measurement of absorption of X-rays at two different energies by different tissues, thereby enabling estimation of bone mineral content (BMC—expressed as grams).

BMD is calculated by dividing BMC by the projected or measured 2-dimensional area evaluated. DXA thereby provides an areal density of a 2-dimensional structure (expressed as grams of mineral per unit area, typically g/cm^2).

Alder Hey Children's NHS Foundation Trust
Bone Densitometry Department

Name: Patient ID: DOB:	Sex: Male Ethnicity: Pediatric	Height: 167.0 cm Weight: 50.9 kg Age: 16

Referring Physician:

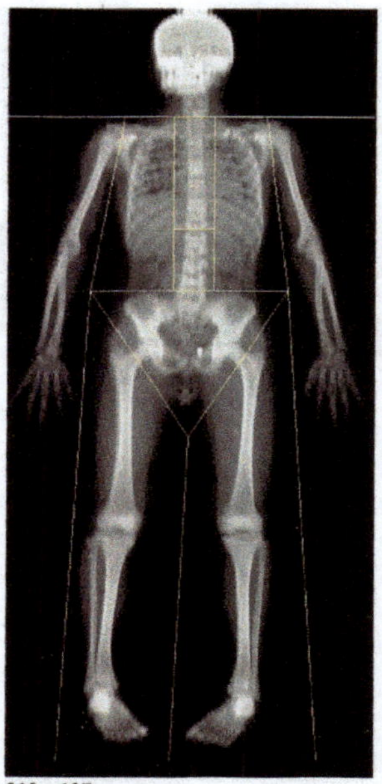

318 x 137

DXA Results Summary:

Region	Area (cm^2)	BMC (g)	BMD (g/cm^2)	T - score	PR (%)	Z - score	AM (%)
L Arm	141.31	91.64	0.649				
R Arm	140.13	99.98	0.714				
L Ribs	104.70	64.13	0.612				
R Ribs	97.62	61.43	0.629				
T Spine	103.92	65.22	0.628				
L Spine	56.68	53.73	0.948				
Pelvis	190.90	191.87	1.005				
L Leg	307.42	286.46	0.932				
R Leg	314.89	293.30	0.931				
Subtotal	1457.57	1207.77	0.829				
Head	251.13	378.24	1.506				
Total	**1708.70**	**1586.00**	**0.928**		**75**	**-1.8**	**85**

Total BMD CV 1.0%

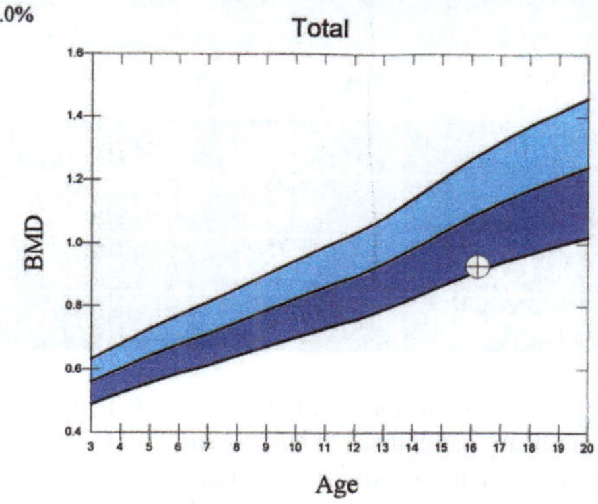

T-score vs. Pediatric Male; Z-score vs. Pediatric Male. Source:Hologic, 2005

Physician's Comment:

Scan Information:

Scan Date: ID:
Scan Type: a Whole Body
Analysis: 2010 11:48 Version 12.7.3.2
Auto Whole Body

HOLOGIC®

Fig. 39 Paediatric DXA study data set. The relevant values are the lumbar spine BMD Z score, the whole body BMC and the whole body bone area. The patient's age and height are also relevant when applying the Molgaard method of interpretation Mølgaard et al. (1997). In the first instance a lumbar spine BMD z score of less than −1 can be considered to be outside the normal range. In our centre the Molgaard method is applied to correct for height and bone size. The decision to treat or intervene must not be made solely on BMD measurements in children and young people

Paediatric BMD is usually measured at the lumbar spine as the bone geometry and size are relatively stable over time; the hip is an alternative site particularly if there is orthopaedic spinal hardware in situ. A whole body scan is also acquired to allow for better analysis with respect to body composition and body area. The region of interest (ROI) within the lumbar spine is from L1 to L4 (Fig. 39). The ROI for the hip includes the femoral neck, greater trochanter and total hip. Less commonly, in the presence of extensive orthopaedic hardware or other artifacts, BMD of the wrist can also be measured. Although the thoracic spine is not included for DXA evaluation the presence of non-lumbar vertebral compression fractures on the lateral spine scanogram has prognostic implication for the diagnosis of osteoporosis in children (Mäkitie et al. 2005).

The interpretation of DXA results obtained on children necessitates an understanding of several key

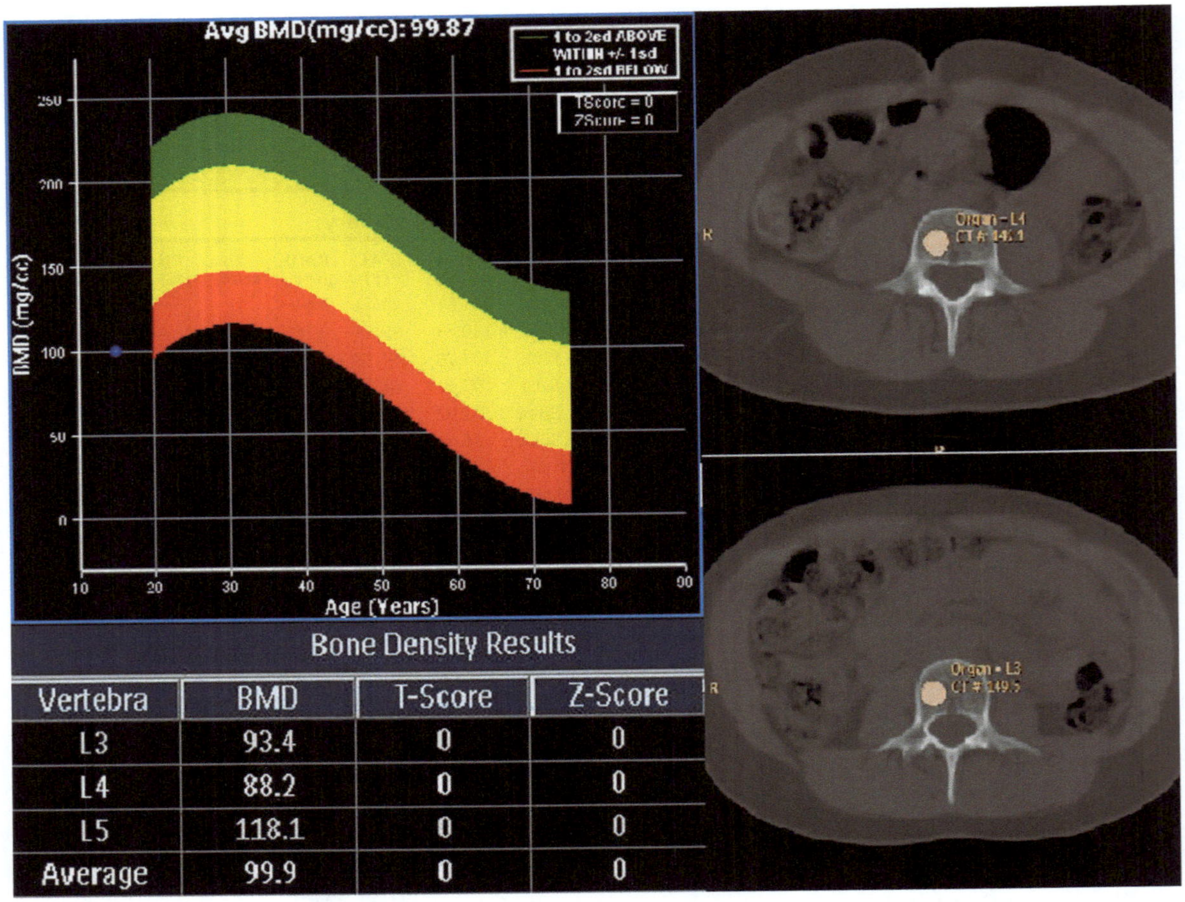

Fig. 40 QCT of the lumbar spine. QCT is largely used in research in paediatrics, since there are no reference ranges available for the paediatric population. Most software applications will provide lumbar spine BMD QCT reference ranges for the adult population. The figure shows the ranges provided for the adult population and the data point for the patient concerned. In our centre the graph is extrapolated to give an estimation of the patient's Lumbar spine BMD, in this case the lumbar spine BMD falls between 1 and 2 standard deviations below normal. This information is not used in isolation, but in relation to the DXA score and the Molgaard interpretation. The decision to treat or intervene must not be made solely on BMD measurements in children and young people

issues which should be borne in mind by both the requesting clinician and reporting radiologist. The reporting radiologist must ensure that the radiographic technique for DXA acquisition technique follow a meticulous protocol. The radiologist cannot simply rely on the DXA generated numerical data set and manufacturers' normative reference data. A detailed knowledge of the concepts of Z-scores and least significant changes is required (Binkovitz and Henwood 2007). Meaningful interpretation of the data must take into account patient-related factors including sex, age, height, weight, pubertal stage, ethnicity, drug and medical history.

The World Health Organisation diagnostic criteria for osteoporosis only apply to Caucasian women and should not be quoted in paediatric practice. In adult females, DXA results are given in the form of a T-score, which represents bone loss since peak bone density in young adulthood, and scores are given as the number of standard deviations away from a mean of zero (where a T-score of greater than minus 1 is normal). In children, results are given in the form of a

Z-score, which is also the number of standard deviations away from a mean of zero, but is related to age matched reference ranges.

DXA is a projection technique and only provides a measure of the areal density of a 2-dimensional structure. As a result the assessment of BMD in children is limited by the fact that the calculated BMD is based on a projected volume of bone rather than a true volume. Consequently, small bones will have an apparently lower areal BMD than larger bones even if the volumetric BMD is the same. One of the limitations of the accuracy of DXA is the inability to account for the large variability in body composition, skeletal size and non-uniform growth in children (Wren et al. 2005).

There are important differences in BMD related to pubertal stage and gender, particularly in adolescence. There are reference ranges for age-related BMD scores but there is, as yet, no prognostic indicator regarding fracture risk and peak BMD. It must therefore be emphasised that decisions regarding treatment of reduced BMD in children should not be made based solely on BMD measurements. The use of robust reference standards is essential. There are numerous published reference standards. A rigorous methodology for evaluating paediatric BMD has been described by Mølgaard et al. (1997). Recently, there have been published paediatric reference standards for BMC which also account for ethnicity (Baxter-Jones et al. 2010). Follow-up DXA should ideally be performed on the same scanner to best assess the serial trend in BMD.

8.1.2 Quantitative Computed Tomography

Quantitative computed tomography (QCT) is a relatively new technique and is an adjunct to DXA. QCT provides a separate 3-dimensional volumetric assessment of cortical and trabecular bone density. This is routinely performed in the lumbar vertebrae (L2–L4) (Fig. 40) but can also be employed peripherally in long bone metaphyses. The role of QCT is not fully established. The main disadvantages of QCT are the lack of normative paediatric reference data and higher radiation doses compared to DXA.

8.1.3 Quantitative Ultrasound

Quantitative ultrasound (QUS) is a newer and less well-established technique which is currently not in widespread clinical use. QUS has been evaluated as an adjunct to DXA or as an alternative method of assessing BMD in children (Fielding et al. 2003; Baroncelli 2008). QUS is portable, less expensive, requires no specific operator training and employs no ionising radiation when compared to DXA. QUS is performed on the calcanei. Measurements obtained include the broadband ultrasound attenuation (BUA) (dB/MHz) and the speed of sound (SOS) (m/s) in a fixed region of interest in the central calcaneal zone. These measures provide an estimate of bone elasticity and microarchitecture.

References

Adams J, Polson DW, Abdulwahid N et al (1985) Multifollicular ovaries: clinical and endocrine features and response to pulsatile gonadotrophin releasing hormone. Lancet 2:1375–1399

Ahmed ML, Warner JT (2007) TW2 and TW3 bone ages: time to change? Arch Dis Child 92:371–372

Argyropoulou MI, Xydis V, Kiortsis DN et al (2004) Pituitary gland signal in preterm infants during the first year of life: an MRI study. Neuroradiology 46:1031–1035

Badouraki M, Christoforidis A, Economou I et al (2008) Sonographic assessment of uterine and ovarian development in normal girls aged 1 to 12 years. J Clin Ultrasound 36:539–544

Baker TG (1963) A quantitative and cytological study of germ cells in human ovaries. Proc R Soc Lond B Biol Sci 158:417–433

Baroncelli GI (2008) Quantitative ultrasound methods to assess bone mineral status in children: technical characteristics, performance, and clinical application. Pediatr Res 63: 220–228

Battaglia C, Regnani G, Mancini F et al (2002) Pelvic sonography and uterine artery color Doppler analysis in the diagnosis of female precocious puberty. Ultrasound Obstet Gynecol 19:386–391

Battaglia C, Mancini F, Regnani G et al (2003) Pelvic ultrasound and color Doppler findings in different isosexual precocities. Ultrasound Obstet Gynecol 22:277–283

Baxter-Jones AD, Burrows M, Bachrach LK et al (2010) International longitudinal pediatric reference standards for bone mineral content. Bone 46:208–216

Berst MJ, Dolan L, Bogdanowicz MM et al (2001) Effect of knowledge of chronologic age on the variability of pediatric bone age determined using the Greulich and Pyle standards. AJR 176:507–510

Beuscher-Willems B (2006) Chapter 13 Female genital tract. In: Schmidt G (ed) Differential diagnosis in ultrasound: a teaching atlas. Thieme Medical Publishers, NY, pp 389–390

Binkovitz LA, Henwood MJ (2007) Pediatric DXA: technique and interpretation. Pediatr Radiol 37:21–31

Bridges NA, Cooke A, Healy MJ et al (1996) Growth of the uterus. Arch Dis Child 75:330–331

Brown MA, Ascher SM (2006) Adnexa. In: Semelka RC (ed) Abdominal-pelvic MRI, 2nd edn. Wiley-Liss, Hoboken, pp 1334–1379

Bull RK, Edwards PD, Kemp PM et al (1999) Bone age assessment: a large scale comparison of the Greulich and Pyle, and Tanner and Whitehouse (TW2) methods. Arch Dis Child 81:172–173

Buzi F, Pilotta A, Dordoni D et al (1998) Pelvic ultrasonography in normal girls and in girls with pubertal precocity. Acta Paediatr 87:1138–1145

Carpenter CT, Lester LL (1993) Skeletal age determination in young children: analysis of 3 regions of the hand/wrist film. J Pediatr Orthop 13:76–79

Clement PB (2002) Anatomy and histology of the ovary. In: Kurman RJ (ed) Blaustein's pathology of the female genital tract. Springer, New York, pp 649–674

Cohen HL, Tice HM, Mandel FS (1990) Ovarian volumes measured by US: bigger than we think. Radiology 177:189–192

Cohen HL, Shapiro MA, Mandel FS, Shapiro ML (1993) Normal ovaries in neonates and infants: a sonographic study of 77 patients 1 day to 24 months old. AJR Am J Roentgenol 160:583–586

Davis JA, Gosink BB (1986) Fluid in the female pelvis: cyclic patterns. J Ultrasound Med 5:75–79

Diaz A, Laufer MR, Breech LL (2006) American Academy of Pediatrics Committee on Adolescence; American College of Obstetricians and Gynecologists Committee on Adolescent Health Care Menstruation in girls and adolescents: using the menstrual cycle as a vital sign. Pediatrics 118:2245–2250

dos Santos Silva I, De Stavola BL, Mann V et al (2002) Prenatal factors, childhood growth trajectories and age at menarche. Int J Epidemiol 31:405–412

Elster AD (1993) Modern imaging of the pituitary. Radiology 187:1–14

Euling SY, Selevan SG, Pescovitz OH et al (2008) Role of environmental factors in the timing of puberty. Pediatrics 121:S167–S171

Farooqi IS, Jebb SA, Langmack G et al (1999) Effects of recombinant leptin therapy in a child with congenital leptin deficiency. N Engl J Med 341:879–884

Fielding KT, Nix DA, Bachrach LK (2003) Comparison of calcaneus ultrasound and dual X-ray absorptiometry in children at risk of osteopenia. J Clin Densitom 6:7–15

Fleischer AC (1999) Sonographic assessment of endometrial disorders. Semin Ultrasound CT MR 20:259–266

Galler JR, Ramsey FC, Salt P et al (1987) Long-term effects of early kwashiorkor compared with marasmus. I. Physical growth and sexual maturation. J Pediatr Gastroenterol Nutr 6:841–846

Ginde AA, Liu MC, Camargo CA Jr (2009) Demographic differences and trends of vitamin D insufficiency in the US population, 1988–2004. Arch Intern Med 169:626–632

Greulich WW, Pyle SI (1959) Radiographic atlas of skeletal development of hand and wrist, 2nd edn. Stanford University Press, Stanford

Griffin IJ, Cole TJ, Duncan KA et al (1995) Pelvic ultrasound measurements in normal girls. Acta Paediatr 84:536–543

Haber HP, Mayer EI (1994) Ultrasound evaluation of uterine and ovarian size from birth to puberty. Pediatr Radiol 24:11–13

Herman-Giddens ME, Slora EJ, Wasserman RC et al (1997) Secondary sexual characteristics and menses in young girls seen in office practice: a study from the Pediatric Research in office settings network. Pediatrics 99:505–512

Herter LD, Golendziner E, Flores JA et al (2002) Ovarian and uterine findings in pelvic sonography. Comparison between prepubertal girls, girls with isolated thelarche, and girls with central precocious puberty. J Ultrasound Med 21:1237–1246

Holm K, Laursen EM, Brocks V et al (1995) Pubertal maturation of the internal genitalia: an ultrasound evaluation of 166 healthy girls. Ultrasound Obstet Gynecol 6:175–181

Ibáñez L, Ferrer A, Marcos MV et al (2000) Early puberty: rapid progression and reduced final height in girls with low birth weight. Pediatrics 106(5):E72

Kadlubar FF, Berkowitz GS, Delongchamp RR et al (2003) The CYP3A4*1B variant is related to the onset of puberty, a known risk factor for the development of breast cancer. Cancer Epidemiol Biomarkers Prev 2:327–331

Kangarloo H, Diament MJ, Gold RH et al (1986) Sonography of adrenal glands in neonates and children: changes in appearance with age. J Clin Ultrasound 14:43–47

Kaplowitz PB, Oberfield SE, the Drug, Therapeutics, Executive Committees of the Lawson Wilkins Pediatric Endocrine Society (1999) Reexamination of the age limit for defining when puberty is precocious in girls in the United States: implications for evaluation and treatment. Pediatrics 104: 936–941

Kaplowitz PB, Slora EJ, Wasserman RC, Pedlow SE, Herman-Giddens ME (2001) Earlier onset of puberty in girls: relation to increased body mass index and race. Pediatrics 108:347–353

Kiortsis D, Xydis V, Drougia AG et al (2004) The height of the pituitary in preterm infants during the first 2 years of life: an MRI study. Neuroradiology 46:224–226

Kitamura E, Miki Y, Kawai M et al (2008) T1 signal intensity and height of the anterior pituitary in neonates: correlation with postnatal time. AJNR Am J Neuroradiol 29:1257–1260

Kulin HE, Bwibo N, Mutie D et al (1982) The effect of chronic childhood malnutrition on pubertal growth and development. Am J Clin Nutr 36:527–536

Landy H, Boepple PA, Mansfield MJ et al (1990) Sleep modulation of neuroendocrine function: developmental changes in gonadotropin-releasing hormone secretion during sexual maturation. Pediatr Res 28:213–217

Lazar L, Pollak U, Kalter-Leibovici O et al (2003) Pubertal course of persistently short children born small for gestational age (SGA) compared with idiopathic short children born appropriate for gestational age (AGA). Eur J Endocrinol 149:425–432

Lee MY, Choi HY, Sung YA et al (2001) High signal intensity of the posterior pituitary gland on T1-weighted images. Acta Radiol 42:129–134

Lee JH, Jeong YK, Park JK et al (2003) "Ovarian vascular pedicle" sign revealing organ of origin of a pelvic mass lesion on helical CT. Am J Roentgenol 181:131–137

López C, Balogun M, Ganesan R et al (2005) MRI of vaginal conditions. Clin Radiol 60:648–662

Maghnie M, Genovese E, Arico M et al (1994) Evolving pituitary hormone deficiency is associated with pituitary vasculopathy: dynamic MR study in children with hypopituitarism, diabetes insipidus, and Langerhans cell histiocytosis. Radiology 193:493–499

Mäkitie O, Doria AS, Henriques F et al (2005) Radiographic vertebral morphology: a diagnostic tool in pediatric osteoporosis. J Pediatr 146:395–401

Marshall WA, Tanner JM (1969) Variations in pattern of pubertal changes in girls. Arch Dis Child 44:291–303

McKiernan JF, Hull D (1981) Breast development in the newborn. Arch Dis Child 56:525–529

Mølgaard C, Thomsen BL, Prentice A et al (1997) Whole body bone mineral content in healthy children and adolescents. Arch Dis Child 76:9–15

Nalaboff KM, Pellerito JS, Ben-Levi E (2006) Imaging the endometrium: disease and normal variants. Radiographics 21:1409–1424

Norjavaara E, Ankarberg C, Albertsson-Wikland K (1996) Diurnal rhythm of 17 beta-estradiol secretion throughout pubertal development in healthy girls: evaluation by a sensitive radioimmunoassay. J Clin Endocrinol Metab 81:4095–4102

Nussbaum AR, Sanders RC, Jones MD (1986) Neonatal uterine morphology, as seen in real time US. Radiology 160: 641–643

Okamoto Y, Tanaka YO, Nishida M et al (2003) MR imaging of the uterine cervix: imaging–pathologic correlation. Radiographics 23:425–445

Oppenheimer DA, Carroll BA, Yousem S (1983) Sonography of the normal neonatal adrenal gland. Radiology 146:157–160

Orsini LF, Salardi S, Pilu G et al (1984) Pelvic organs in premenarcheal girls: real-time ultrasonography. Radiology 153:113–116

Polhemus DW (1953) Ovarian maturation and cyst formation in children. Pediatrics 11:588–594

Porcu E (2004) Imaging in pediatric and adolescent gynecology. In: Sultan C (ed) Pediatric and adolescent gynecology. Evidence-based clinical practice endocrine development, vol 7. Basel, Karger, pp 9–22

Powls A, Botting N, Cooke RW, Pilling D (1996) Growth impairment in very low birthweight children at 12 years: correlation with perinatal and outcome variables. Arch Dis Child Fetal Neonatal Ed 75:F152–F157

Rathaus V, Grunebaum M, Konen O et al (2003) Minimal pelvic fluid in asymptomatic children: the value of the sonographic finding. J Ultrasound Med 22:13–17

Roche AF, Chumlea WC, Thissen D (1988) Assessing the skeletal maturity of the hand-wrist: FELS method. Charles C Thomas, Springfield

Salardi S, Orsini LF, Cacciafi E et al (1985) Pelvic ultrasonography in premenarcheal girls: relation to puberty and sex hormone concentration. Arch Dis Child 60:819–822

Seigel MJ (2010) Female Pelvis. In: Pediatric sonography. Siegel MJ (Ed). 4th edn LWW pp 511–533

Stanhope R, Adams J, Jacobs HS et al (1985) Ovarian ultrasound assessment in normal children, idiopathic precocious puberty, and during low dose pulsatile gonadotrophin releasing hormone treatment of hypogonadotrophic hypogonadism. Arch Dis Child 60:116–119

Stavrou I, Zois C, Ioannidis JP et al (2002) Association of polymorphisms of the oestrogen receptor alpha gene with the age of menarche. Hum Reprod 17:1101–1105

Stranzinger E, Strouse PJ (2008) Ultrasound of the pediatric female pelvis. Semin Ultrasound CT MRI 29:98–113

Takeuchi M, Matsuzaki K, Nishitani H (2010) Manifestations of the female reproductive organs on MR Images: changes induced by various physiologic states. Radiographics 30:e39

Tanner JM (1975) Growth and endocrinology of the adolescent. In:Gardner LI (ed) Endocrine and genetic diseases of childhood and adolescents, 2nd edn. Philadelphia, WB Saunders, p 14

Tanner JM, Whitehouse RH, Cameron N et al (1975) Assessment of skeletal maturity and prediction of adult height (TW2 method), 2nd edn. Academic Press, London

Tanner JM, Healy MJR, Goldstein H, Cameron N (2001) Assessment of skeletal maturity and prediction of adult height (TW3 method). WB Saunders, London

Thodberg HH (2009) Clinical review: an automated method for determination of bone age. J Clin Endocrinol Metab 94: 2239–2244

Thodberg HH, Sävendahl L (2010) Validation and reference values of automated bone age determination for four ethnicities. Acad Radiol 17:1425–1432

Timor-Tritsch I (2006) Relevant Pelvic Anatomy. In: Timor-Tritsch I, Goldstein SR (eds) Ultrasound in Gynecology, 2nd edn. Churchill Livingstone, New York, pp 69–70

Umek WH, Morgan DM, Ashton-Miller JA et al (2004) Quantitative analysis of uterosacral ligament origin and insertion points by magnetic resonance imaging. Obstet Gynecol 103:447–451

Veening MA, van Weissenbruch MM, Roord JJ et al (2004) Pubertal development in children born small for gestational age. J Pediatr Endocrinol Metab 17:1497–1505

Winter JS, Faiman C, Hobson WC et al (1975) Pituitary-gonadal relations in infancy. I. Patterns of serum gonadotropin concentrations from birth to four years of age in man and chimpanzee. J Clin Endocrinol Metab 40:545–551

Winter JS, Hughes IA, Reyes FI et al (1976) Pituitary-gonadal relations in infancy: 2. Patterns of serum gonadal steroid concentrations in man from birth to two years of age. J Clin Endocrinol Metab 42:679–686

Wren TA, Liu X, Pitukcheewanont P et al (2005) Bone densitometry in pediatric populations: discrepancies in the diagnosis of osteoporosis by DXA and CT. J Pediatr 146: 776–779

Xita N, Tsatsoulis A, Stavrou I et al (2005) Association of SHBG gene polymorphism with menarche. Mol Hum Reprod 11:459–462

Ziereisen F, Heinrichs C, Dufour D et al (2001) The role of Doppler evaluation of the uterine artery in girls around puberty. Pediatr Radiol 31:712–719

Delayed and Precocious Puberty

Laurence J. Abernethy, Joanne C. Blair, Julie B. Smith, and Mohammed A. Didi

Contents

1	**Introduction**	116
2	**Clinical Assessment of the Girl with Abnormal Puberty**	117
3	**Radiological Investigations for Assessment of the Stage of Pubertal Development**	118
4	**Delayed Puberty**	119
4.1	Biochemical Investigation	119
4.2	Hypogonadotropic Hypogonadism	119
4.3	Hypergonadotropic Hypogonadism	127
5	**Precocious Puberty**	130
5.1	Classification of Precocious Puberty	130
5.2	Biochemical Investigation	132
5.3	Ultrasound Investigation of True Precocious Puberty	133
5.4	Cranial Imaging Evaluation of Central Precocious Puberty	134
5.5	Radiological Investigations for Pseudo-precocious Puberty	136
5.6	Investigation of Girls with Virilisation	140
References		141

L. J. Abernethy (✉) · J. B. Smith
Department of Radiology,
Alder Hey Children's NHS Foundation Trust,
Liverpool L12 2AP, UK
e-mail: laurence.abernethy@alderhey.nhs.uk

J. C. Blair · M. A. Didi
Department of Endocrinology,
Alder Hey Children's NHS Foundation Trust,
Liverpool L12 2AP, UK

Abstract

Delayed and precocious puberty are distressing conditions that can have serious long-term effects, and may also be the presenting manifestation of serious underlying medical conditions affecting the hypothalamic-pituitary-gonadal axis. An understanding of the various disorders of sexual development is essential for rational radiological investigation and the interpretation of its findings. True (central) precocious puberty and precocious pseudopuberty must be distinguished from the variants of precocious sexual development that may have similar early clinical features (isolated premature menarche, isolated premature thelarche and thelarche variant, and isolated premature adrenarche). Before initiating radiological investigations, full clinical assessment is essential. Radiological investigations are important in both delayed and precocious puberty to provide additional indicators of the stage of puberty. The most important radiological indicators of stage of puberty are radiographic estimation of bone age, and ultrasound of the pelvis. Ultrasound assessment of the stage of development of the uterus and ovaries is a valuable tool in the diagnosis of precocious puberty in girls and in differentiating between true precocious puberty and other types of early puberty. Serial ultrasound is also useful to assess the response to treatment. Delayed and precocious puberty may be caused by intracranial pathology which disrupts the hypothalamic-pituitary axis. True precocious puberty in girls is idiopathic or familial in over 80% of cases, but cranial MRI is necessary to exclude CNS

G. Mann et al. (eds.), *Imaging of Gynecological Disorders in Infants and Children*, Medical Radiology. Diagnostic Imaging, DOI: 10.1007/174_2011_202,

abnormalities. Hypothalamic hamartoma is the most common intracranial tumour identified in true precocious puberty. CNS lesions that may result in either delayed or precocious puberty include neurofibromatosis type 1 (usually in association with an optic pathway glioma), craniopharyngioma, and suprasellar lesions such as arachnoid cysts and epidermoid cysts.In pseudo-precocious puberty, pelvic ultrasound should be undertaken to assess the stage of development of the uterus and ovaries; the ovaries should also be carefully examined for evidence of an autonomously functioning ovarian cyst or tumour that secretes oestrogen (granulosa-theca cell tumours are the most common). A comprehensive ultrasound examination of the whole of the abdomen should also be undertaken, with particular attention to the adrenals for evidence of an adrenal tumour or diffuse bilateral hypertrophy.

Abbreviations

GnRH	Gonadotropin-Releasing Hormone
TSH	Thyroid-stimulating hormone
MAS	McCune-Albright syndrome
MFO	Multifollicular ovary
TBI	Traumatic brain-injury
DI	Diabetes insipidus
ACTH	Adrenocorticotropic Hormone
GH	Growth hormone
SOD	Septo-optic dysplasia
cAMP	Cyclic adenosine monophosphate
STK11	Serine/threonine kinase 11
JGCT	Juvenile granulosa cell tumour
FIGO	The International Federation of Gynecology and Obstetrics
VWGS	Van Wyk-Grumbach syndrome
Gsα	Guanine-nucleotide-binding protein α-subunit
PJS	Peutz-Jeghers syndrome
SLCT	Sertoli-Leydig cell tumour
PCO	Polycystic ovary morphology
KAL1	Anosmin-1
FGFR1	Basic fibroblast growth factor receptor 1
PROK2	Prokineticin-2
PROKR2	Prokineticin-2 receptor
CHD7	Chromodomainhelicase-DNA-binding protein 7
FGF8	Fibroblast Growth Factor 8
CHARGE	Colobomata, Heart defect, choanal Atresia, Retarded growth and development, Genital hypoplasia and Ear abnormalities and/or deafness
LCH	Langerhans cell histiocytosis
IV	Intravenous
CNS	Central nervous system
CAH	Congenital Adrenal Hyperplasia
ACT	Adrenocortical tumours
OPG	Optic pathway glioma
DHEAS	Dehydroepiandrosterone sulphate
17 OHP	17-hydroxyprogesterone
MR	Magnetic Resonance
NF-1	Neurofibromatosis type 1
BMI	Body mass-index
CT	Computed Tomography
MRI	Magnetic Resonance Imaging
CSF	Cerebrospinal fluid
LH	Luteinising hormone
FSH	Follicle stimulating hormone
POU1F1	POU class 1 homeobox 1
PROP1	PROP paired-like homeobox 1
HESX1	HESX homeobox 1
LHX3	LIM homeobox 3 LHX3
LHX4	LIM homeobox 4 LHX4
SOX2	SRY (sex determining region Y)-box 2 sox-2
SOX3	SRY (sex determining region Y)-box 3
TBX19	T-box 19

1 Introduction

Puberty is the process in which the body undergoes the complex transition from childhood to maturity, and is a time of profound physical and emotional change. Delayed or precocious puberty is distressing and can have serious long-term effects. It may also be the presenting manifestation of serious underlying medical conditions affecting the hypothalamic-pituitary-gonadal axis.

Most girls enter puberty between the ages of 8 and 13 years. Normal puberty occurs when pulsatile secretion of gonadotropin releasing hormone (GnRH) by the hypothalamus results in release of gonadotropins, follicle stimulating hormone (FSH) and luteinising hormone (LH), from the anterior lobe of the pituitary. In early puberty, pulsatile GnRH secretion mainly occurs during sleep; an adult pattern of pulsatile secretion of GnRH throughout the day develops subsequently. Rising gonadotropin levels stimulate oestrogen production by the ovaries, causing secondary sexual development. Androgen production by the adrenals and ovaries stimulates the growth of axillary and pubic hair. The normal sequence of events is breast development, (thelarche), followed by the appearance of pubic and axillary hair (adrenarche) then a growth spurt and finally menstruation (menarche). These physical changes take place in a predictable sequence, but the time taken for any given individual to progress through these stages may vary between 18 months and 5 years. Normal puberty is described in detail in chapter entitled "Normal Growth and Puberty".

In normal girls, all of the functional and anatomical components necessary for sexual development are present, but there is a central restraining mechanism which prevents release of GnRH before the age of 8 years. Diseases which interfere with this central restraining mechanism result in true (central) precocious puberty.

An understanding of the precise clinical definition of the various disorders of sexual development is essential for rational radiological investigation and the interpretation of its findings. Gonadotropin-dependent or 'true' precocious puberty results from premature but normal activation of the hypothalamic-pituitary-gonadal axis. Gonadotropin-independent or pseudo-precocious puberty results from autonomous sex steroid production or exposure to exogenous sex steroids. Other variants of precocious sexual development include isolated premature menarche, isolated premature thelarche and thelarche variant and isolated premature adrenarche.

Puberty is considered to be delayed in the absence of secondary sexual characteristics in girls aged 13 years and above.

2 Clinical Assessment of the Girl with Abnormal Puberty

Before initiating radiological investigations, full clinical assessment is essential. Clinical assessment of girls with delayed or precocious puberty should begin with a detailed clinical history.

A systematic history should be completed in girls presenting with delayed puberty as this may be the presenting feature of undiagnosed chronic disease, most commonly Crohn's disease or coeliac disease. Note should be made of exposure to alkylating agents and treatment with pelvic radiotherapy as both therapies may result in ovarian damage. Cranial irradiation may result in loss of pituitary function. Patients with under or over activity of the thyroid can present with either delayed or precocious puberty.

In girls with precocious puberty the history should elicit whether or not puberty is consonant i.e., whether development follows for the normal sequence of breast growth, followed by pubic and axillary hair growth and finally menarche as loss of consonance suggests a diagnosis of gonadotropin-independent puberty. In all patients the history should pay particular attention to features of central nervous system pathology including perinatal problems (periventricular haemorrhage, hydrocephalus), neurological deficit (cerebral palsy) and any symptoms to suggest an intracranial tumour (headaches, vomiting or visual disturbance).

Examination should start with accurate measurement of the patient's height and weight. The height centile or standard deviation score of a girl with delayed puberty will be below the target height centile or standard deviation score, calculated from the formula:

$$\text{Target height} = \frac{\text{mother's height} + (\text{father's height} - 13\ \text{cm})}{2}$$

In general, a child who has entered the period of rapid pubertal growth due to premature exposure to sex steroids will have a height centile or standard deviation score that rests above the target height. There are two important exceptions to this observation: (1) girls with precocious puberty due to hypothyroidism in whom thyroid insufficiency inhibits growth and (2) girls presenting with precocious pubic and axillary hair growth and acne due to Cushing's syndrome in whom excess cortisol inhibits growth hormone secretion and action.

The patient's nutritional status is assessed most simply from body mass index (BMI). Puberty is often delayed in competitive athletes with low BMI, but this can also be the presentation of anorexia nervosa or chronic inflammatory disease. Obese patients with delayed puberty are more likely to have a structural lesion of the central nervous system, an abnormality of ovarian function or an anatomical abnormality of the female reproductive tract. Hypothyroidism should also be considered in girls who are short, overweight and delayed in their pubertal development.

Examination should proceed with assessment of the stage of the puberty according to the Tanner standards (also see chapter "Normal Growth and Puberty"). Careful inspection for dysmorphic features is important as a number of genetic syndromes are associated with abnormally early or late puberty, for example William's syndrome in which puberty occurs early, and Turners and Noonan syndrome in which puberty is delayed. Examination of the skin may reveal café au lait patches which are typically large, irregular and rarely cross the midline in McCune Albright Syndrome or may be accompanied by axillary and inguinal freckling and cutaneous neurofibromas in neurofibromatosis type 1.

Girls presenting with pubic and axillary hair growth as the first feature of puberty should be examined for cliteromegaly. Most girls with isolated pubic and axillary hair growth have exaggerated adrenarche, a variant of puberty which is discussed more detail in chapter "Normal Growth and Puberty", however the presence of cliteromegaly excludes this diagnosis and a source of pathological androgen secretion should be identified (Street et al. 1997). Examination is completed by examination of the chest and abdomen and fundoscopy for features of chronic disease that may influence the timing and tempo of puberty.

3 Radiological Investigations for Assessment of the Stage of Pubertal Development

Radiological investigations are important in both delayed and precocious puberty to provide additional indicators of the stage of puberty. The most important radiological indicators of stage of puberty are radiographic estimation of bone age and ultrasound of the pelvis. MRI appearances of the pituitary and breast ultrasound, may occasionally give further useful information.

Radiographic estimation of bone age involves taking an X-ray of the non-dominant hand and wrist to determine skeletal age compared to chronological age. A difference of more than two standard deviations above or below the mean is suggestive of early or delayed puberty, respectively. Different methods are used, including those of (Tanner et al. 1983; Greulich and Pyle 1959) and the FELS method (Roche et al. 1988). Serial estimation of bone age is often helpful in monitoring progress and the response to treatment.

Ultrasound assessment of the stage of development of the uterus and ovaries is a valuable tool in the diagnosis of precocious puberty in girls and in differentiating between true precocious puberty and other types of early puberty. Serial ultrasound is also useful to assess the response to treatment. Knowledge of the normal developmental ultrasound appearances and access to age-specific normal values for uterine length and ovarian volumes are essential (see chapter "Normal Growth and Puberty"). Ovarian volume and morphology and uterine length are key indicators of maturation and should be compared to age-specific normal values (Griffin et al. 1995). The presence of a definite endometrial echo is an important marker of pubertal development, and if present its thickness should be measured.

Breast ultrasound is occasionally helpful to distinguish developing breast tissue from adipose tissue in obese girls, and to exclude other pathology in unilateral or asymmetrical breast enlargement.

MRI shows changes in the size and appearances of the anterior lobe of the pituitary in pre-pubertal and pubertal children. The height of the anterior lobe of the pituitary increases with age (Argyropolou et al. 1991). The upper surface of the anterior lobe of the pituitary is normally flat throughout childhood (Fig. 1a), but around the time of puberty it becomes convex (Fig. 1b). After puberty it regains a flat configuration. This physiological change in the shape of the anterior pituitary gland can be identified in central precocious puberty, whether idiopathic or secondary to intracranial pathology, and in pregnancy and conditions such as untreated hypothyroidism, and should not be mistaken for a pituitary adenoma.

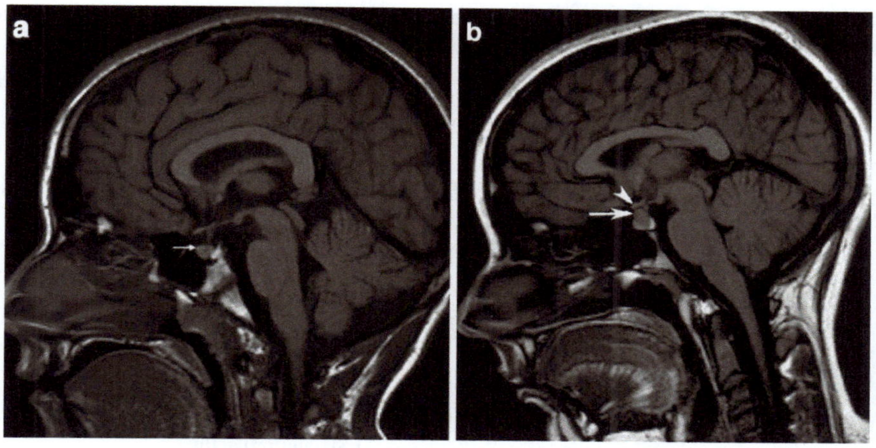

Fig. 1 **a, b** Normal pituitary anatomy. Sagittal T1-weighted unenhanced MR images of the pituitary fossa. **a** The upper surface of the anterior lobe of the pituitary is normally flat (*arrow*) throughout childhood and following completion of puberty. **b** Around the time of puberty the upper border becomes convex and the craniocaudal height of the anterior pituitary may increase due to physiological hypertrophy (*arrow*), the optic chiasm is indicated by the *arrowhead*

4 Delayed Puberty

Puberty is generally considered to be delayed, and should be investigated, in girls who have developed no secondary sexual characteristics by the age of 13 years. However, racial and geographic differences also need to be taken into account (see chapter "Normal Growth and Puberty"). Delayed puberty is often idiopathic or constitutional, and is probably due to genetic factors. Causes of delayed puberty are given in Table 1.

4.1 Biochemical Investigation

Biochemical investigation of delayed puberty should: (1) exclude underlying chronic disease and (2) assess the integrity of the hypothalamic-pituitary-ovarian axis. Patients in whom the gonadotropin levels are low and respond poorly to GnRH stimulation (hypogonadotropic hypogonadism) should undergo CNS imaging, while those in whom gonadotropin levels are high (hypergonadotropic hypogonadism) should be investigated for causes of premature ovarian failure, including consideration of Turner syndrome, gonadal dysgenesis, defects of androgen biosynthesis and mutations of the LH receptor.

4.2 Hypogonadotropic Hypogonadism

4.2.1 Imaging of the Brain

Both precocious and delayed puberty may be caused by any intracranial pathology which disrupts the hypothalamic-pituitary axis (Table 1). Constitutional delay of puberty is much less common in girls than in boys. Where it does occur, a family history is often elicited. Delayed puberty is also associated

Table 1 Causes of delayed puberty

Idiopathic (Constitutional)
Hypogonadotropic hypogonadism
• Chronic systemic disorders (e.g., inflammatory bowel disease and cystic fibrosis)
• Anorexia nervosa
• Intense athletic training
• Idiopathic hypopituitarism
• Pituitary agenesis
• Pituitary stalk interruption syndrome (PSIS)
• Developmental midline brain abnormalities
– Septo-optic dysplasia
– Holoprosencephaly
– Kallman syndrome
• Tumours
– Craniopharyngioma
– Optic and hypothalamic glioma
– Langerhans cell histiocytosis
Hypergonadotropic hypogonadism
• Gonadal dysgenesis
– Turner syndrome
– XX gonadal dysgenesis
• Pelvic radiotherapy
• Chemotherapy
• Surgical oophorectomy
• Bilateral ovarian torsion
• Auto-immune oophoritis

Table 2 Radiological, endocrine and phenotypic features of patients with mutations of genes encoding transcription factors important in the regulation of pituitary development

Gene	Radiological characteristics	Endocrinopathy	Associated anomalies
POU1F1	Small or normal anterior pituitary	GH, TSH and prolactin deficiencies	
PROP1	Small, normal or enlarged anterior pituitary	GH, TSH, LH, FSH, prolactin and ACTH deficiencies	
HESX1	Anterior pituitary hypoplasia, absent infundibulum, ectopic posterior pituitary, agenesis of corpus callosum	Isolated growth hormone deficiency and combined pituitary hormone deficiencies	Septo-optic dysplasia
LHX3	Small, normal or enlarged anterior pituitary	Growth hormone, TSH, LH, FSH and prolactin deficiencies	Short cervical spine, limited rotation
LHX4	Small anterior pituitary	Growth hormone, TSH, LH, FSH and prolactin deficiencies	
SOX3	Anterior pituitary hypoplasia, infundibular hypoplasia, ectopic posterior pituitary	Panhypopituitarism and isolated growth hormone deficiency	Mental retardation
SOX2	Anterior pituitary hypoplasia	LH and FSH deficiencies	Bilateral anopthalmia/micropthalmia, learning difficulties, oesophageal atresia, sensorineural hearing loss
TBX19		Neonatal ACTH deficiency	

Kelberman and Dattani (2007)

with congenital midline malformations of the brain, such as septo-optic dysplasia and holoprosencephaly by virtue of the hypopituitarism that may be associated with these conditions. An MRI brain scan is therefore indicated in any child in whom biochemical investigations reveal abnormally low levels of gonadotropins.

4.2.1.1 Congenital Abnormalities of the Hypothalamic Pituitary Structures

Pituitary Hypoplasia and Pituitary Stalk Interruption Syndrome

Morphological changes in the appearance of the pituitary and hypothalamus are associated with isolated growth hormone deficiency and combined anterior pituitary hormone deficiencies. The aetiology of these developmental abnormalities is uncertain. Perinatal insults such as breech presentation and neonatal hypoxia have been reported to occur with increased frequency in affected patients (Fujisawa et al. 1987; Kikuchi et al. 1988) leading to speculation that traumatic ischaemic injury to the pituitary stalk or median eminence results in hypopituitarism. However, it has also been suggested that this relationship reflects an increased susceptibility to perinatal abnormalities in infants with abnormalities of the pituitary. The recognition of familial cases and associated congenital abnormalities lent support to the hypothesis that developmental abnormalities of the pituitary gland occurred in the prenatal period.

Pituitary development occurs at a very early stage of embryogenesis. Normal development is dependent on the complex interplay between multiple transcription factors and signalling molecules that regulate cell proliferation and differentiation. In recent years there has been an explosion in our understanding of the regulation of pituitary development, and from this the recognition of genetic abnormalities result in developmental abnormalities of the pituitary. These are summarised in Table 2.

Patients who are found to have isolated growth hormone deficiency in early childhood may acquire deficiencies of other anterior pituitary hormones over time. This may present in adolescent years as delayed puberty as a consequence of hypogonadal hypogonadism or hypothyroidism due to TSH deficiency. In some of these patients, MRI shows evidence of

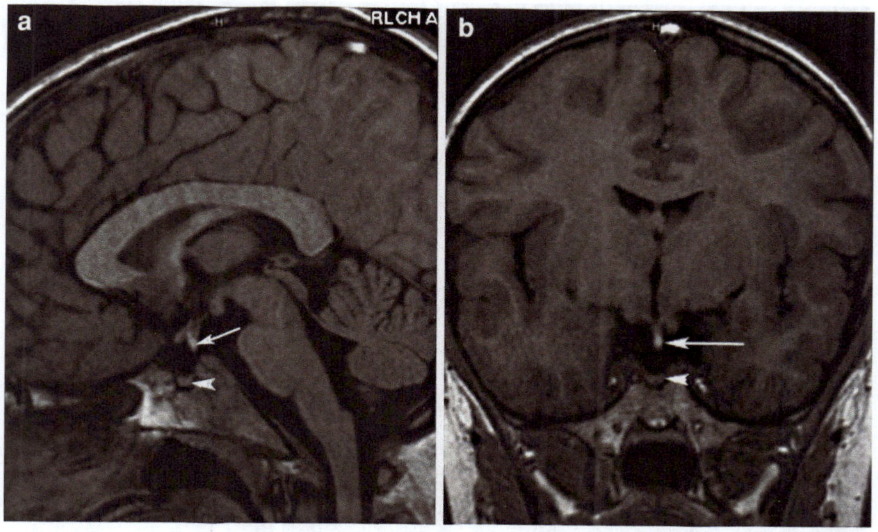

Fig. 2 **a**, **b** Pituitary stalk interruption syndrome. **a** Sagittal and **b** coronal T1-weighted MR images. The anterior pituitary is normally located, but of small size (*arrowhead*). The normal high signal of the posterior pituitary (bright spot) is absent from the pituitary fossa. The pituitary stalk is truncated and there is a nodule of high signal intensity (the ectopic posterior pituitary) just below the hypothalamus (*arrow*). (Reproduced with permission from Abernethy (1998)—Elsevier Publishers Ltd)

pituitary stalk interruption syndrome, manifest as an ectopic location of the normal high signal of the posterior pituitary gland and absence of a normal pituitary infundibulum (Fig. 2). Others show a hypoplastic anterior pituitary with a normally located posterior pituitary (Garel and Leger 2007).

Agenesis of the pituitary is part of the hydranencephaly facial cleft syndrome. The pituitary may also be ectopic in cases of complex craniofacial anomalies, particularly when associated with a large, persistent craniofacial canal; this is a midline, vertical defect within the basisphenoid, involving the floor of the sella turcica. In such cases, the pituitary may be located in the roof of the pharynx; if this is not recognised, the ectopic pituitary may be surgically excised in mistake for a mucosal lesion.

Septo-Optic Dysplasia

Septo-optic dysplasia (SOD), or DeMorsier syndrome is a rare condition with a highly heterogeneous phenotype. It is a developmental abnormality related to holoprosencephaly. There is an association with schizencephaly. Affected infants present with visual impairment and pituitary deficiency. The diagnosis is made in patients with two or more of the following developmental abnormalities: (1) optic nerve hypoplasia (2) midline radiological abnormalities and (3) pituitary insufficiency. The aetiology of the condition is probably multifactorial in most patients. Cases are reported to cluster in inner city areas with high rates of teenage pregnancy and unemployment (Patel et al. 2006). A link between SOD and young maternal age has been reported by some authors (Arslanian et al. 1984) and a preponderance of primigravida mothers has been reported by others (Izenberg et al. 1984). A minority of cases are familial and both autosomal recessive and dominant modes of inheritance are reported.

Mutations of the HESX1 gene have been reported in patients with familial and sporadic SOD. HESX1 is a transcription factor that is expressed early in pituitary development. Affected patients generally have anterior pituitary hypoplasia or aplasia and the posterior pituitary bright spot is often ectopic or absent. Growth hormone deficiency occurs most commonly, although deficiency of all pituitary hormones has been reported (Kelberman and Dattani 2007). The prevalence of HESX1 gene mutations in patients with SOD is low, occurring in fewer than 1% of a large cohort of over 800 patients (McNay et al. 2007).

CT or MRI show that the interventricular septum is absent, and the frontal horns of the lateral ventricles are dilated and square in configuration (Fig. 3). The optic nerves and chiasm are typically small, but may appear normal. The hypothalamus and pituitary are hypoplastic.

Kallmann Syndrome

Kallmann Syndrome (Maestre de San Juan-Kallmann syndrome/Morsier-Gauthier Syndrome) is a rare heterogeneous disorder defined by the association of an impaired sense of smell and hypogonadotropic hypogonadism. Kallmann syndrome occurs most commonly

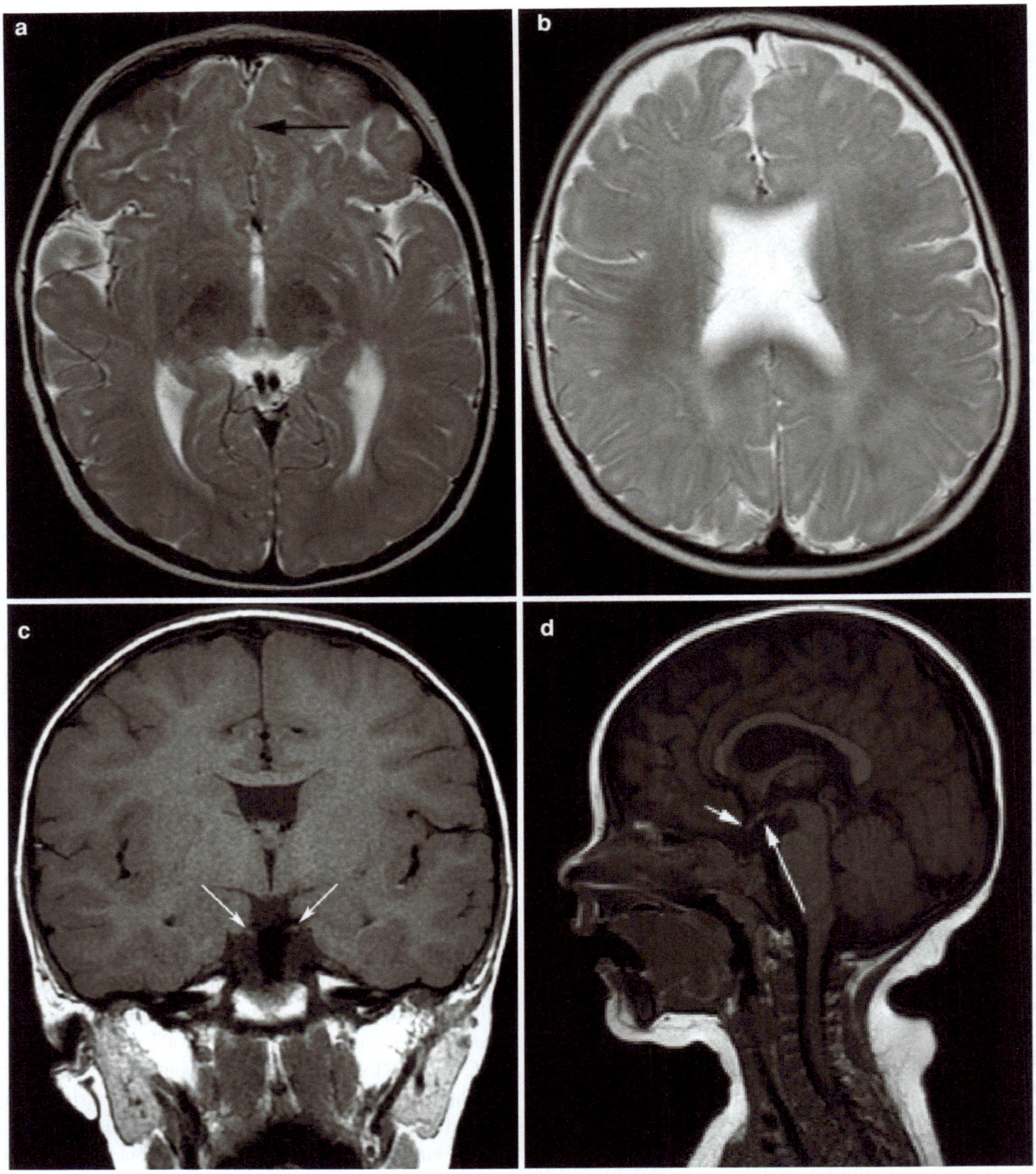

Fig. 3 **a–d** Septo-optic dysplasia. **a**, **b** Axial T2-weighted imaging, **a** showing a deficient anterior falx (*black arrow*) and **b** absence of the leaflets of the septum pellucidum **c** Coronal T1-weighted image, **c** the retrobulbar optic nerves are hypoplastic (*arrows*). **d** Sagittal T1-weighted image showing a small optic chiasm (*short arrow*), absence of the pituitary stalk and anterior pituitary (*arrow*), with an ectopic posterior pituitary (*long arrow*)

Table 3 Clinical subtypes of Kallmann's syndrome (Ks)

KS Subtype	Mode of inheritance	Gene symbol	Protein	Chromosomal locus	Non-endocrine phenotypes
1	XR	KAL1	Anosmin-1	8p11.2–p11.1	Short stature chondrodysplasia punctata mental retardation, steroid sulfatase deficiency synkinesia renal agenesis (male) sensorineural hearing loss high-arched palate
2	AD	FGFR1	Basic fibroblast growth factor receptor 1	Xp22.3	Cleft lip and/or palate dental agenesis synkinesia brachydactyly syndactyly agenesis of corpus callosum
3	AD/AR	PROK2	Prokineticin-2	3p21.1	Pectus excavatum
4	AD/AR	PROKR2	Prokineticin-2 receptor	20p13	seizures synkinesia high-arched palate pes planus sensorineural hearing loss
5	AD	CHD7	Chromodomain-helicase-DNA-binding protein 7	8q12	CHARGE syndrome cleft lip and/or palate idiopathic scoliosis dental agenesis auricular dysplasia sensorineural deafness semicircular canal aplasia short stature
6	AD	FGF8	Fibroblast growth factor 8	10 q24	Cleft lip and/or palate Hearing loss hypertelorism camplodactyly

XR X-linked recessive *AD* Autosomal dominant *AR* Autosomal recessive
Adapted from Pallais et al. (2010)

in boys and the male to female ratio ranges from 4:1 to 5:1. Approximately 1 in 50,000 females are affected.

Kallmann syndrome results from the disordered migration of gonadotropin-releasing hormone (GnRH) neurons in the developing forebrain from the olfactory area to arcuate nucleus of the hypothalamus, resulting in varying degrees of FSH and LH deficiency. The development of the olfactory placode, the precursor of the olfactory bulbs is also abnormal.

The diagnosis of Kallmann syndrome in prepubertal children can be difficult to ascertain. Clinical genetics and diagnostic imaging play an important role in confirming the diagnosis. Most cases of Kallmann syndrome are sporadic but in around one quarter of cases a specific pattern of inheritance can be demonstrated including X-linked, autosomal recessive and autosomal dominant transmissions. Mutations of several distinct genes (KAL-1, FGFR1, PROKR2 and PROK2) which encode proteins responsible for mediating neuronal migration of olfactory cells from the olfactory placode and GnRH-producing neurons have been defined. Six distinct clinical subtypes of Kallmann syndrome are recognised (Table 3).

The principle clinical features of Kallmann syndrome are:

- Primary amenorrhea in girls with normal karyotype.
- Delayed or incomplete puberty—in adolescent females little or no breast development is seen. Normal onset of pubic hair growth is present under the influence of adrenal androgens (Tanner stages 2–3).

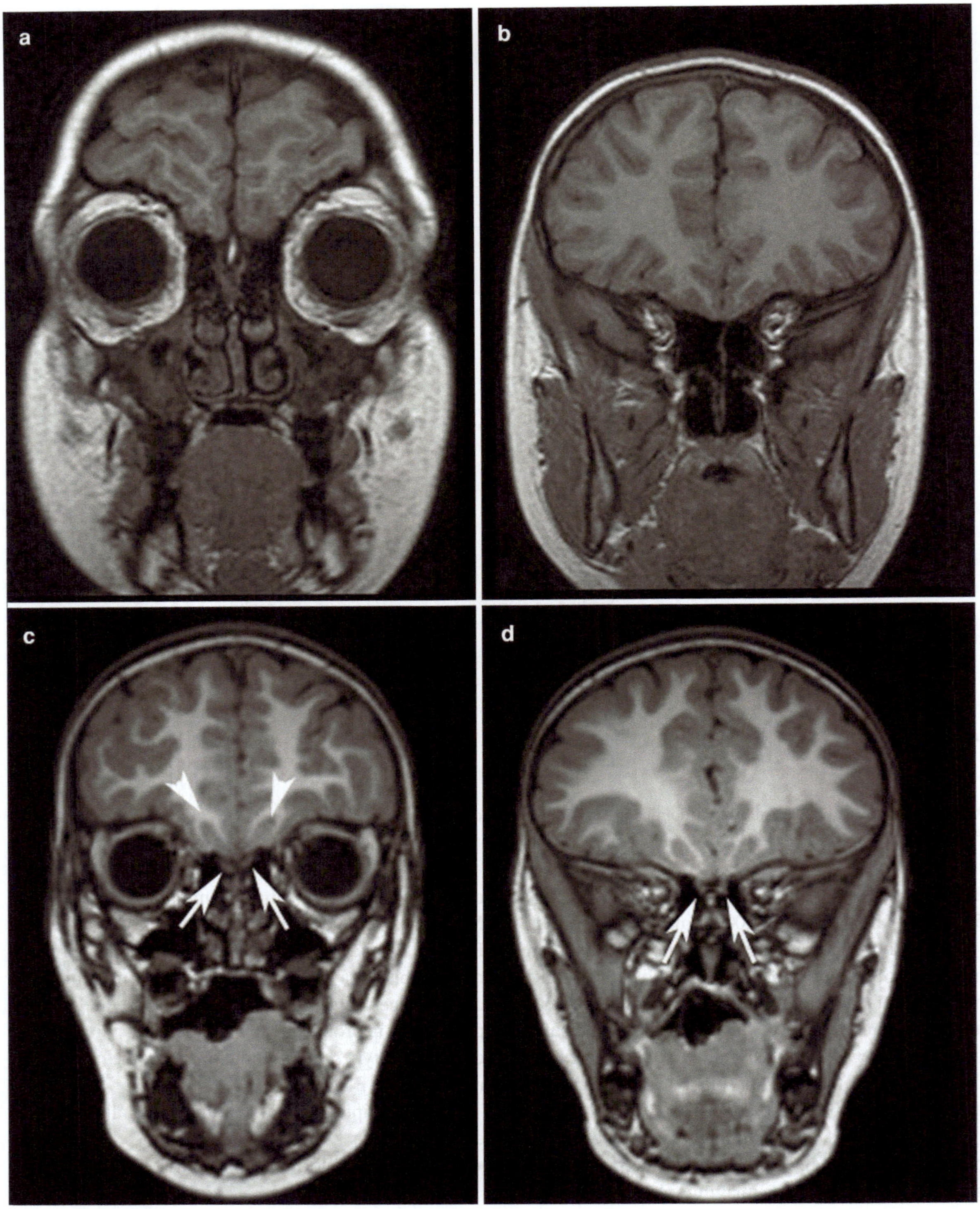

Fig. 4 Kallman syndrome. **a–b** Coronal T1-weighted MR images of an anosmic 14 year old with bilateral absence of the olfactory bulbs, and shallow/absent interrupted olfactory sulci. **c–d** comparison imaging from a normal patient with intact olfactory gyri (arrow heads) and olfactory bulbs(arrows)

- An impaired sense of smell—impairment may range from a reduced sense of smell (hyposmia) to complete absence (anosmia). The patient may be unaware of the impairment until formal clinical testing of olfaction is undertaken.

Body proportions are eunuchoidal. Skeletal maturation may be delayed; however the linear rate of growth is typically normal. The pubertal growth spurt is usually absent. Other specific associations of Kallmann syndrome are summarised in Table 3.

Deficient hypothalamic GnRH secretion underlies a markedly abnormal pattern of gonadotropin secretion. Diagnosis is established when the levels of gonadotropin and gonadal steroids remain in the pre-pubertal range in the absence of other anterior pituitary hormone deficiencies. The gonadotropin response to the standard GnRH stimulation test is markedly blunted.

The main role of imaging is to exclude pituitary or hypothalamic causes of hypogonadotropic hypogonadism and to identify structural abnormalities of the olfactory apparatus. The appearance of the pituitary gland and hypothalamus is normal in Kallmann syndrome. MRI is the investigation of choice. Dedicated imaging of the olfactory tracts is indicated. High resolution coronal T2-weighed fast spin echo and T1-W volumetric magnetic resonance imaging is best suited to evaluate olfactory tracts. Recognised imaging findings include anomalous, hypoplastic or aplastic olfactory sulci and hypoplastic or aplastic olfactory bulbs (Suzuki et al. 1989; Truwit et al.1993) (Fig. 4). Evaluation should take into consideration the normal maturation and age-related variation of the olfactory apparatus (Schneider and Floemer 2009).

4.2.1.2 Acquired Abnormalities of the Hypothalamus and Pituitary

Craniopharyngioma

Craniopharyngioma is a relatively uncommon, but important tumour in childhood, accounting for up to 10% of all intracranial neoplasms and 80% of tumours affecting the hypothalamic-pituitary region (Kaatsch et al. 2001; May et al. 2006). Presentation is commonly with headaches, visual disturbance, vomiting and growth arrest. Symptoms of raised intracranial pressure occur if the lesion encroaches on the foramen of Monro causing hydrocephalus.

There is evidence of pituitary dysfunction in more than 70% of patients at diagnosis (Sklar 1994; de Vries et al. 2003a; Devile et al. 1996). Growth hormone deficiency occurs most commonly and gonadotropin deficiency is reported in 40–50% of patients at presentation (Sklar 1994; Devile et al. 1996). Adolescent patients typically present with delayed puberty (de Vries et al. 2003a) although precocious puberty has also been described (de Vries et al. 2003b).

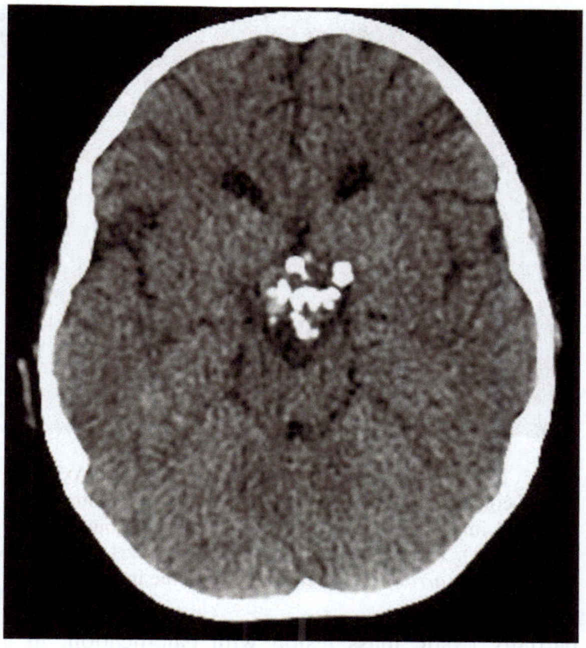

Fig. 5 Craniopharyngioma. Axial non-contrast CT showing a calcified suprasellar tumour mass

Craniopharyngiomas arise from remnants of squamous epithelium of the craniopharyngeal duct, and usually occur between the sella turcica and the floor of the third ventricle, although some are situated within the pituitary fossa, or rarely in ectopic locations such as within the sphenoid bone. The lesion is characteristically partly cystic; the cystic elements contain a fluid rich in cholesterol.

Craniopharyngiomas in childhood typically contain calcification, which is visible on skull X-rays in 85% of cases. CT shows calcification in almost all childhood cases (Fig. 5). The cystic elements are variable in their CT attenuation, depending on their content of cholesterol and protein. The degree of enhancement with intravenous contrast is also variable. However, the typical (and almost conclusively diagnostic) CT appearance is of an enhancing,

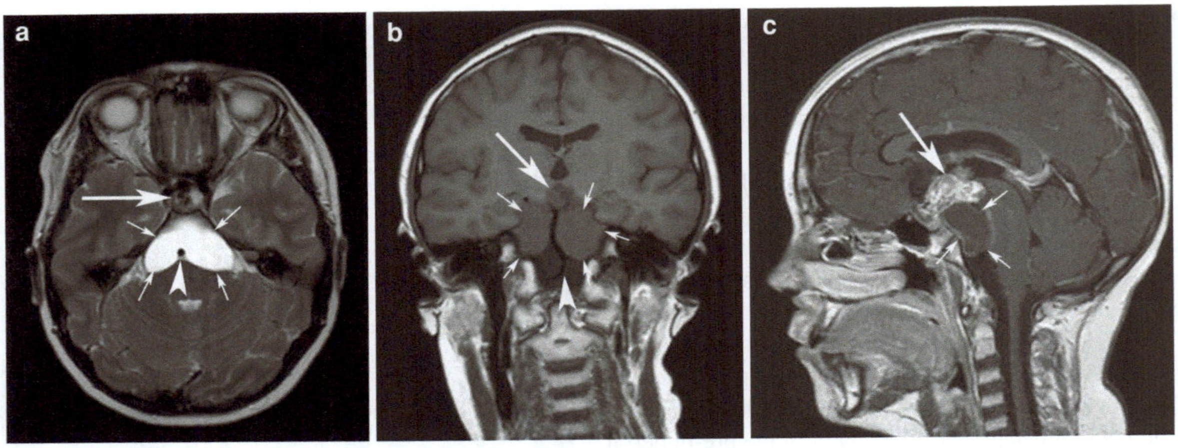

Fig. 6 **a–c** Retrochiasmatic craniopharyngioma. **a** Axial T2 **b** non-contrast coronal T1 and **c** sagittal postcontrast T1-weighted images of an enhancing craniopharyngioma tumour (*long arrow*). The cystic component (*short arrows*) encases the basilar artery (*arrowhead*) and extends into the interpeduncular cistern. The cyst isointense to CSF on T2-weighted imaging but of slightly increased signal on T1-W imaging. Cyst protein, cholesterol crystal and methaemoglobin content may cause high signal on T1-weighted images

partially cystic mass lesion with calcification, in a suprasellar position. Tumours in which there is hypothalamic involvement, retrochiasmatic extension or that exceed 4 cm in height in the midline are associated with a poor prognosis.

The appearances of craniopharyngiomas on MRI are variable. Routine spin-echo sequences may fail to demonstrate calcification. On T1 weighted images, signal characteristics are very variable, although the fluid content of the cystic components may show high signal due to the presence of cholesterol crystals. Sagittal and coronal images are valuable for demonstrating extension of the tumour inferiorly into the pituitary fossa, superiorly into the suprasellar cistern and third ventricle and laterally in relation to the cavernous sinuses and carotid arteries (Fig. 6). Volumetric MRI is an important adjunct to stereotactic tumour biopsy.

Post-traumatic hypopituitarism

Post–traumatic hypopituitarism has been studied extensively in adult patients, however data reporting the prevalence and natural history of the disease in childhood and adolescence are sparse. Three retrospective studies have been published to date and together they suggest that growth hormone deficiency occurs most commonly followed by gonadotropin, TSH and ACTH deficiency, respectively (Niederland et al. 2007; Einaudi et al. 2006; Poomthavorn et al. 2008). Precocious puberty has also been reported (Einaudi et al. 2006; Poomthavorn et al. 2008).

In a study of 22 subjects who had sustained a TBI of 0.7–7.25 years prior to endocrine assessment, one subject had precocious puberty, one had GHD, one hypogonadism and one patient was deficient for all anterior pituitary hormones (Einaudi et al. 2006).

Langerhans cell histiocytosis

Langerhans cell histiocytosis (LCH), a condition previously known as 'Letterer-Siwe' disease, Hand-Schüller-Christian disease, histiocytosis X and eosinophilic granuloma, is characterised by tissue destruction in areas of clonal proliferation of abnormal dendritic cells accompanied by an infiltrate of lymphocytes, neutrophils and eosinophils. The classical clinical description refers to the triad of diabetes insipidus, skull lesions, and exophthalmos. The hypothalamo-pituitary region is affected in isolation or as part of disseminated disease with multiple bone and soft tissue lesions in 15–50% of patients (Bernstrand et al. 2005; Amato et al. 2006; Nanduri et al. 2000). Diabetes insipidus (DI) is the most common manifestation of pituitary involvement; however anterior pituitary function can also be affected. In a study of 144 patients with multisystem LCH, 50 patients had an endocrinopathy of whom 49 had DI, 21 had growth hormone insufficiency, seven had gonadotropin deficiency, five had TSH deficiency and one patient had ACTH deficiency. Precocious puberty was reported in one male patient (Nanduri et al. 2000).

CT and MRI show thickening of the pituitary stalk in 75% of patients at diagnosis of DI, however this persists

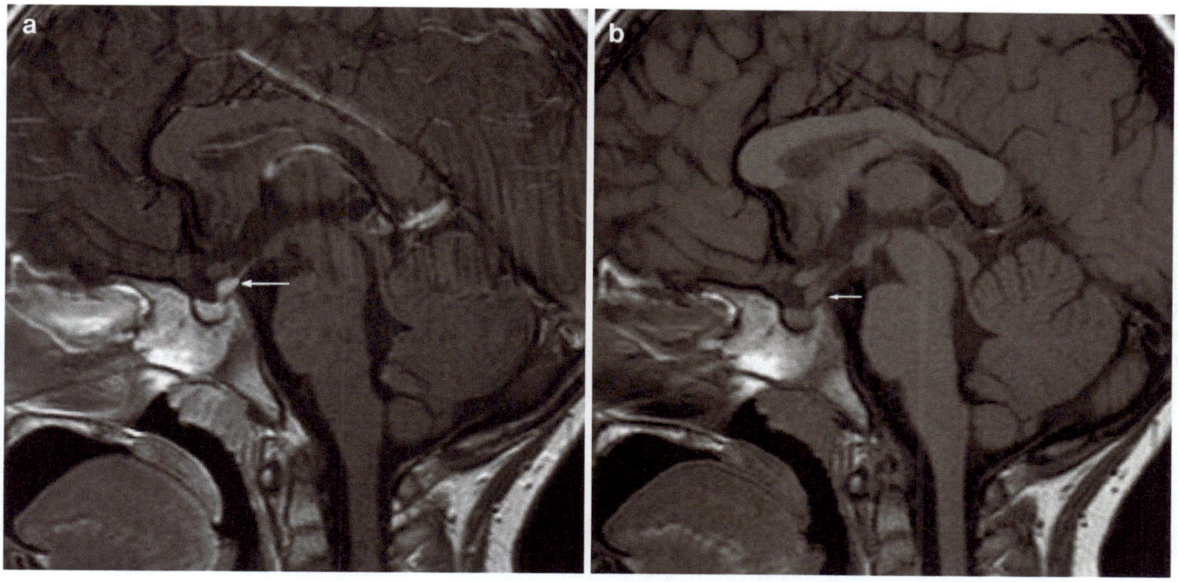

Fig. 7 a, b Langerhans cell Histiocytosis. Sagittal T1-weighted images of the pituitary fossa **a** showing diffuse thickening of the pituitary stalk, **b** which shows uniform enhancement following IV contrast

in only 25% of patients after 5 years (Grois et al. 2004). MRI shows absence of the usual high signal in the posterior pituitary, but as noted above, this is nonspecific and may be observed in DI of any cause (Fig. 7). Both techniques may show adjacent bone lesions in the base of the skull. A radiographic skeletal survey should form part of the workup (Fig. 8). Occasionally there is focal disease elsewhere in the brain.

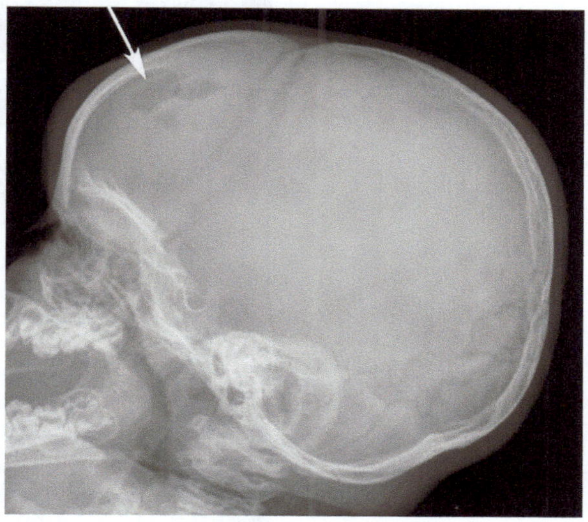

Fig. 8 Langerhans cell Histiocytosis. Lateral skull X-ray obtained as part of a radiographic skeletal survey depicting lytic bone lesions in the frontal region

4.3 Hypergonadotropic Hypogonadism

The differential diagnosis of delayed puberty in girls with elevated gonadotropins includes (1) primary ovarian failure, (2) gonadal dysgenesis, (3) defects in androgen biosynthesis and (4) defects of the LH receptor. The majority of girls who present in this manner have primary ovarian failure as part of the phenotype of Turner syndrome. A small minority of patients will be found to have a female phenotype, delayed puberty and elevated gonadotropins in which the karyotype is 46XY. This scenario arises in patients with gonadal dysgenesis, biosynthetic defects of androgen synthesis and abnormalities of the LH receptor. A pelvic ultrasound can be helpful in directing investigation as the girl with Turner syndrome or complete gonadal dysgenesis is likely to have a small, immature uterus, whereas the uterus will be absent in the girl with an androgen biosynthetic defect due to the normal testicular secretion of anti-Müllerian hormone. However, it is important to note that the uterus can be difficult to visualise in the prepubertal girl. Imaging with a full urinary bladder and use of tissue harmonic imaging and/or high-resolution ultrasound is helpful in difficult cases.

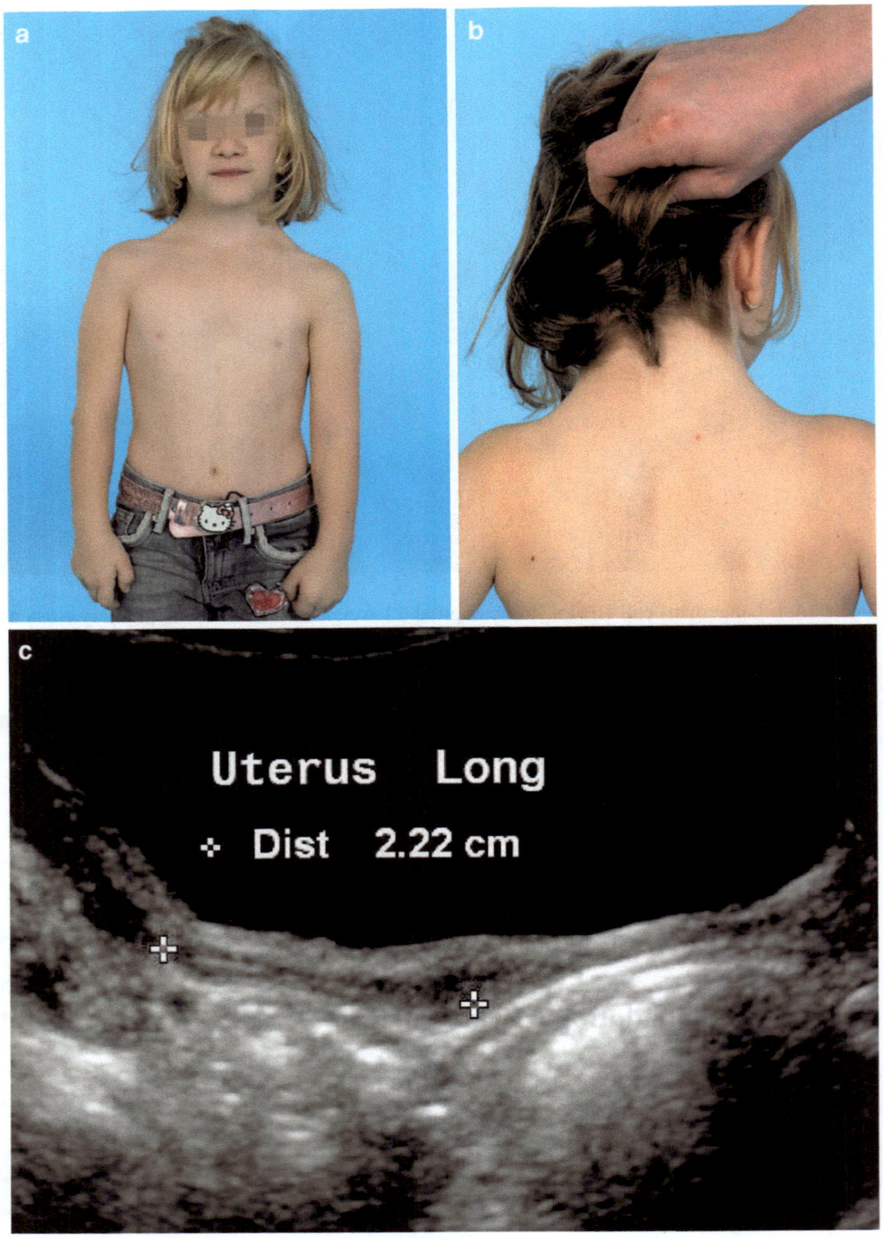

Fig. 9 **a–c** Clinical and sonographic features of Turner's syndrome. **a–b** Frontal and Posterior view showing the characteristic webbed neck and shield-shaped (*broad chest with widely spaced nipples*) of Turner syndrome. **c** Longitudinal sonogram showing an immature 'tubular' uterus, the ovaries were not identified on ultrasound

4.3.1 Turner Syndrome

Turner syndrome (Ullrich-Turner syndrome) occurs in females with an absent or structurally abnormal second X chromosome. Approximately 1 in 2,500 live born females are affected and the presentation is varied. The diagnosis should be suspected in girls with unexplained short stature, pubertal delay or amenorrhoea in the presence of a spectrum of characteristic clinical features. These include short stature with impaired growth velocity, high-arched palate, shield chest, cubitus valgus, nail hypoplasia, congenital lymphoedema of the neck, hands and feet and distinct facial features with a small mandible, low hairline and low-set ears (Fig. 9a, b). It is important to note that many patients show none or only very subtle dysmorphic features and the diagnosis should not be

Table 4 Spectrum of clinical features found in Turner syndrome

Gynaecological	Ovarian dysgenesis (streak ovary) Premature ovarian failure Gonadoblastoma
Endocrine	Absent pubertal development Amenorrhoea Hypothyroidism Impaired glucose tolerance Type 2 diabetes mellitus Dsylipidaemia
Cardiovascular	Bicuspid aortic valve Aortic coarctation Aortic root dilatation Elongated transverse aortic arch Mitral valve prolapse Hypoplastic left heart syndrome Partial anomalous pulmonary connection Persistent left superior vena cava Renal artery stenosis
Gastrointestinal	Inflammatory bowel disease Intestinal lymphangectasia Coeliacs disease
Hepatobiliary	Liver dysfunction
Cutaneous	Fetal cystic hygroma and Lymphoedema (resulting in webbed neck) Naevi Keloid Melanoma Vitiligo Alopecia areata
Renal	Horseshoe kidney Malrotation of kidney Collecting system anomalies
Auditory	Otitis media Sensorineural hearing loss
Musculoskeletal	Short stature Scoliosis Madelung deformity Short IV metacarpal

From Ho et al. (2004) and Bondy (2007)

discounted in girls in whom the only phenotypic characteristic is short stature. Patients are at increased risk of cardiovascular and renal anomalies and other associated clinical features which are summarised in Table 4. Echocardiography and ultrasound of the renal tract is indicated at diagnosis.

Approximately 50% are monosomic (45,X), 5–10% have chromosomal duplication and the remainder have mosaicism (45,X/46XX or 45X, 46XY) (Sybert and Mccauley 2004). Approximately 30% of affected females have Y chromosome material and this is associated with an increased risk of gonadoblastoma (Mazzanti et al. 2005) (Fig. 4.6) and ovarian dysgerminoma. For this reason prophylactic laparoscopic gonadectomy is recommended in those with Y chromosome material.

Sexual maturation usually fails to occur although 10–20% of girls have spontaneous breast development and a smaller proportion of girls will experience menarche. Spontaneous puberty and menarche occur most commonly in girls with mosaic karyotypes.

On ultrasound examination the uterus is prepubertal (Fig. 9c). The ovaries are typically small and may be difficult to visualise. A study of the pelvic ultrasound appearances of girls with Turner syndrome related to age and karyotype reported that those with detectable ovaries showed an initial increase in ovarian volume at about 9 years of bone age (Mazzanti et al. 1997). This increase was sustained and more apparent only after 14 years of age, appearing later than age-matched control subjects. Girls with mosaicism had the highest proportion of bilateral detectable ovaries and the greatest total ovarian volume. Approximately 50% of these patients had spontaneous breast appearance and 40% had spontaneous menarche (Mazzanti et al. 1997). Nomograms for uterine and ovarian volume have been developed from a cohort of girls aged 12–18 years with Turner's syndrome compared to age-matched controls using transabdominal ultrasound (Haber and Ranke 1999). An increase of uterine volume and visualisation of ovaries has been demonstrated in Turner's syndrome patients receiving growth hormone therapy (Sampaolo et al. 2003).

4.3.2 Gonadal Dysgenesis

Normal male development is mediated via hormonal pathways dependent upon normal Leydig and Sertoli cell function. Abnormalities in the development of these cells result in dysgenetic or 'streak' gonads and failure of normal male development. The dysgenetic gonad consists almost entirely of fibrous tissue with no visible Leydig cells, germ cells, Sertoli cells, tubules or follicles. When both gonads are dysgenetic the phenotype is invariably female. The term 'Swyers syndrome' is applied to patients with a 46XY karyotype and a female phenotype. Approximately 10–20% of patients have a mutation in the SRY gene (Harley et al. 2003). Girls present with delayed puberty, primary amenorrhoea and elevated

Table 5 Causes of female precocious puberty

True precocious puberty: gonadotropin dependent
Idiopathic
Tumours of the central nervous system
Cerebral palsy
Head injury
Following meningitis
CAH
Primary hypothyroidism
Pseudo-precocious puberty: GnRH independent
Isolated precocious thelarche
Ovarian cysts
Oestrogen-secreting tumours of the ovary or adrenals
McCune-Albright syndrome
Iatrogenic
Isolated virilisation
Isolated precocious adrenarche
Non-classical congenital adrenal hyperplasia
Androgen-secreting adrenal or ovarian neoplasm
Cushing's disease/syndrome
Iatrogenic
Isolated vaginal bleeding
Hypothyroidism
McCune-Albright syndrome
Isolated autonomous ovarian cysts
Vaginal rhabdomyosarcoma
Vaginal streptococcal infection
Trauma, including sexual abuse

gonadotropins. On ultrasound examination a rudimentary uterus is typically present which excludes complete androgen insensitivity syndrome. The streak gonads are usually not visualised. The streak gonads are at high risk of neoplastic change and as such should be removed shortly after diagnosis.

Mixed gonadal dysgenesis is a term applied to patients with 45X0 and 46XY mosaicism. The phenotype of these individuals is extremely variable ranging from a Turner syndrome like phenotypic female to a male phenotype with a penile urethra. Short stature is common in childhood with late or absent pubertal development. Fallopian tubes and a uterus may be present. Asymmetric gonadal differentiation is seen in the form of both a streak gonad and testis. Chromosomal analysis of the streak gonad often reveals an XY cell line. Some patients may have mild virilisation manifested only by prepubertal cliteromegaly. Gonadectomy is indicated because of the risk of malignancy.

4.3.3 Biosynthetic Defects of Androgen Synthesis

Biosynthetic defects of androgen synthesis typically present in the neonatal period with abnormal genital development. A small minority of patients with mutations of the gene encoding 17β-hydroxysteroid dehydrogenase type 3 present with a normal female phenotype and delayed puberty with primary amenorrhoea. On ultrasound examination the uterus is absent as anti-Müllerian hormone is secreted normally.

Any cause of delayed puberty will also result in primary amenorrhoea, but primary amenorrhoea in a girl with otherwise normal pubertal development should raise suspicion of pelvic pathology such as haematometrocolpos or a genitourinary malformation. In this situation, pelvic ultrasound is the most appropriate initial imaging investigation, supplemented by MRI of the pelvis in complex cases (see chapter "Structural Abnormalities of the Female Reproductive Tract").

5 Precocious Puberty

Precocious puberty is defined as the development of secondary sexual characteristics in girls who are younger than 8 years of age. Untreated precocious puberty can result in premature physeal closure with premature attainment of final height resulting in short stature which may adversely influence psychosocial development (Baumann et al. 2001). Table 5 summarises a classification precocious puberty.

5.1 Classification of Precocious Puberty

5.1.1 True Precocious Puberty

True precocious puberty results from premature but normal activation of the hypothalamic–pituitary–gonadal axis. Most cases are idiopathic or familial, but up to 20% of cases are secondary to intracranial pathology (Table 5).

Gonadotropin-dependent precocious puberty can be treated with GnRH analogues. In girls with early puberty (onset of secondary sexual characteristics between the age of 8 and 9 years) there appears to be no significant difference in final height in girls who are treated compared to those who are untreated, and both treated and untreated girls generally attain a final adult height that is within the target height range (Lazar et al. 2002). The tempo of puberty is slowed, however, with the mean age at menarche being 12.8 years in a study of 63 treated girls, compared to 10.8 years in 63 untreated girls (Lazar et al. 2002). In this scenario the primary indication for treatment is psychosocial difficulties associated with early pubertal development. Girls in whom the onset of puberty is before the age of 8 years appear to benefit more with regard to growth and final adult height has been reported to be significantly greater that predicted adult height at the start of treatment (Klein et al. 2001). Gain in body fat mass has been widely reported (Paterson et al. 2004), however it has also been reported that girls treated with these agents are overweight at the start of treatment (Paterson et al. 2004; Heger et al. 1999).

On cessation of treatment, puberty is reinitiated and menarche is reported to occur on average 16 months following the cessation of treatment (Carel et al. 2009). Infertility has not been reported.

5.1.2 Pseudo-Precocious Puberty

Gonadotropin-independent or pseudo-precocious puberty results from autonomous sex steroid production or exposure to exogenous sex steroids. Onset is usually rapid and characterised by low FSH and LH levels. Most cases in girls are caused by excessive oestrogen production (Table 5).

5.1.3 Exaggerated Adrenarche

The zona reticularis of the adrenal gland produces adrenal androgens between 5 and 7 years of age and sometimes produces a growth spurt and apocrine sweating. In a minority of children this is sufficient to produce axillary and pubic hair. This has been termed premature adrenarche. There are no other signs of puberty. Exaggerated adrenarche is described in detail in chapter "Normal Growth and Puberty".

5.1.4 Premature Isolated Menarche

5.1.4.1 Isolated Premature Menarche

Rarely girls present with premature menarche in the absence of other secondary sexual characteristics. The diagnosis of isolated premature menarche is one of exclusion, as a number of serious pathologies can present in this manner, including neoplastic lesions of the female reproductive tract and McCune Albright syndrome. Vaginal bleeding may be cyclical or sporadic. Pelvic ultrasound is important to exclude other causes of vaginal bleeding, such as trauma, infection, foreign bodies, and vaginal tumours such as rhabdomyosarcoma (see "Menstrual Disorders and Vaginal Discharge "). Ultrasound examination reveals a normal pre-pubertal uterus. Typically the endometrial echo is not well developed. In most girls there is a normal pre-pubertal response to the GnRH test. Final adult height appears to be normal (Pinto and Garden 2006).

5.1.5 Premature Thelarche

Premature thelarche (isolated premature thelarche) is a benign, self-limiting condition of unilateral or bilateral breast development, without any other accompaniment of puberty or further progression through puberty. It usually occurs before the age of 2 years and onset after the age of 4 years is rare. Breast tissue may show some cyclical tendency with increase and decrease in breast size. Premature thelarche is confirmed by normal growth with appropriate bone age and absence of other signs of puberty. The aetiology is unknown although small transient ovarian cysts may be implicated. The natural history is of fairly static breast development before true puberty eventually ensues at the normal time. It usually needs no investigation beyond clinical examination, growth assessment and pelvic ultrasound. Breast ultrasound is useful in demonstrating normal breast bud development and can provide appropriate reassurance.

5.1.6 Thelarche Variant

Thelarche variant also described as atypical premature thelarche or non-classical premature thelarche, refers to a spectrum of findings, between premature thelarche, and true precocious puberty. It has been described as

Table 6 Ultrasound appearances in different types of premature development of secondary sexual characteristics

	Uterus	Ovaries	Adrenals
True precocious puberty	Adult size and shape Thickened endometrium	Pubertal	Normal
Pseudo-precocious puberty	Variable	Pre-pubertal ± cyst or tumour	±tumour
Premature thelarche	Prepubertal	Prepubertal, but isolated follicles may be present	Normal
Premature adrenarche	Prepubertal	Prepubertal	Normal

Table 7 Published sonographic criteria outlining cut-off values for the diagnosis of precocious puberty

Uterine volume (cm^3)	Uterine length (cm)	Uterine AP depth (cm)	Uterine transverse Diameter (cm)	Uterine cross-sectional area (cm^2)	Ovarian volume (cm^3)	Ovarian circumference (cm)	Source
>1.8	>3.6				>1.2		Haber and Mayer (1994)
3.0	>4.0			4.5	1.0		Herter et al. 2002
>1.96	>3.4	0.8	>1.5			>4.5	de Vries et al. (2006)

'a slowly progressive variant of precocious puberty in girls' (Stanhope and Brook 1990). Girls generally present later than those with premature thelarche and breast development is progressive and may be accompanied by advanced growth and skeletal maturation with occasional progression to central precocious puberty (Nanduri et al. 2000). Ovarian volumes are larger than the pre-pubertal range. Other signs of puberty may be present such as pubic and axillary hair.

5.2 Biochemical Investigation

The aim of biochemical investigation is to determine whether puberty is mediated by the hypothalamic–pituitary–gonadal axis (central precocious puberty) or due to autonomous hormone secretion or exposure to exogenous sex hormone (pseudo- precocious puberty). On completion of these investigations the clinician should be able to direct the radiologist to the most likely source of sex steroid secretion in patients in whom exogenous steroid exposure has been excluded. The choice of investigation will be determined by the clinical findings. Girls with consonant precocious puberty are most likely to have gonadotropin-dependent puberty, and investigation should be targeted to define pituitary function. Investigations should include thyroid hormone levels, basal and stimulated gonadotropins and serum oestradiol. Patients with established puberty demonstrate an LH-dominant response to GnRH stimulation (Pescovitz et al. 1988). Patients in whom the first feature of puberty is pubic or axillary hair growth or acne should be investigated for androgen excess.

Patients with discordant puberty, in whom the first features are pubic and axillary hair growth, acne and body odour are most likely to have exaggerated adrenarche, a variant of normal puberty (also see chapter "Normal Growth and Puberty"), however non-classical congenital adrenal hyperplasia (CAH) and androgen secreting tumours may also present in this manner. In all patients adrenal androgens 17-hydroxyprogesterone (17 OHP), androstendione, dehydroepiandrosterone-sulphate (DHEAS) and testosterone should be measured and compared to reference ranges appropriate for pubertal status. Girls with exaggerated adrenarche have levels higher than the age-related reference range but normal for stage of pubic hair growth. Patients with cliteromegaly should be aggressively investigated for androgen secreting tumours and non-classical congenital adrenal hyperplasia. Baseline endocrinology should include measurement of adrenal androgens. A twenty–four hour urinary steroid profile gives greater detail of adrenal hormone production and the ratio of urinary metabolites may be diagnostic of a biosynthetic defect in the girl with non-classical congenital adrenal hyperplasia. Further information can be obtained by the measurement of 17 OHP and androstendione following stimulation (250 μg synacthen IV) and plotting these values on established nomograms (New et al. 1983).

Where uncertainty exists, patients with androgen secreting tumours can be differentiated from those with non-classical congenital adrenal hyperplasia by the low-dose dexamethasone suppression test (0.5 mg dexamethasone every 6 h for 48 h). Patients with congenital adrenal hyperplasia, in whom androgen production is regulated by the pituitary, suppress androgen secretion following dexamethasone administration. Patients with androgen secreting tumours have autonomous androgen secretion and androgen levels do not suppress following dexamethasone (Street et al. 1997).

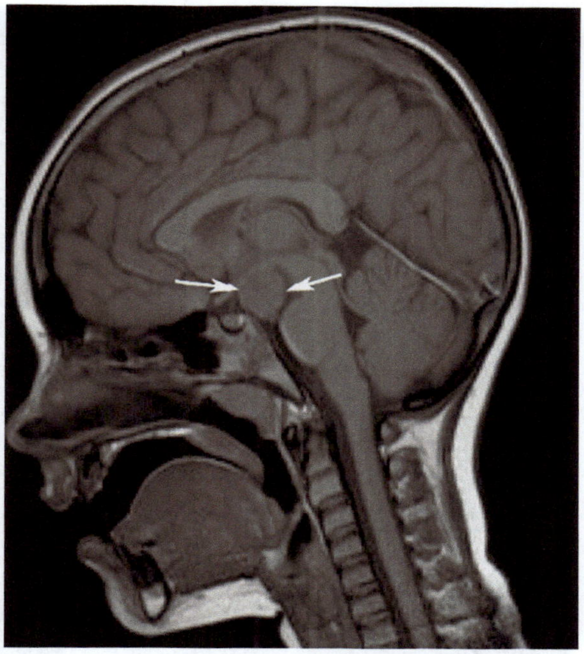

Fig. 10 Hypothalamic hamartoma. Sagittal T1-weighted midline image shows a large hamartoma (*arrows*) within floor of the third ventricle

5.3 Ultrasound Investigation of True Precocious Puberty

Table 6 summarises the different ultrasound appearances seen in the various types of precocious sexual development. In true precocious puberty the uterus and ovaries are pubertal in appearance due to early activation of the hypothalamic–pituitary–gonadal axis. As sex steroid production is independent in the other types of precocious sexual development, the appearances are prepubertal, the exception being in pseudo-precocious puberty where the appearances depend on the underlying cause. In pseudo-precocious puberty ultrasound must exclude an oestrogen secreting ovarian or adrenal tumour. Autonomously functioning ovarian cysts and congenital adrenal hyperplasia are other important causes of pseudo-precocious puberty (Fahmy et al. 2000).

5.3.1 Pelvic Ultrasound

A variety of sonographic parameters have been evaluated in the assessment of precocious puberty including uterine length, fundal anteroposterior diameter, uterine transverse dimension, uterine volume, ovarian length, ovarian circumference and mean ovarian volume. These parameters have all been shown to be increased in girls with central precious puberty compared with age-matched healthy controls (Herter et al. 2002; Haber and Mayer 1994; de Vries et al. 2006) (Table 7). Significant differences in these parameters have been reported between healthy girls and age-matched girls with central precocious puberty (Buzzi et al. 1998; de Vries et al. 2006) but not in girls with isolated premature thelarche. The presence of a definite endometrial echo is a highly specific (100%) measure of pubertal maturation with a high positive predictive value (100%) (de Vries et al. 2006). The minimum evaluation of pubertal maturation using pelvic US should include documentation of uterine length and morphology, the presence and thickness of the endometrial stripe, and, the ovarian volume and follicular morphology.

5.3.2 Pelvic Colour Doppler Ultrasound

There are few studies evaluating the utility of pelvic colour Doppler analysis in the evaluation of

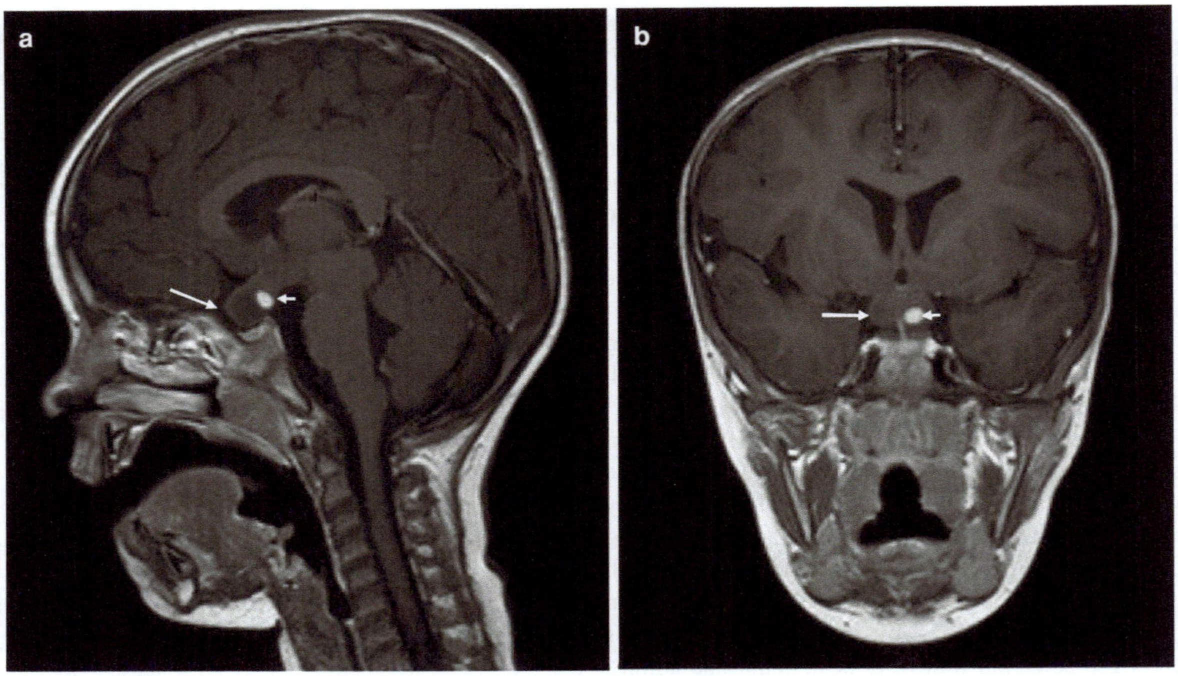

Fig. 11 **a**, **b** Optic pathway glioma (OPG). **a** Sagittal and **b** coronal T1-weighted post contrast images of a large OPG extending into the hypothalamus (*arrow*) with a solid enhancing nodule (*short arrow*)

precocious puberty. The presence of a low uterine artery pulsatility index (<2.5) has been shown to indicate a high diagnostic value for true precocious puberty (Battaglia et al. 2002).

5.3.3 Breast Ultrasound

In addition to recognising racial variations in the timing of the attainment of normal pubertal landmarks (see chapter "Normal Growth and Puberty"); additional difficulty arises when distinguishing between adipose 'pseudobreast tissue' from true premature breast development in thelarche or central precocious puberty in children with high body mass index. In general pubertal landmarks occur earlier in children who are overweight (Rosenfield et al. 2009). Bone age may be advanced in obese girls (Klein et al. 1998). Ultrasound of the breast plays an important role in assessing this subset of children.

5.3.4 Cranial Imaging Evaluation of True Precocious Puberty

True precocious puberty in girls is idiopathic or familial in over 80% of cases. Cranial MRI is necessary to confirm this and excludes CNS abnormalities (Ng et al. 2003). The response to GnRH stimulation has been shown to be of no value in predicting an underlying intracranial space occupying lesion (Ng et al. 2005).

Some of the intracranial conditions which cause delayed puberty in some children may paradoxically result in precocious puberty in other patients. CNS lesions which may result in either delayed or precocious puberty include neurofibromatosis type 1 (usually in association with an optic pathway glioma), craniopharyngioma and suprasellar lesions such as arachnoid cysts and epidermoid cysts.

5.4 Cranial Imaging Evaluation of Central Precocious Puberty

5.4.1 Hypothalamic Hamartoma

Hypothalamic hamartoma is the most common intracranial tumour identified in patients with true precocious puberty. These are benign tumours which are usually small and slow growing. Hypothalamic hamartomas usually present with precocious puberty, often in early childhood. They do not usually cause

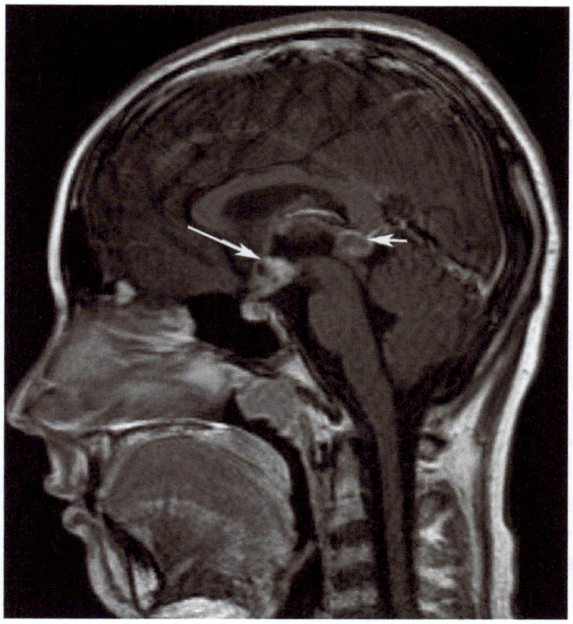

Fig. 12 Germinoma. Sagittal T1-weighted post contrast image showing synchronous pineal (*arrow*) and suprasellar (*long arrow*) enhancing germinomas

neurological symptoms, but may cause gelastic seizures, characterised by outbursts of inappropriate laughter. This lesion is also known as hamartoma of the tuber cinereum; the lesion is always located on the floor of the third ventricle, anterior to the mamillary bodies (Barral et al. 1988). Its size varies from a few millimetres to several centimetres; it can extend into the posterior fossa behind the dorsum sellae. On CT it appears as a mass which is homogenous, similar in attenuation to normal brain, and shows no contrast enhancement. Small lesions are therefore easily missed. MRI is much more sensitive; appearances on MRI are characteristic, even when the lesion is small. The lesion appears as a homogenous mass, its signal intensity usually following that of normal gray matter on all sequences, although the lesion may show high signal on T2-weighted images (Fig. 10). There is no enhancement with intravenous gadolinium. However, differentiation of hamartomas from small hypothalamic or optic gliomas may be impossible on radiological appearances.

5.4.2 Pallister-Hall Syndrome

In Pallister-Hall syndrome, hypothalamic hamartoma is associated with imperforate anus, polydactyly, craniofacial anomalies and bifid epiglottis. MRI may demonstrate other CNS abnormalities including pituitary aplasia, absence of the olfactory nerves, agenesis of the corpus callosum and holoprosencephaly. Affected children may have associated hypopituitarism.

5.4.3 Optic and Hypothalamic Glioma

These are slowly progressing neoplasms which are usually classified as pilocytic astrocytomas. Hypothalamic gliomas may present with a variety of endocrine abnormalities including diabetes insipidus, obesity and precocious or delayed puberty. Optic pathway gliomas (OPG) usually cause visual disturbance. Up to 50% of cases are associated with neurofibromatosis type 1 (NF-1).

The typical MRI appearances of OPG include tubular or tortuous enlargement of the optic nerve, enlargement of the optic chiasm, and diffuse infiltration of the posterior optic pathways. These lesions are often of the same or slightly lower intensity in comparison with cortical gray matter on T1-weighted images; T2-weighted images show slightly increased intensity. There is variable enhancement following intravenous gadolinium. Signal characteristics are, however, not specific; germinomas and sarcoid granulomas may have similar appearances.

Some optic and hypothalamic gliomas are very large at presentation, involving the optic chiasm and hypothalamus, with solid and cystic components, and intense enhancement of the solid component (Fig. 11).

OPG associated with NF-1 more often involves the optic nerves, and less often involves the posterior optic pathways. Involvement of both optic nerves is characteristic of NF-1. Cystic components are more common in non-NF-1 OPG (Chateil et al. 2001). OPG and brainstem gliomas associated with NF-1 are histologically identical with pilocytic astrocytomas in non-NF1 patients but tend to have a much more benign prognosis. The majority of OPG in NF-1 are diagnosed before the age of 6 years and show no progression over many years of follow-up, and some may regress spontaneously, but a small minority of tumours are more aggressive.

Precocious puberty in NF-1 is usually secondary to an OPG involving the hypothalamus, but may rarely be caused by the rare association of NF-1 and McCune-Albright Syndrome (polyostotic fibrous dysplasia), reflecting the close genetic linkage between these two conditions.

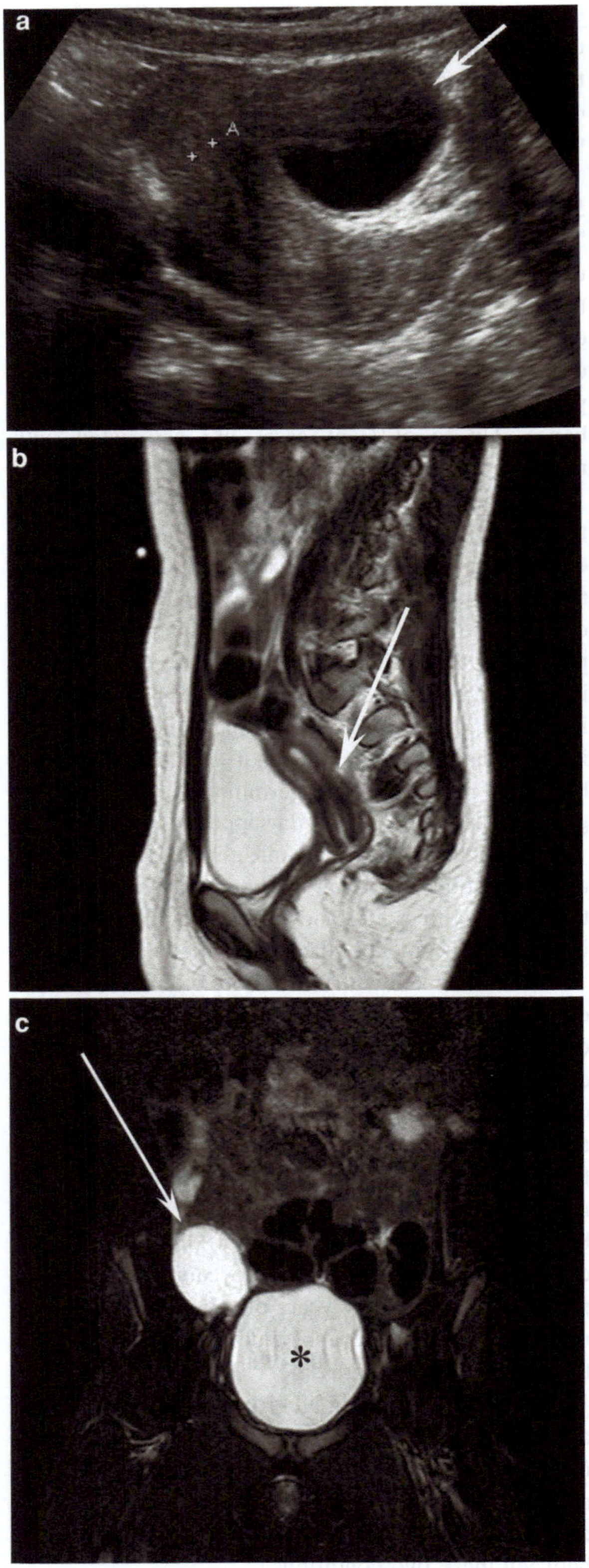

◂**Fig. 13** **a–c** Imaging from a 3-year old girl with gonadotropin-independent (pseudo-precocious) puberty secondary to an autonomous ovarian cyst. **a** Longitudinal ultrasound from referring hospital showing a bulky post-pubertal uterus with an oestrogen stimulated endometrium (between callipers) and adjacent anechoic ovarian cyst (*arrow*). **b** Sagittal T2-weighted image showing the uterus (*arrow*) and **c** coronal T2 fat-suppressed image showing the cyst (*arrow*) and urinary bladder (*asterisk*). There were no clinical features of McCune–Albright syndrome in this child

5.4.4 Germinoma

Germinomas in the hypothalamus are rare. CT and MRI typically show a lobulated mass in the floor of the third ventricle; it may invade or compress the optic chiasm and pituitary stalk. On CT, the lesion is well defined, and may show similar or increased attenuation in comparison with gray matter, with no calcification. There is usually uniform enhancement following contrast. On MRI scans, the lesions are isointense or hypointense on T1-weighted images; they show moderately high signal on T2-weighted images. There is normally uniform enhancement with gadolinium. Germinomas may occur in the pineal and the hypothalamus; synchronous tumours are sometimes found at both sites (Fig. 12). Metastatic spread through the cerebrospinal fluid may produce multiple tumour deposits over the surface of the brain and spine; small arachnoid deposits can be readily demonstrated on T1-weighted images with gadolinium enhancement.

5.4.5 Pituitary Adenoma

It is a common misconception that a likely cause for precocious puberty is a pituitary adenoma. Pituitary adenomas rarely present in childhood. Physiological enlargement of the anterior pituitary is frequently observed in true precocious puberty, and should not be misinterpreted as a pituitary tumour. Prolactinomas may rarely present with precocious puberty or more commonly with primary or secondary amenorrhoea. Gonadotropin secreting pituitary adenomas are exceptionally rare.

5.5 Radiological Investigations for Pseudo-precocious Puberty

Abdominopelvic ultrasound will normally be undertaken to assess the stage of development of the uterus and ovaries; the ovaries should also be carefully

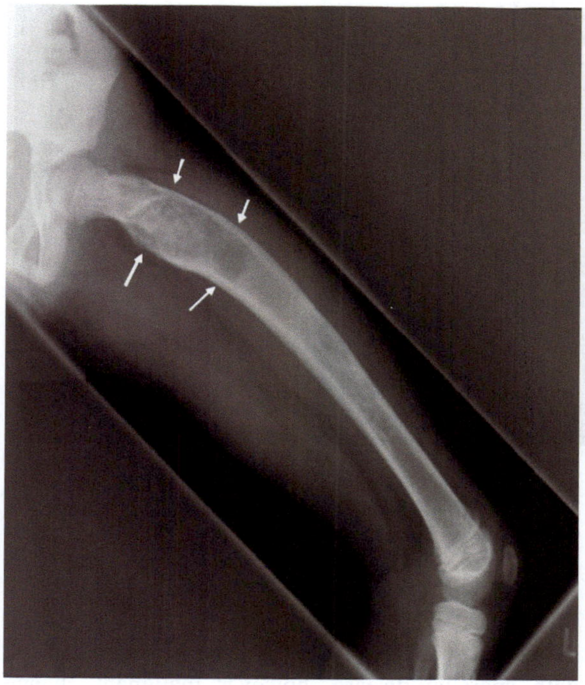

Fig. 14 Polyostotic fibrous dysplasia in McCune Albright syndrome. Radiograph of an unfused skeleton. There are several geographic lesions showing narrow zone of transition, throughout the diaphysis of the femur. The largest lesion in the proximal femur (*arrows*) shows classical features including mild expansion, ground-glass matrix without aggressive features such as periosteal reaction, soft tissue mass or pathological fracture

examined for evidence of an autonomously functioning ovarian cyst or tumour that secretes oestrogen (granulosa-theca cell tumours are the most common). A comprehensive ultrasound examination of the whole of the abdomen should also be undertaken, with particular attention to the adrenals for evidence of an adrenal tumour or diffuse bilateral hypertrophy.

5.5.1 Autonomously Functioning Ovarian Cyst

Occasionally an ovarian cyst may autonomously secrete sufficient oestrogen to stimulate the endometrium to induce premature menstrual bleeding. US reveals an ovarian cyst in the presence of oestrogenised uterus with post-pubertal dimensions and a thickened endometrial stripe (Fig. 13). Most cases of autonomous ovarian hyperfunction are idiopathic and self-limiting but similar findings may be seen in McCune-Albright syndrome (see Sect. 5.5.3). If an ovarian cyst is complex in the context of pseudo-precocious puberty then ovarian malignancy should be considered and further investigation is mandatory (see Sect. 5.4.2 and " Gynaecological Neoplasia").

5.5.2 McCune-Albright Syndrome

McCune-Albright syndrome (MAS) is a sporadic disorder classically described as the triad of polyostotic fibrous dysplasia, café au lait macules and endocrine dysfunction (typically pseudo-precocious puberty). Beyond this classic triad, numerous partial or atypical presentations have been reported.

The molecular aetiology of MAS is based on post-zygotic mutations of the cyclic AMP regulating protein, guanine-nucleotide-binding protein α-subunit ($G_s\alpha$). Post-zygotic activating mutations of the *GNAS1* gene lead to a mosaic distribution of cells bearing constitutively active cyclic AMP (Lumbroso et al. 2004). Mutations of $G_s\alpha$ result in intracellular accumulation of cyclic AMP resulting in cell proliferation and autonomous cell function (Weinstein et al. 1991). These cells include osteoblasts, melanocytes, thyroid, gonad and specific pituitary cells and account for the heterogeneous nature of MAS. MAS is an example of somatic mosaicism in which a wide spectrum of disease is possible. Clinical manifestations of the condition reflect the specific tissues that carry the mutant gene and the ratio of mutant to normal cells in each affected tissue.

In pre-pubertal girls MAS most commonly presents as isolated vaginal bleeding in the presence of suppressed gonadotropins and elevated oestradiol for age. Elevated oestrogen results from autonomous secretion from an ovarian cyst. Although the ovary is the site most commonly affected in childhood, the thyroid, adrenal and specific pituitary cells can also be affected.

The diagnosis is essentially clinical and requires the presence of at least two features of the triad of polyostotic fibrous dysplasia, café au lait skin pigmentation and autonomous endocrine function. Ninety-five percent of cases are female and can present at any age. Average age of puberty is 3 years. Affected individuals are at risk of multiple endocrinopathies including thyrotoxicosis, Cushing's syndrome, acromegaly, hyperparathyroidism, growth hormone excess, hyperprolactinaemia,

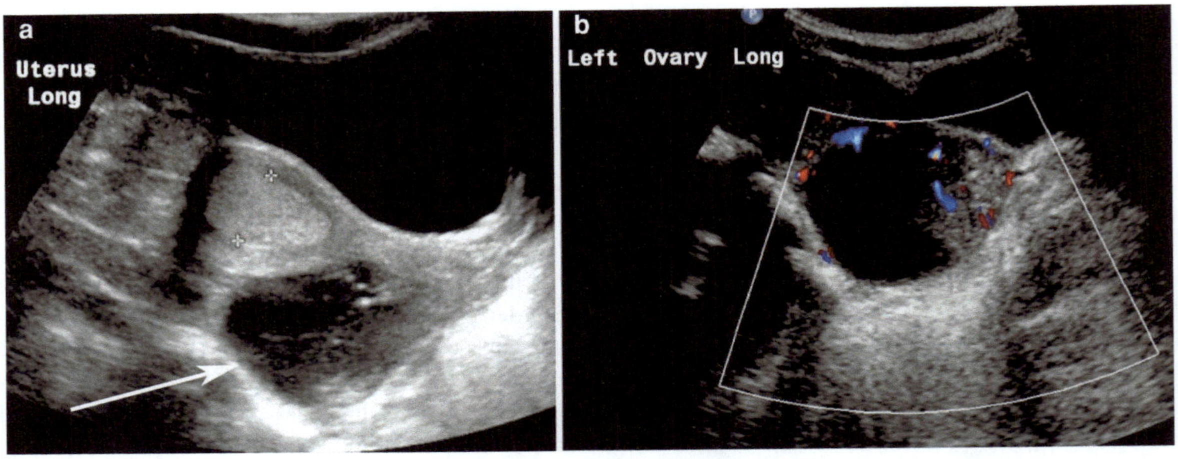

Fig. 15 **a**, **b** Sertoli-Leydig cell tumour (SLCT). US imaging from a 2-year old girl with Peutz-Jeghers syndrome and pseudo-precocious puberty. **a** Longitudinal US showing the relationship of a SLCT (*arrow*) to the uterus – note the oestrogen stimulated uterus seen as a thickened endometrial echogenic stripe (*between callipers*). **b** Colour Doppler US indicating flow to the solid components of the tumour

and hypophosphatemic rickets due to renal phosphate wasting.

When MAS is suspected, a radio-isotope bone scan or a radiographic skeletal survey is appropriate to search for evidence of polyostotic fibrous dysplasia. Typically, multiple bone lesions with the characteristic amorphous ground-glass appearance are identified at several different sites on radiographs (Fig. 14).

5.5.3 Functional Ovarian Tumours

Ovarian tumours in young girls arise most commonly from the sex cord stroma (granulosa, theca and interstitial cells or stromal fibroblasts). They are rare tumours, accounting for 5 to 8% of all ovarian neoplasms.

Ovarian sex cord stromal tumours occur with increased frequency in patients with Peutz-Jeghers syndrome (PJS), an autosomal dominant disorder comprising of characteristic mucocutaneous melanin pigmentation, gastrointestinal hamartomatous polyposis with a predilection to intussusception and haemorrhage, and increased risk of neoplasia. Mutations (germline deletions) of the tumour suppressor gene STK11 (19p13.3) are responsible for most cases of malignancy in PJS. Ovarian neoplasms are extremely rare but include Sertoli-Leydig cell tumours (SLCT) and sex cord tumours with annular tubules. SLCT may result in pseudo-precocious puberty with pubertal levels of sex steroids and suppressed levels of gonadotropins (Fig. 15). Patients with PJS are more likely to have bilateral disease than patients with sporadic disease, however malignant change occurs less frequently. Most cases are benign and treatment is effected with primary resection.

The juvenile variant of granulosa-theca ovarian tumours (JGCT—Juvenile granulosa cell tumour) is extremely rare. JGCT are usually found in premenarchal girls and occasionally in women up to the age of 30 years. The association of JGCT and isosexual pseudo-precocious puberty results from hypersecretion of androstenedione from thecal cells which is then converted to oestradiol by the granulosa cells. Elevated oestrogen levels result in premature breast development and uterine bleeding. Rapid onset of precocious puberty is an indicator of tumour (Cronjé et al. 1998). FSH and LH levels are typically markedly diminished. Serum inhibin levels may be useful as a specific tumour marker to monitor treatment response and for the detection of occult local relapse.

Virilisation is a recognised, albeit extremely rare feature of JGCT (Kalfa et al. 2010). Maffucci's and Ollier's syndrome are also rare associations of JGCT.

There are no diagnostic features which are specific for JGCT. Imaging appearances include a multilocular or occasionally a solid adnexal mass which may undergo intratumoural haemorrhage, necrosis or result in adnexal torsion. Calcifications are rare. The diagnosis should be considered in a girl with precious puberty and an adnexal mass.

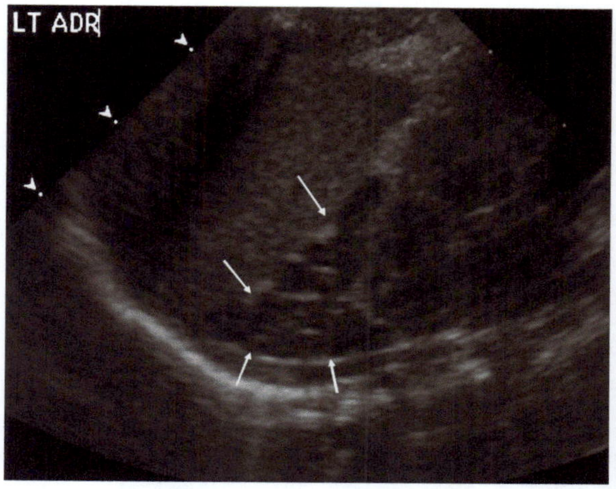

Fig. 16 Classical congenital adrenal hyperplasia. Ultrasound showing an enlarged, lobulated adrenal gland with characteristic 'cerebriform' morphology. The ultrasound and clinical features of non-classical forms of congenital adrenal hyperplasia may sometimes be indistinguishable from polycystic ovarian syndrome

JGCT are typically large at presentation but usually confined to the ovary. In a retrospective review of 40 girls with JGCT, Plantaz et al. (1992) found at diagnosis that 94% had abdominal signs related to tumour mass and 68% had clinical features of precocious puberty. All girls with precocious puberty had FIGO stage 1A disease. Tumour capsule breach and ascites occurs in around 10% of cases and bilateral disease is exceedingly rare. Staging is principally based on surgical findings. The prognosis in most cases is very good. Surgical treatment is aimed at preserving fertility and endocrine function. JGCT rarely demonstrates malignant behaviour, typically in those with a delay in diagnosis with early transperitoneal spread, early relapse following surgery and poor overall prognosis (Outwater et al. 1998).

5.5.4 Primary Hypothyroidism

Rarely, severe untreated primary hypothyroidism may present with cystic ovarian enlargement and precocious puberty, this is known as Van Wyk-Grumbach syndrome (VWGS). Its mechanism has been attributed to the cAMP mediated dose-dependent action of TSH upon FSH receptors inducing ovarian follicular hyperstimulation in hypothyroidism (Anasti et al. 1995).

The presence of enlarged multicystic ovaries in a girl with precocious puberty can erroneously raise the possibility of an oestrogen secreting tumour such as

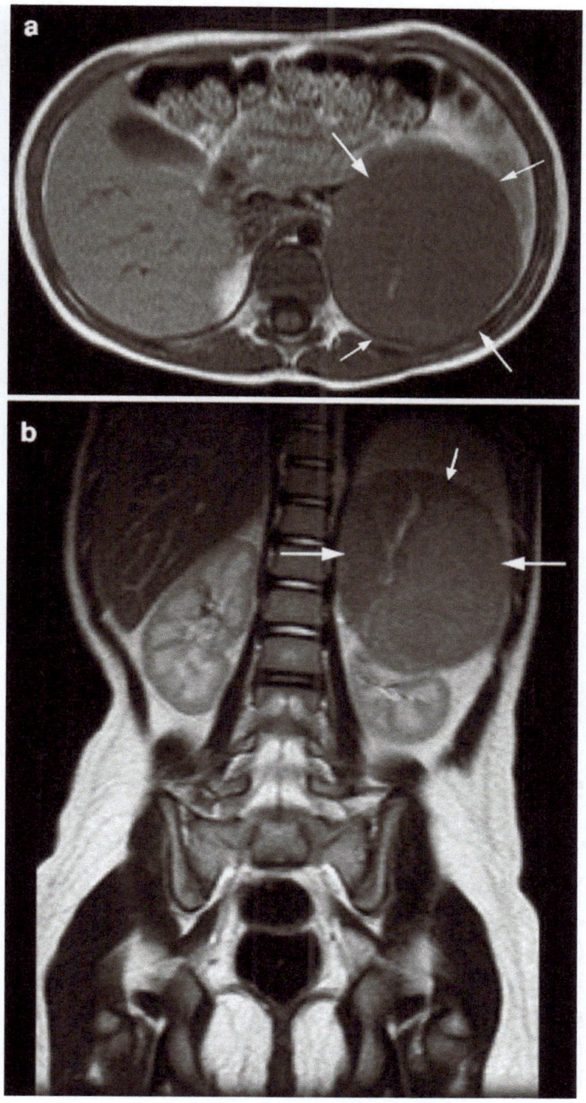

Fig. 17 **a**, **b** Virilising adrenal tumour. **a** Axial T1-weighted and **b** coronal T2-weighted images of large solid adrenal tumour mass abutting the left kidney (*between arrows*). No distant metastases or nodal disease were present. Symptoms resolved following surgical resection

juvenile granulosa-theca cell tumour. Correlation with thyroid function tests is essential in these cases to avoid unnecessary investigation and delay in medical therapy (Browne et al. 2008). Short stature and delayed bone age distinguish VWGS from other causes of precocious puberty. Cranial MRI may show hypertrophy of the anterior lobe of the pituitary. Reversion to the pre-pubertal state follows treatment by thyroid hormone replacement.

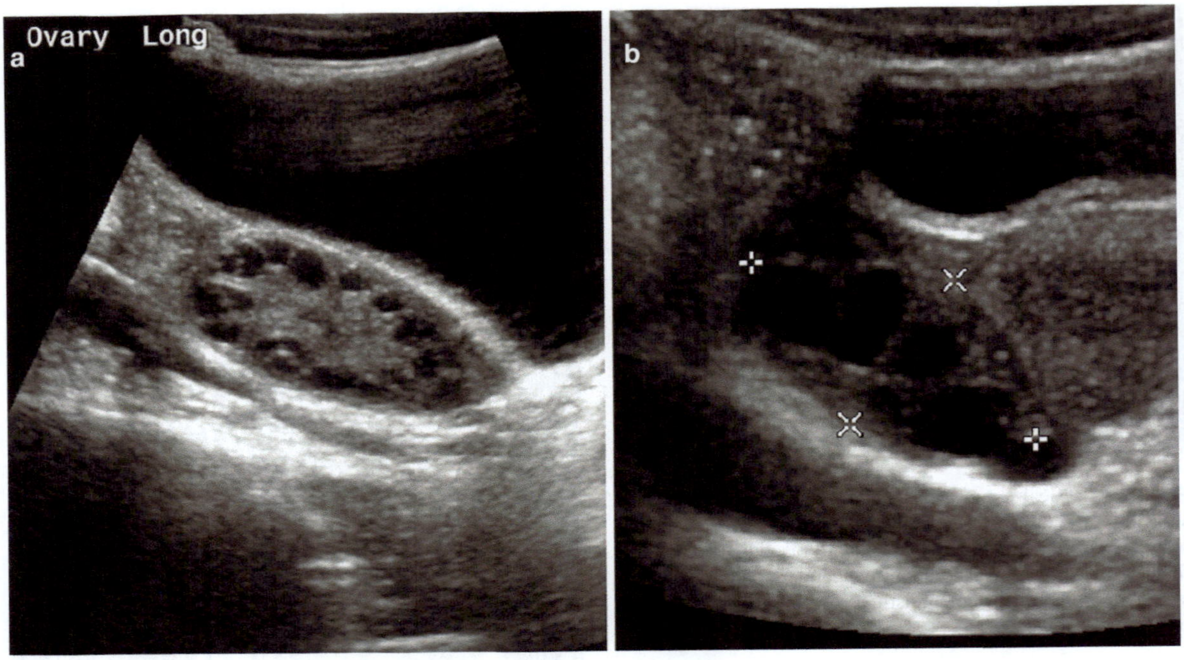

Fig. 18 **a, b** Ultrasound appearances of **a** Polycystic ovarian (PCO) and **b** multifollicular ovarian (MFO) morphology

5.6 Investigation of Girls with Virilisation

Virilisation in girls is rare, but particularly distressing as affected girls develop male sexual characteristics (hirsutism, acne, deepening of voice, cliteromegaly, increased muscle mass and temporal balding). Congenital adrenal hyperplasia (non-salt wasting) is the most common cause. The differential diagnosis includes functional ovarian tumours (see Sect. 5.4.2).

5.6.1 Congenital Adrenal Hyperplasia

Congenital adrenal hyperplasia is an autosomal recessive disorder in which there is complete or partial deficiency of one of the enzymes involved in the synthesis of steroid hormones. In 90% of cases the deficient enzyme is 21-hydroxylase, with 11-beta hydroxylase deficiency accounting for most of the rest. Glucocorticoid deficiency stimulates secretion of adrenocorticotropic hormone (ACTH) by the anterior pituitary, resulting in adrenal hyperplasia and excessive production of adrenal androgens. The vast majority of these cases are detected in the neonatal period. If ambiguous genitalia are not identified at birth, affected girls will later present (usually between 2–4 years) with the effects of androgen excess, increased height, development of pubic hair with or without clitoral enlargement and advanced bone age. Enlargement of the adrenal gland may be identified in ultrasound in about 50% of cases. The adrenal cortex is enlarged, whereas the adrenal medulla remains normal (Fig. 16). In some cases the enlarged adrenal cortex has a lobulated, convoluted, "cerebriform" appearance.

5.6.2 Adrenocortical Tumours (ACT)

Adrenal carcinomas and adenomas can both present with pseudo-precocious puberty. Ninety percent of ACT affecting young children are functional and the majority of children present with clinical features of androgen excess: accelerated growth and skeletal maturity, acne, pubic hair growth and cliteromegaly. Oestrogen secretion occurs very rarely and also induces accelerated growth and skeletal maturity with breast development and vaginal bleeding in girls. Glucocorticoid excess results in the clinical characteristics of Cushing's syndrome in a minority of patients (Fig. 17). Adenomas are usually smaller, solid and well defined, whereas carcinomas tend to be larger and more complex in appearance. In general, lesions larger than 5 cm in diameter are considered suspicious for malignancy, but no imaging modality can reliably distinguish between benign and malignant adrenal masses. Even on histological examination the distinction between adenomas and carcinomas can be very difficult in many cases.

Referral to medical genetics is mandatory as 50–80% of childhood ACTs have an inherited basis. Li-Fraumeni syndrome, a dominantly inherited condition that results from mutations of the p53 gene, is found in approximately 50% of children. Affected patients are at increased risk of a number of other malignancies in early adult life including sarcomas, brain tumours, breast cancer and lung cancer. Childhood ACT may be the first presentation of Li-Fraumeni syndrome in a family. The prevalence of ACT is increased in a number of other genetic conditions including Beckwith-Wiedemann syndrome, isolated hemihypertrophy, Carney complex and multiple endocrine neoplasia type 1. It is important that these diagnoses are not overlooked as all are associated with an increased risk of malignant and/or benign tumours of other organs.

Idiopathic hirsutism and polycystic ovarian syndrome are also considered as virilising disorders, and may occasionally be confused with heterosexual precocious puberty. The ultrasound appearances of polycystic ovaries (increased ovarian stroma and peripheral distribution of numerous small follicles) should not be confused with multi-follicular appearance of a stimulated ovary where follicles are scattered throughout the ovary (Fig. 18). Polycystic ovarian syndrome is discussed in detail in chapter "Menstrual Disorders and Vaginal Discharge".

References

Abernethy LJ (1998) Imaging of the pituitary in children with growth disorders. Eur J Radiol 26:102–108

Amato MC, Elias LL, Elias J et al (2006) Endocrine disorders in pediatric—onset Langerhans cell histiocytosis. Horm Metab Res 38:746–751

Anasti JN, Flack MR, Froehlich J et al (1995) A potential novelmechanism for precocious puberty in juvenile hypothyroidism. J Clin Endocrinol Metab 80:276–279

Argyropolou M, Perignon F, Brunelle F et al (1991) Height of normal pituitary gland as a function of age evaluated by MRI in children. Pediatr Radiol 21:247–249

Arslanian SA, Rothfus WE, Foley TP (1984) Hormonal, metabolic, and neuroradiologic abnormalities associated with septo-optic dysplasia. Acta Endocrinol 107:282–288

Barral V, Brunelle F, Brauner R et al (1988) MRI of hypothalamic hamartomas in children. Pediatr Radiol 18: 449–452

Battaglia C, Regnani G, Mancini F et al (2002) Pelvic sonography and uterine artery color doppler analysis in the diagnosis of female precocious puberty. Ultrasound Obstet Gynecol 19:386–391

Baumann DA, Landolt MA, Wetterwald R et al (2001) Psychological evaluation of young women after medical treatment for central precocious puberty. Horm Res 56: 45–50

Bernstrand C, Sandstedt B, Ahström L et al (2005) Long-term follow-up of Langerhans cell histiocytosis: 39 years' experience at a single centre. Acta Paediatr 94:1073–1084

Bondy CA (2007) Turner syndrome study group. Care of girls and women with Turner syndrome: a guideline of the Turner syndrome study group. J Clin Endocrinol Metab 92:10–25

Browne LP, Boswell HB, Crotty EJ et al (2008) Van Wyk and Grumbach syndrome revisited: imaging and clinical findings in pre- and postpubertal girls. Pediatr Radiol 38:538–542

Buzzi F, Pilotta A, Dordoni D et al (1998) Pelvic ultrasonography in normal girls and in girls with pubertal precocity. Acta Paediatr 87:1138–1145

Carel JC, Eugster EA, Rogol A et al ESPE-LWPES GnRH Analogs Consensus Conference Group (2009) Consensus statement on the use of gonadotropin-releasing hormone analogs in children. Pediatrics 123:e752–e762

Chateil J, Sousotte C, Pedespan J et al (2001) MRI and clinical differences between optic pathway tumours in children with and without neurofibromatosis. Br J Radiol 74:24–31

Cronje′ HS, Niemand I, Bam RH et al (1998) Granulosa and theca cell tumors in children: a report of 17 cases and literature review. Obstet Gynecol Surv 53:240–247

de Vries L, Lazar L, Phillip M (2003a) Craniopharyngioma: presentation and endocrine sequelae in 36 children. J Pediatr Endocrinol Metab 16:703–710

de Vries L, Weintrob N, Phillip M (2003b) Craniopharyngioma presenting as precocious puberty and accelerated growth. Clin Pediatr 42:181–184

de Vries L, Horev G, Schwartz M et al (2006) Ultrasonographic and clinical parameters for early differentiation between precocious puberty and premature thelarche. Eur J Endocrinol 154:891–898

DeVile CJ, Grant DB, Hayward RD et al (1996) Growth and endocrine sequelae of craniopharyngioma. Arch Dis Child 75:108–114

Einaudi S, Matarazzo P, Peretta P et al (2006) Hypothalamo-hypophysial dysfunction after traumatic brain injury in children and adolescents: a preliminary retrospective and prospective study. J Pediatr Endocrinol Metab 19: 691–703

Fahmy JL, Kaminsky CK, Kaufman F et al (2000) The radiological approach to precocious puberty. Br J Radiol 73:560–567

Fujisawa I, Kikuchi K, Nishimura K et al (1987) Transection of the pituitary stalk: development of an ectopic posterior lobe assessed with MR imaging. Radiology 165:487–489

Garel C, Leger J (2007) Contribution of magnetic resonance imaging in non-tumoral hypopituitarism in children. Horm Res 67:194–202

Greulich WW, Pyle SI (1959) Radiographic atlas of skeletal development of the hand and wrist, 2nd edn. Stanford University Press, Stanford, California

Griffin IJ, Donaldson TJ, Duncan KA et al (1995) Pelvic ultrasound measurements in normal girls. Acta Paediatr 84:536–543

Grois N, Prayer D, Prosch H et al (2004) Course and clinical impact of magnetic resonance imaging findings in diabetes insipidus associated with Langerhans cell histiocytosis. Pediatr Blood Cancer 43:59–65

Haber HP, Mayer EI (1994) Ultrasound evaluation of uterine and ovarian size form birth to puberty. Pediatr Radiol 24:11–13

Haber HP, Ranke MB (1999) Pelvic ultrasonography in Turner syndrome: standards for uterine and ovarian volume. J Ultrasound Med 18:271–276

Harley VR, Clarkson MJ, Argentaro A (2003) The molecular action and regulation of the testis-determining factors, SRY (sex-determining region on the Y chromosome) and SOX9 [SRY-related high-mobility group (HMG) box 9]. Endocr Rev 24:466–487

Heger S, Partsch CJ, Sippell WG (1999) Long-term outcome after depot gonadotropin-releasing hormone agonist treatment of central precocious puberty: final height, body proportions, body composition, bone mineral density, and reproductive function. J Clin Endocrinol Metab 84: 4583–4590

Herter LD, Golendziner E, Flores JA et al (2002) Ovarian and uterine findings in pelvic sonography. Comparison between prepubertal girls, girls with isolated thelarche, and girls with central precocious puberty. J Ultrasound Med 21: 1237–1246

Ho VB, Bakalov VK, Cooley M (2004) Major vascular anomalies in Turner syndrome. Circulation 110:1694–1700

Izenberg N, Rosenblum M, Parks JS (1984) The endocrine spectrum of septo-optic dysplasia. Clin Pediatr 23:632–636

Kaatsch P, Rickert CH, Kühl J et al (2001) Population-based epidemiologic data on brain tumors in German children. Cancer 92:3155–3164

Kalfa N, Méduri G, Philibert P et al (2010) Unusual virilization in girls with juvenile granulosa cell tumors of the ovary is related to intratumoral aromatase deficiency. Horm Res Paediatr 74:83–91

Kelberman D, Dattani MT (2007) Hypothalamic and pituitary development: novel insights into the aetiology. Eur J Endocrinol 157:S3–S14

Kikuchi K, Fujisawa I, Momoi T et al (1988) Hypothalamic-pituitary function in growth hormone-deficient patients with pituitary stalk transection. J Clin Endocrinol Metab 67:817–823

Klein KO, Larmore KA, de Lancey E et al (1998) Effect of obesity on estradiol level, and its relationship to leptin, bone maturation, and bone mineral density in children. J Clin Endocrinol Metab 83:3469–3475

Klein KO, Barnes KM, Jones JV et al (2001) Increased final height in precocious puberty after long term treatment with LHRH agonists: the National Institutes of Health experience. J Clin Endocrinol Metab 86:4711–4716

Lazar L, Kauli R, Pertzelan A et al (2002) Gonadotropin-suppressive therapy in girls with early and fast puberty affects the pace of puberty but not total pubertal growth or final height. J Clin Endocrinol Metab 87:2090–2094

Lumbroso S, Paris F, Sultan C (2004) Activating Gsalpha Mutations: Analysis of 113 Patients with Signs of McCune-Albright Syndrome - A European Collaborative Study. J Clin Endocrinol Metab 89:2107–2113

May JA, Krieger MD, Bowen I et al (2006) Craniopharyngioma in childhood. Adv Pediatr 53:183–209

Mazzanti L, Cacciari E, Bergamaschi R et al (1997) Pelvic ultrasonography in patients with Turner syndrome: Age-related findings in different karyotypes. J Pediatr 131: 135–140

Mazzanti L, Cicognani A, Baldazzi L et al (2005) Gonadoblastoma in Turner syndrome and Y-chromosome-derived material. Am J Med Genet A 135:150–154

McNay DE, Turton JP, Kelberman D et al (2007) HESX1 mutations are an uncommon cause of septooptic dysplasia and hypopituitarism. J Clin Endocrinol Metab 92:691–697

Nanduri VR, Bareille P, Pritchard J et al (2000) Growth and endocrine disorders in multisystem Langerhans' cell histiocytosis. Clin Endocrinol 53:509–515

New MI, Lorenzen F, Lerner AJ et al (1983) Genotyping steroid 21-hydroxylase deficiency: hormonal reference data. J Clin Endocrinol Metab 57:320–326

Ng SM, Kumar Y, Cody D, Smith CS, Didi M (2003) Cranial MRI scans are indicated in all girls with central precocious puberty. Arch Dis Child 88:414–418

Ng SM, Kumar Y, Cody D, Smith CS, Didi M (2005) The gonadotrophins response to GnRH test is not a predictor of neurological lesion in girls with central precocious puberty. J Pediatr Endocrinol Metab 18:849–852

Niederland T, Makovi H, Gál V et al (2007) Abnormalities of pituitary function after traumatic brain injury in children. J Neurotrauma 24:119–127

Outwater EK, Wagner BJ, Mannion C et al (1998) Sex cord-stromal and steroid cell tumors of the ovary. Radiographics 18:1523–1546

Pallais JC, Au M, Pitteloud N et al (2010) Kallmann syndrome. In: Pagon RA, Bird TC, Dolan CR, Stephens K (eds). GeneReviews [Internet]. Seattle (WA): University of Washington, Seattle; 1993–2007 May 23 [updated 2010 Apr 8] Accessed Aug 2010

Patel L, McNally RJ, Harrison E et al (2006) Geographical distribution of optic nerve hypoplasia and septo-optic dysplasia in Northwest England. J Pediatr 148:85–88

Paterson WF, McNeill E, Young D, Donaldson MD (2004) Auxological outcome and time to menarche following long-acting goserelin therapy in girls with central precocious or early puberty. Clin Endocrinol (Oxf) 61:626–634

Pescovitz OH, Hench KD, Barnes KM et al (1988) Premature thelarche and central precocious puberty: the relationship between clinical presentation and the gonadotropin response to luteinizing hormone-releasing hormone. J Clin Endocrinol Metab 67:474–479

Pinto SM, Garden AS (2006) Prepubertal menarche: a defined clinical entity. Am J Obstet Gynecol 195:327–329

Plantaz D, Flamant F, Vassal G et al (1992) Granulosa cell tumors of the ovary in children and adolescents. Multicenter retrospective study in 40 patients aged 7 months–22 years]. Arch Fr Pediatr 49:793

Poomthavorn P, Maixner W, Zacharin M (2008) Pituitary function in paediatric survivors of severe traumatic brain injury. Arch Dis Child 93:133–137

Roche AF, Chumlea WC, Thissen D (1988) Assessing the skeletal maturity of the hand-wrist: FELS method. Charles C Thomas, Springfield, Illinois

Rosenfield RL, Lipton RB, Drum ML (2009) Thelarche, Pubarche, and Menarche attainment in children with normal and elevated body mass index. Pediatrics 123:84–88

Sampaolo P, Calcaterra V, Klersy C et al (2003) Pelvic ultrasound evaluation in patients with Turner syndrome during treatment with growth hormone. Ultrasound Obstet Gynecol 22:172–177

Schneider JF, Floemer F (2009) Maturation of the olfactory bulbs: MR imaging findings. Am J Neuroradiol 30:1149–1152

Sklar CA (1994) Craniopharyngioma: endocrine abnormalities at presentation. Pediatr Neurosurg 21(Suppl 1):18–20

Stanhope R, Brook CC (1990) Thelarche variant: a new syndrome of precocious sexual maturation? Acta Endocrinol 123:481–486

Street ME, Weber A, Camacho-Hübner C et al (1997) Girls with virilisation in childhood: a diagnostic protocol for investigation. J Clin Pathol 50:379–383

Suzuki M, Takashima T, Kadoya M et al (1989) MR imaging of olfactory bulbs and tracts. Am J Neuroradiol 10:955–957

Sybert VP, McCauley E (2004) Turner's syndrome. New Eng J Med 351:1227–1238

Tanner JM, Whitehouse RH, Cameron N et al (eds) (1983) Assessment of skeletal maturity and prediction of adult height (TW2 method), 2nd edn. Academic Press, London

Truwit CL, Barkovich AJ, Grumbach MM et al (1993) MR imaging of Kallmann syndrome: a genetic disorder of neuronal migration affecting the olfactory and genital systems. Am J Neuroradiol 14:827–838

Weinstein LS, Shenker A, Gejman PV et al (1991) Activating mutations of the stimulatory G protein in the McCune-Albright syndrome. N Engl J Med 325:1688–1695

Menstrual Disorders and Vaginal Discharge

Urmi Das and Gurdeep S. Mann

Contents

1	**Introduction**	146
2	**Menstrual Disorders**	146
3	**Amenorrhoea**	146
3.1	Definitions and Summary of Causes	146
3.2	History and Examination	148
3.3	Endocrine Investigation	149
4	**Specific Causes of Amenorrhoea**	149
4.1	Amenorrhoea of Hypothalamic Origin	149
4.2	Amenorrhoea of Pituitary Origin	152
4.3	Thyroid Dysfunction	155
4.4	Amenorrhoea of Ovarian Origin	155
4.5	Amenorrhoea of Adrenal Origin	160
4.6	Disorders of the Genital Outflow Tract	161
4.7	Vaginal Bleeding and Vaginal Discharge in Childhood	166
4.8	Vaginal Foreign Body	167
4.9	Neoplasms	167
4.10	Vascular Malformations	168
References		169

U. Das (✉)
Department of Paediatric Endocrinology and Diabetes,
Alder Hey Children's Hospital NHS Foundation Trust,
Liverpool, UK
e-mail: urmi.das@alderhey.nhs.uk

G. S. Mann
Department of Paediatric Radiology,
Alder Hey Children's Hospital NHS Foundation Trust,
Liverpool, UK

Abstract

Disorders of menstruation in adolescents are the second most common symptom group after vulvovaginitis and pelvic discharge referred to the paediatric and adolescent gynaecology service. In general, menstrual disorders and problems related to pelvic discharge are benign and self-limiting and diagnostic imaging is not routinely required. However, a number of important conditions merit further clinical evaluation. This chapter considers the role of diagnostic imaging in these disorders.

Abbreviations

PCOS	Polycystic ovarian syndrome
LCH	Langerhans cell histiocytosis
E2	E2-Oestradiol
GnRH	Gonadotropin-Releasing Hormone
TSH	Thyroid-stimulating hormone
TFT	Thyroid function tests
IHH	Idiopathic Hypogonadotropic Hypogonadism
MFO	Multifollicular ovary
ICA	Internal carotid artery
PTHP	Post traumatic hypopituitarism
TBI	Traumatic brain injury
RCC	Rathke's cleft cyst
NIH	National Institute of Health
ESHRE	European Society for Reproduction and Embryology
ASRM	American Society for Reproductive Medicine
AES	Androgen Excess Society
PCO	Polycystic ovary morphology
POF	Premature ovarian failure

G. Mann et al. (eds.), *Imaging of Gynecological Disorders in Infants and Children*, Medical Radiology. Diagnostic Imaging, DOI: 10.1007/174_2010_123, © Springer-Verlag Berlin Heidelberg 2012

POI	Primary ovarian insufficiency
BPES	Blepharophimosis-ptosis-epicanthus inversus syndrome
FMRI	Fragile X Mental Retardation-1 gene
NCAH	Nonclassic Congenital Adrenal Hyperplasia
CAH	Congenital Adrenal Hyperplasia
ACT	Adrenocortical tumours
MEN 1	Multiple Endocrine Neoplasia type 1
IVC	Inferior vena cava
MRKH	Mayer-Rokitansky–Küster–Hauser
MURCS	Müllerian duct aplasia, Renal dysplasia, Cervical Somite anomalies
CAIS	Congenital androgen insensitivity syndrome
MR	Magnetic Resonance
PAIS	Partial androgen insensitivity syndrome
MAIS	Mild androgen insensitivity syndrome
SPAIR	Spectral Adiabatic Inversion Recovery
TSE	Turbospin Echo
PELVIS	Perineal haemangioma, external genitalia malformations, lipomyelomeningocele, vesicorenal abnormalities, imperforate anus and skin tag
SACRAL	Spinal dysraphism, anogenital anomalies, cutaneous anomalies, and renal and urologic anomalies associated with angioma of lumbosacral localisation)
AR	Androgen receptor
US	Ultrasound
CT	Computed Tomography
MRI	Magnetic Resonance Imaging
StAR	Steroidogenic acute regulatory protein
LH	Luteinising hormone
FSH	Follicle stimulating hormone
DXA	Dual-emission X-ray absorptiometry
AR	Androgen receptor

1 Introduction

Disorders of menstruation in adolescents are the second most common symptom group after vulvovaginitis and pelvic discharge referred to the paediatric and adolescent gynaecology service (Garden 1998). In general, menstrual disorders and problems related to pelvic discharge are benign and self-limiting and diagnostic imaging is not routinely required. However, a number of important conditions merit further clinical evaluation. This chapter considers the role of diagnostic imaging in these disorders.

2 Menstrual Disorders

Menarche, the onset of menstrual bleeding represents a key milestone in female development heralding the onset of reproductive maturity and the near completion of physical growth. The onset of menstruation is an extremely salient and intensely experienced event in the life of an adolescent (Koff and Rierdan 1996) and any change in menstrual pattern can evoke extreme anxiety.

Following menarche menstrual cycles are frequently anovulatory due to immaturity of the hypothalamic-pituitary-ovarian axis and it takes 2–5 years for regular cycles to be established. (Legro et al. 2000; Apter et al. 1978). Normal menstrual periods occur cyclically at intervals of between 18 and 40 days.

Disorders of menstruation in adolescence are commonplace. Frequently menstrual periods may be heavy or painful (dysmenorrhoea). Menstruation may be irregular (oligomenorrhoea) or absent (amenorrhoea). It is important to remember that any perceived abnormality of menstruation could be associated with an intrauterine or extrauterine pregnancy. Dysfunctional uterine bleeding is a heterogeneous disorder in which there is abnormal uterine bleeding in the absence of an underlying structural abnormality or organic pathology. A classification of menstrual bleeding disorders in adolescents is outlined in Table 1.

3 Amenorrhoea

Amenorrhoea is the absence or cessation of menstruation and is a manifestation of an underlying clinical disorder which requires further evaluation.

3.1 Definitions and Summary of Causes

Amenorrhoea is traditionally classified according to the timing of onset and subdivided into primary and

Table 1 Classification of menstrual disorders in adolescents

Disorder	Description	Pathologies
Amenorrhoea	Primary—absence of menstruation Secondary—cessation of menstruation	Summarised in Table 2.
Hypomenorrhoea	Decreased volume or duration of flow of menstrual bleeding (usually assessed by tampon usage) occurring at regular intervals	Physiologic—early postmenarchal menses Psychogenic—stress Premature ovarian failure Endocrine (hypothyroid, prolactinoma) Uterine (hypoplasia, synechiae) Cervical stenosis Oral contraceptives Polycystic ovarian syndrome (PCOS)
Oligomenorrhoea	Irregular menstrual bleeding occurring at intervals exceeding 35 days	Complication of pregnancy Functional ovarian cysts PCOS
Hypermenorrhoea (Menorrhagia)	Increased volume or duration of flow of menstrual bleeding occurring at time of regular menstrual cycle	Endometrial pathology (polyp, endometritis) Anovulation Oligoovulation Blood dyscrasia Hypothyroidism
Metrorrhagia	Variable volume (not excessive) of uterine bleeding occurring frequently at irregular intervals	Complication of pregnancy Anovulation Oligoovulation Blood dyscrasia Wide differential of benign and malignant pelvic pathology Hypothyroidism
Menometrorrhagia	Prolonged or excessive bleeding at irregular intervals	As metrorrhagia
Dysfunctional uterine bleeding	Abnormal uterine bleeding in the absence of organic disease	
Polymenorrhoea	Abnormal frequency of menstrual periods occurring at short intervals of less than 21 days duration	Psychogenic—stress Sexually transmitted diseases Endometriosis
Dsymenorrhoea	Painful period	
Intermenstrual bleeding	Uterine bleeding between regular menstrual cycles	Anovulation Oligoovulation Wide differential of benign and malignant pelvic pathology
Postcoital bleeding	Bleeding following sexual intercourse	Usually indicative of cervical pathology
Cryptomenorrhoea	Presence of menstrual symptoms in the absence of visible menstruation	Obstruction of the genital outflow tract

secondary amenorrhoea. A wide range of pathologies present as either primary or secondary amenorrhoea.

The term 'primary amenorrhoea' is applied to patients who have never have had a menstrual period. Primary amenorrhoea is defined as the absence of menstruation by 16 years of age in the presence of normal secondary sexual characteristics or by 14 years of age when there are no visible secondary sexual characteristics. This definition of primary amenorrhoea is two standard deviations from the mean age when secondary sexual characteristics and menstruation should normally occur. The median age of menarche is between 12 and 13 years, and the mean interval between thelarche and menarche is approximately 2 years. About 90% of females menstruate by the time they have attained Tanner stage 4 breast and pubic hair development. Inevitably there is overlap in the discussion of primary amenorrhoea with aetiologies which preclude menstrual outflow (Structural Abnormalities of the Female Reproductive Tract), disorders of sexual differentiation (Disorders of Sex Development) and pubertal delay (Delayed and precocious puberty). Guidelines for the investigation of primary amenorrhoea recommend that girls/young women who have not menstruated by the age or 15 years or within 5 years of thelarche should be investigated (Herman-Giddens et al. 1997).

The term 'secondary amenorrhoea' is applied to those who have experienced menarche but have had no menstrual bleeds for at least three consecutive months and who are not pregnant or breast feeding. Secondary amenorrhoea occurs more commonly than primary amenorrhoea and many of the causes of secondary amenorrhoea may also present as primary amenorrhoea. The principle causes of amenorrhoea by anatomical compartment are summarised in Table 2. Thyroid dysfunction and hyperprolactinaemia are more common causes of secondary amenorrhoea. Ovarian failure, lesions of the hypothalamic-pituitary axis including eating disorders and hyperandrogenic states such as polycystic ovarian syndrome (PCOS) are less common.

Table 2 Summary of principle causes of amenorrhoea by anatomic compartment

Hypothalamic	Excessive weight loss/exercise
	Constitutional delay in growth and puberty†
	Anorexia nervosa/bulimia nervosa
	Tumour
	Kallmann syndrome†
	Infiltration—Langerhans cell histiocytosis (LCH), tuberculosis, sarcoidosis, Wegener's granulomatosis
	Irradiation
Pituitary gland	Tumour (adenoma/macroprolactinoma)
	Idiopathic
	Empty sella syndrome
	Drug induced hyperprolactinaemia
	Infiltration—LCH, haemosiderosis
	Hypophysitis—granulomatous, lymphocytic, xanthomatous
	Abscess
	Sheehan's syndrome
	Irradiation
	Resection
	Traumatic brain injury
Thyroid gland	Hypothyroidism
	Hyperthyroidism
Adrenal	Tumour
	Virilising congenital adrenal hyperplasia
	Nonclassical congenital adrenal hyperplasia
	Lipoid congenital adrenal hyperplasia
	Cushing disease
	Addison disease
Ovarian	Polycystic ovarian syndrome
	Premature ovarian failure
	Gonadal agenesis/dysgenesis†
	Autoimmune oophoritis
	Oopherectomy
	Torsion
	Irradiation
	Gonadotoxic drugs
Uterine	Agenesis†
	Synechiae (Asherman's syndrome)
	Pregnancy
	Hysterectomy

(continued)

3.2 History and Examination

A thorough history and clinical examination of a girl with primary and secondary amenorrhoea may point the underlying cause and help to target relevant clinical and radiological investigation. To establish

Table 2 (continued)

Cervical	Agenesis†
	Stenosis
Vagina	Agenesis†
	Transverse septum†
	Imperforate hymen†
	Foreign body
Other	Pregnancy
	Lactation
	Congenital androgen insensitivity syndrome†

† cause of primary amenorrhoea only

the cause of amenorrhoea it is essential to determine whether secondary sexual characteristics are present (Fig. 1); if these are present then pregnancy must first be excluded. The presence of breast development indicates the presence of a functioning hypothalamic-pituitary-gonadal axis.

3.3 Endocrine Investigation

Before imaging is undertaken a number of baseline endocrine investigations should be performed as these will direct further investigations. This should include measurement of LH, FSH, oestradiol, thyroid hormones and prolactin. Androgens should be measured in either serum or urine in patients presenting with clinical features of androgen excess. Cortisol levels should be evaluated in patients with the clinical stigmata of Cushing's syndrome. Gonadotropin and oestradiol levels are low in patients with disorders of the hypothalamus or pituitary (hypogonadotropic hypogonadism). Patients with disorders of the ovary have elevated gonadotropin levels in the presence of low oestradiol levels (hypergonadotropic hypogonadism). Prolactin levels can be elevated in patients with structural abnormalities of the hypothalamic-pituitary axis, and are highest in patients with prolactinomas. Prolactin is also elevated in patients with renal and liver impairment. Iatrogenic hyperprolactinaemia occurs in patients taking a number of mediations including the oral contraceptive pill, antihistamines, antipsychotics, antidepressants, and antihypertensives. Oligomenorrhoeic adolescents with polycystic ovary syndrome have high LH and androgen concentrations and normal concentrations of FSH (Franks 1995; Ehrmann 2005). Patients with structural abnormalities of the reproductive tract have normal endocrine profiles.

4 Specific Causes of Amenorrhoea

4.1 Amenorrhoea of Hypothalamic Origin

4.1.1 Weight/Stress/Exercise/Chronic Illness Related Amenorrhoea

Profound weight loss, malnutrition, stress, chronic ill health or excessive sustained exercise may cause sufficient debilitation to compromise hypothalamic function. Suppression of the hypothalamic-pituitary-ovarian axis results in impaired oestradiol secretion and amenorrhoea associated with immature patterns of LH secretion. Amenorrhoea can occasionally antedate weight loss. Subfertility is commonplace and osteoporosis is a long-term complication.

Eating Disorders

Anorexia nervosa is a complex multifactorial eating disorder consisting of a failure to maintain an adequate body weight, altered body image with a strong aversion to weight gain. Patients with anorexia may present with delayed puberty but more commonly with secondary amenorrhoea following sudden weight loss. Young females between the ages of 15 and 30 years are affected most commonly.

Treatment of anorexia nervosa includes attaining a target body weight, typically expressed as a minimal ideal body mass index, sufficient to enable progress through puberty if pubertal delay is present or resumption of ovulatory menstrual cycles and reproductive potential. Serum oestradiol measures may help to predict return to menstruation; however, the current gold standard for evaluation of a healthy body weight in females with eating disorders is pelvic ultrasound (Treasure et al. 1988; Lai et al. 1994; Key et al. 2002; Mason et al. 2007). Pelvic ultrasound is the best descriptor of pelvic maturity and can be used to estimate the degree of weight gain required in order to achieve resumption of menstruation. An algorithmic approach using pelvic ultrasound findings has been advocated by Mason et al. to assess clinical progress (Mason et al. 2007). As with pubertal disorders, pelvic ultrasound should be used to document

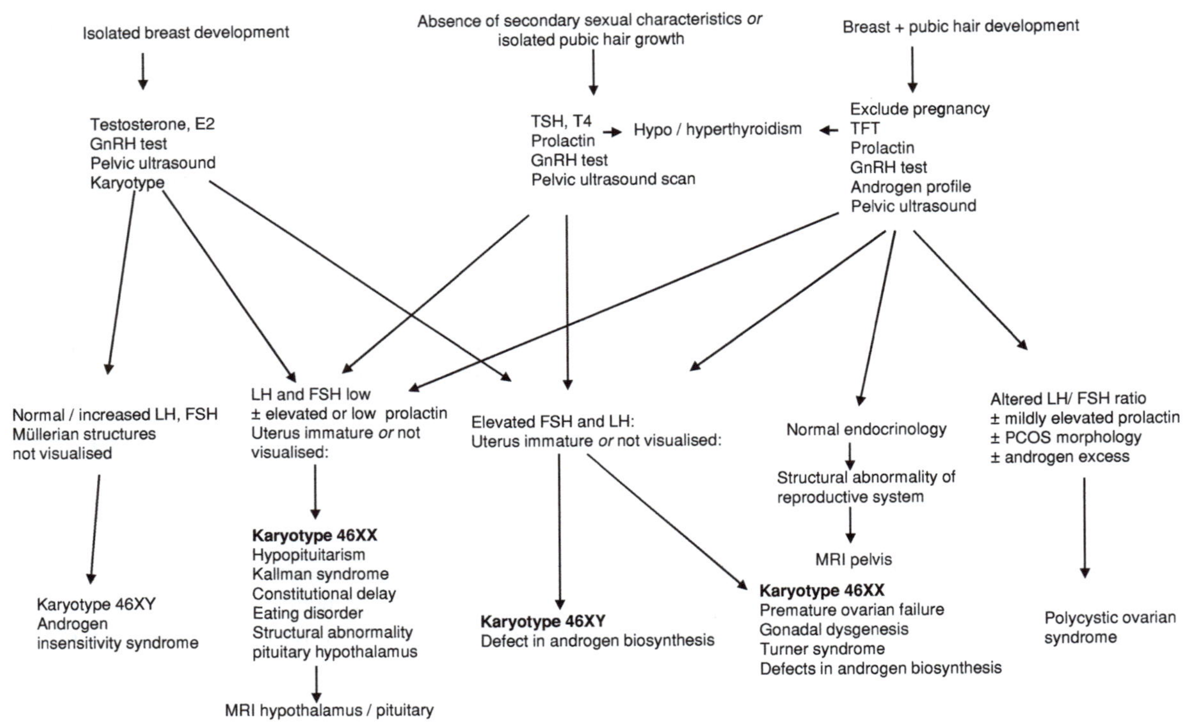

Fig. 1 Investigation of girls with amenorrhoea. Algorithm-diagram for the investigation of amenorrhoea based on the presence, or the absence of secondary sexual characteristics

the size and morphology of the uterus, the thickness and uniformity of the endometrial stripe and the size (preferably volume) and content (stromal and follicular) of the ovaries. Changes in these appearances provide an overview of recent oestradiol levels.

In disorders of weight loss, indicators of hypo-oestrogenism include

- Reduction in uterine length to pre-pubertal dimensions (2.0–3.3 cm) (Buzi et al. 1999).
- Endometrial stripe thickness measuring <3 mm which may be undetectable in the immature pelvis (Shulman et al. 1989; Bakos et al. 1993).
- Changes in ovarian volume and morphology.

Ovarian volume increases throughout pubertal maturation with an increase in stromal volume, follicle count and size. During puberty the ovaries may demonstrate mutlifollicular morphology (Fig. 2) characterised by greater than six follicles of 4 mm in diameter (Adams et al. 1985). Ovarian maturity is attained when a dominant ovarian follicle is demonstrated. An increase of ovarian volume in response to weight gain has been reported in patients with eating disorders (Treasure et al. 1985). Conversely with weight loss ovarian volume diminishes. Ovarian volume $< 2\ cm^3$ is indicative of pelvic immaturity (Mason et al. 2007).

4.1.2 Constitutional Delay of Growth and Puberty

Individuals with constitutionally delayed puberty are characterised by short stature, delayed attainment of secondary sexual characteristics and delayed fusion of the epiphyses but with stable linear bone growth velocity. This results in a delay in the attainment of final height which is within the normal range for the parental heights and a temporary delay in menarche. A positive family history is typical.

4.1.3 Space Occupying Lesions and Infiltration of the Hypothalamus

Space occupying lesions of the hypothalamus are rare but include hamartomas (Fig. 3), Langerhans cell histiocytosis (LCH), astrocytoma, glioma, dermoid and epidermoid cysts. The hypothalamus may be indirectly affected by tumours of pituitary origin (craniopharyngioma, germinoma and suprasellar

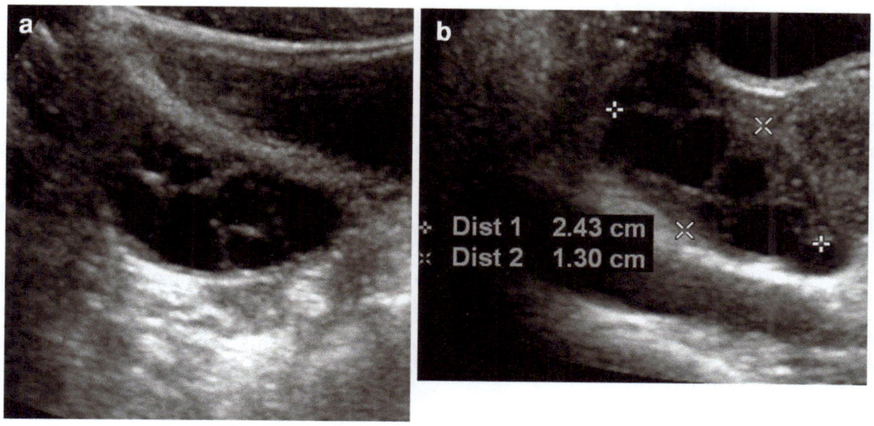

Fig. 2 Multifollicular ovaries. Longitudinal transabdominal images **a** and **b** (between callipers) of multifollicular ovaries (MFO). MFO contain between 6 and 10 follicles per ovary measuring up to 10 mm in diameter, which are distributed throughout the ovary with no stromal hypertrophy

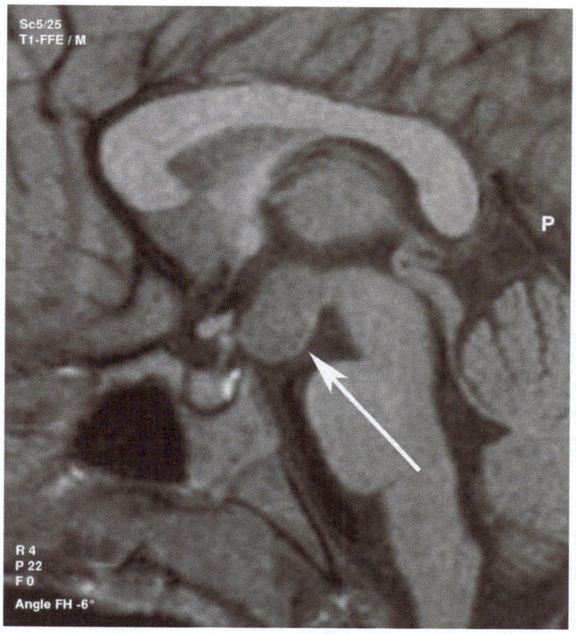

Fig. 3 Hypothalamic hamartoma. Sagittal T1-weighted midline image depicting a large hamartoma (*white arrow*) which is iso-intense to cortical grey matter. This showed no contrast enhancement

Table 3 Comparison of clinical features of hypothalamic and pituitary tumours

	Hypothalamic tumour	Pituitary tumour
Visual field defect	±	±
Cranial nerve palsies	Often	±
Diabetes insipidus	±	±
Anterior pituitary hormone hypersecretion		+
Anterior pituitary hormone hyposecretion	±	±
Hyperprolactinaemia	+	±
Precocious puberty	±	
Autonomic dysfunction	±	

tumours such as an optic glioma). Hypothalamic hamartoma is a rare cause of amenorrhoea and more often a cause of precocious puberty.

The clinical effects of a hypothalamic space occupying lesions relate to mass effect and endocrine dysfunction resulting from destruction of hypothalamic tissue. Associated endocrine dysfunction may include hyperprolactinaemia, anterior pituitary hormone hyposecretion and panhypopituitarism. Symptoms related to mass effect include headache, visual field defect, cranial nerve palsies and disturbance of autonomic functions such as the regulation of appetite, temperature, water–electrolyte metabolism, circulation, emotional state and sleep–wake cycle. A comparison of the clinical features related to hypothalamic and sellar tumours is summarised in Table 3.

4.1.4 Idiopathic Hypogonadotropic Hypogonadism

Idiopathic hypogonadotropic hypogonadism (IHH) is a condition in which the pulsatile secretion of

Table 4 Key diagnostic features of idiopathic hypogonadotropic hypogonadism

Low or normal FSH/LH in the context of low circulating oestrogen (E2 oestradiol levels)
Normal serum ferritin levels
Normal pituitary function
Normal MRI of the pituitary and hypothalamus

Table 5 Causes of hyperprolactinaemia

PROLACTIN ≤ 500–1000 mIU/l	Idiopathic
	Breast feeding
	Hypothyroidism
	Medications (oral contraceptive pill, antihistamine H2 blocker, antipsychotics, antidepressants, antihypertensives)
	Germ cell tumour
	Gonadoblastoma
	Bronchogenic carcinoma, renal carcinoma
	Liver failure
	Renal failure
PROLACTIN > 1000 mIU/L	Empty sella syndrome
	Pituitary adenoma

gonadotropin-releasing hormone (GnRH) from the hypothalamic neurones is absent or abnormal.

Adolescent females present with amenorrhoea. Physical examination reveals little or no breast development (Tanner stage 3 or less). Body habitus is typically eunuchoid (arm span exceeds height by 6 cm or more). Skeletal maturation is usually delayed with an absence of a distinct adolescent pubertal growth spurt but linear growth velocity is preserved. Treatment includes replacement of sex hormones and hormonal induction of fertility. The diagnostic features of IHH are outlined in Table 4.

4.2 Amenorrhoea of Pituitary Origin

4.2.1 Hyperprolactinaemia

Hyperprolactinaemia is the most common pituitary cause of amenorrhoea, but is rarely seen in those presenting with primary amenorrhoea. Numerous causes are recognised which are summarised in Table 5. Tonic inhibition of prolactin secretion from the anterior pituitary gland is mediated by hypothalamic dopamine. Hyperprolactinaemia results from

- Depletion of hypothalamic dopamine (tumour, infiltration, drugs)
- Defective hypothalamic dopamine transport (pituitary stalk lesion)
- Insensitivity of anterior pituitary lactotrophs to dopamine (drugs)
- Stimulation of lactotrophs (seen in primary hypothyroidism due to thyrotropin releasing hormone secretion—this is associated with enlargement of the pituitary gland simulating a pituitary adenoma)

Two specific conditions associated with high levels of prolactin secretion which merit further discussion are pituitary adenomas—specifically prolactinoma and empty sella syndrome.

4.2.2 Pituitary Adenoma

Tumours affecting the pituitary gland of children and adolescents are uncommon, the majority occur in adolescents. Pituitary adenomas may be non-functioning, functioning (hormone-secreting) and classified according to size; micro (< 10 mm) or macro (≥ 10 mm). A particular feature of pituitary adenomas in adolescents is a higher proportion of functional tumours as compared with the adult population.

Prolactinoma

Prolactin secreting tumours (prolactinoma) suppress pulsatile gonadotropin-releasing hormone secretion. Clinical symptoms related to a prolactinoma include pubertal delay, galactorrhoea (30–50%); oligomenorrhoea and weight gain (Steele et al. 2010). This may account for a higher proportion of delayed presentations in males with symptoms principally related to mass effect such as headache, ophthalmoplegia and visual field defect; gynaecomastia is a clue to the diagnosis. In cases where symptoms predominately relate to mass effect a craniopharyngioma may be suspected initially. Persistent elevation of serum prolactin merits investigation with MRI of the brain including dedicated views of the hypothalamic-pituitary axis (Figs. 4 and 5). When a sellar or suprasellar mass lesion is demonstrated it is the authors current practice to obtain at least a limited unenhanced axial CT collimated to include the lesion and pituitary fossa in order to document tumour calcification and bony sellar morphology. First-line treatment is medical with dopamine agonists such as bromocriptine or

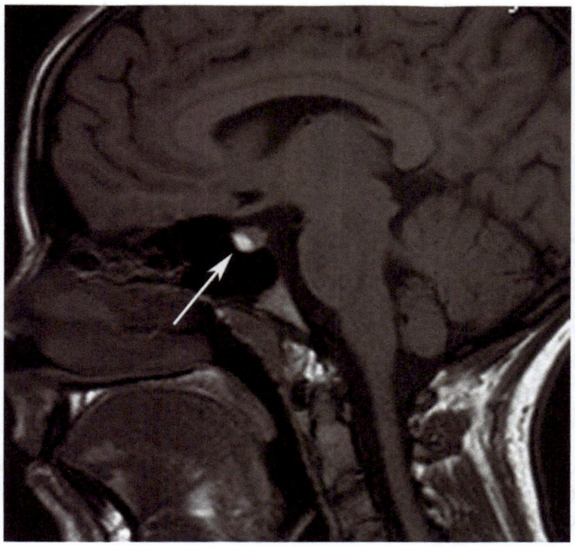

Fig. 4 Prolactinoma. MRI of a pituitary microadenoma. Sagittal T1-gradient echo image showing a discrete hyperintense nodule within the anterior pituitary in a girl with hyperprolactinaemia (*arrow*). Her symptoms abated with dopamine agonist therapy

cabergoline. Radiotherapy, surgery or both is reserved for refractory cases (Gillam et al. 2006; Steele et al. 2010).

Pituitary Apoplexy

Pituitary apoplexy is a well recognised albeit rare condition in children, and results from haemorrhage into and/or infarction related to a pituitary tumour. Tumours are generally macroadenomas. Typical symptoms include sudden-onset severe headache, visual deficit, ophthalmoplegia, impaired consciousness, with or without endocrine dysfunction related to disturbance of the pituitary gland and mass effect upon the hypothalamus (see Table 3) including amenorrhoea and pubertal arrest.

MRI is the investigation of choice. Infarctive pituitary apoplexy is seen as low signal intensity on T1- and T2-weighted MRI sequences. Gadolinium enhanced sequences may show rim enhancement and enhancement of viable tumour but non-enhancement of the infarcted areas (Ostrov et al. 1989). Restricted diffusion in tumours relates to tumour cellularity, but has also been described as a feature of infarctive apoplexy (Rogg et al. 2002). Restricted diffusion does not differentiate from an abscess. MRI appearances of haemorrhagic pituitary apoplexy are variable but tend to follow a predictable course. In the acute phase (Days 1–2), haemorrhage is typically high signal intensity on T1-weighted images and of low signal intensity on T2-weighted images (Bonneville et al. 2006). In sub-acute haemorrhage (Days 3–15) signal intensity changes evolve result from degradation of haemoglobin into methaemoglobin, with high signal on both T1- and T2-weighted sequences. Beyond 15 days sedimentation of blood products may result in a fluid level within the mass, a feature that is highly suggestive of haemorrhagic pituitary apoplexy (Piotin et al. 1990).

4.2.3 Empty sella Turcica

In this disorder intrasellar herniation of suprasellar subarachnoid space results from a deficient diaphragma sellae (Fig. 6). The primary form rarely gives rise to endocrine disturbance. Secondary empty sella turcica is a rare complication of surgery or radiotherapy. Anterior pituitary hormone deficiencies may result with associated slowing of growth and failure of pubertal development or pubertal arrest. The regulation of cortisol and thyroid hormones may also be disturbed. Imaging reveals a cerebrospinal fluid filled sella with no visible anterior or posterior pituitary tissue. The pituitary stalk typically extends into the floor of the sella.

4.2.4 Infiltrative Lesions

Inflammatory lesions of the pituitary gland (hypophysitis) are rare and mimic pituitary tumours based on their clinical and imaging features. Aetiologies are classified as lymphocytic (Langerhan's cell histiocytosis, ruptured Rathke's cleft cyst) (Fig. 7), granulomatous (Sarcoidosis, Wegener's granulomatosis, tuberculous) and xanthomatous based on histopathologic findings. These subtypes are indistinguishable on imaging. Other infiltrative lesions of the pituitary gland include non-Hodgkin's lymphoma and leukaemia. Symptoms range from headache, diabetes insipidus, visual disturbance, anterior pituitary dysfunction and amenorrhoea/galactorrhoea syndrome. Treatment relates to the specific underlying cause.

4.2.5 Traumatic Brain Injury

Post traumatic hypopituitarism (PTHP) has been recognised for many years. More than 50 years ago autopsy data from 102 patients who succumbed to severe head injuries reported haemorrhage and

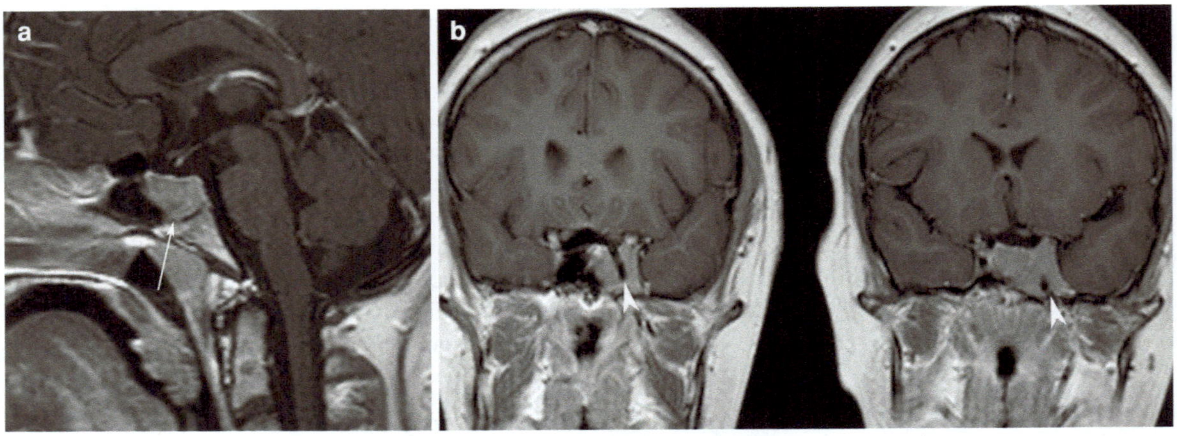

Fig. 5 Invasive prolactinoma. **a** Sagittal and **b** coronal enhanced T1 weighted MRI showing a left sided pituitary adenoma that has eroded the sella floor (*arrow*) and encased the cavernous segment of the left internal carotid artery (ICA) (*arrowhead*). As tumour lies lateral to the left ICA, tumour extension into the left cavernous sinus is implied

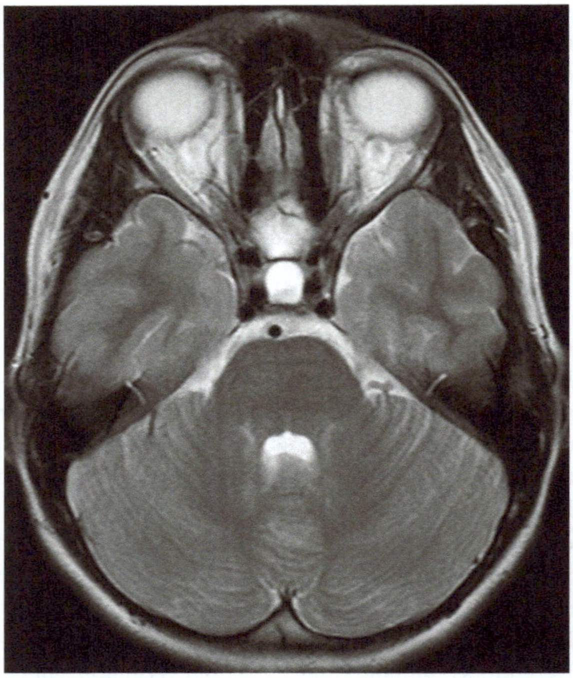

Fig. 6 Empty sella. Axial T2-weighted MRI showing absence of anterior and posterior pituitary tissue

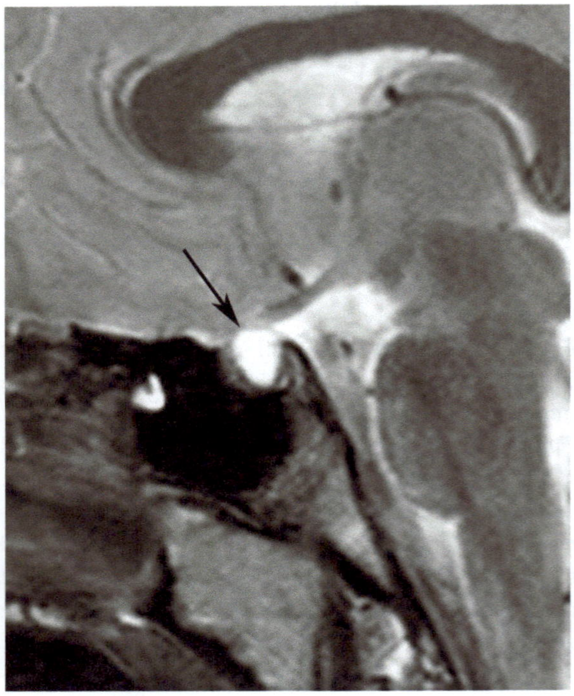

Fig. 7 Rathke's cleft cyst (RCC). Sagittal T2-weighted MR image of an iso-intense cyst (*black arrow*) seen arising in the typical location for an RCC in the pars intermedia between the anterior pituitary and posterior pituitary bright spot

necrosis of the pituitary stalk in 27 and 6% of subjects, respectively, of the anterior pituitary in 4 and 22% of subjects, respectively, and haemorrhage of the posterior pituitary was reported in 20% of subjects (Ceballos 1966). However, it is only in recent years that prospective studies have started to define the prevalence and natural history of the condition in adult life. Data reporting outcomes following traumatic brain injury (TBI) in children are now being reported, however, data from robust prospective studies are yet to become available.

In general somatotropes (growth hormone producing cells), appear to be most vulnerable to injury and growth hormone deficiency is reported more commonly than other anterior pituitary hormones. Gonadotropes are also vulnerable to injury and transient hypogonadotropic amenorrhoea (low FSH and LH) has been described following TBI (Cytowic et al. 1986). Recovery of gonadotrope function appears to be the rule. In a study of 52 adult subjects gonadotropin deficiency was reported 20 subjects in the acute phase, but persisted in only two patients 1 year following injury. However, a further two subjects, with normal gonadotropin deficiency at the time of injury, became gonadotropin deficient in the first year following injury (Tanriverdi et al. 2006). Deficiencies of TSH and ACTH are reported less frequently (Blair 2010). Precocious puberty has been reported in relation to TBI (Blendonohy and Philip 1991). Data from paediatric studies suggest that the prevalence of PTHP in childhood is lower than in adult life (Khadr et al. 2010; Moon et al. 2010).

There are few detailed studies describing the imaging findings in PTHP and these are confined to adults. These retrospective reviews of patient cohorts rely on a history recalling TBI as a cause of PTHP. In a comprehensive review of the literature reported between 1970 and 1998, Benvenga et al. (2000) identified a total of 367 cases where anterior pituitary dysfunction was reported. The diagnostic imaging findings of 76 cases with PTHP whom under went CT and/or MRI was reviewed. The most common findings were haemorrhage of the hypothalamus (29%) which would account for the high incidence of diabetes insipidus following TBI, haemorrhage of the posterior pituitary lobe (26%) and haemorrhage of the posterior pituitary lobe (25%). These findings would result in increased pituitary volume in the acute phase of TBI. Other findings included pituitary stalk interruption (4%) and infarction of the posterior pituitary (1.3%). Pituitary infarction may eventually manifest as an empty sella or Rathke's cleft cyst.

4.3 Thyroid Dysfunction

In adolescents with hypothyroidism LH and FSH levels are normal but a raised TSH may stimulate hyperprolactinaemia. Hyperthyroidism may present with primary or secondary amenorrhoea.

4.4 Amenorrhoea of Ovarian Origin

4.4.1 Polycystic Ovarian Syndrome

Polycystic ovarian syndrome is a common endocrinopathy with heterogenic manifestations and multiple diagnostic criteria. The aetiology of PCOS is uncertain. Approximately 5–10% of women of reproductive age are affected.

Clinical Features

PCOS presents in adolescence and is characterised by features of menstrual dysfunction with anovulation or oligoovulation leading to amenorrhoea, oligomenorrhoea and irregular menstrual cycles. This is combined with signs and symptoms of androgen excess including hirsutism, acne and male pattern alopecia. Hirsutism of PCOS is usually slowly progressive. Sudden-onset or rapidly progressive hirsutism and/or virilisation should prompt consideration of an alternate diagnosis such as a virilising adrenal or ovarian tumour or a disorder of sexual differentiation. PCOS is a disorder of folliculogenesis. Affected individuals are usually subfertile and fail to develop dominant ovarian follicles.

Metabolic derangements associated with PCOS are collectively referred to as the 'metabolic syndrome'. These include insulin resistance, hyperinsulinaemia, dyslipidaemia and impaired glucose tolerance with an increased risk of developing type 2 diabetes. A high proportion of patients are centrally obese and hypertension occurs with increased frequency. These factors increase the long-term risk of significant cardiovascular complications and early identification and management of these risk factors is important.

Diagnostic Criteria

No precise definition of PCOS exists. Various expert groups have convened and published consensus diagnostic criteria. These are summarised in Table 6. The first established in 1990 by the National Institute of Health (NIH) (Zawadski and Dunaif 1992) concentrated on the clinical and biochemical features of PCOS with no specific criteria related to diagnostic imaging. More recent consensus guidelines recognise the improvements in ultrasound technology which can reliably depict the characteristic morphological changes in the ovaries seen in PCOS, these features referred to as 'polycystic ovarian morphology'(PCO) are discussed below. The 2003 Rotterdam criteria, co-

Table 6 Summary of published diagnostic ultrasound criteria for polycystic ovarian syndrome

	NIH consensus criteria (1990)	Rotterdam (ESHRE/ASRM) criteria (2003)	AES criteria (2006)
Inclusion criteria	All the following criteria:	2 of 3 of the following criteria:	All the following criteria:
	Chronic anovulation	Oligoovulation and/or anovulation	Ovarian dysfunction: oligoovulation and/ or polycystic ovarian morphology
	Clinical and/or biochemical features of hyperandrogenism	Clinical and/or biochemical features of hyperandrogenism	Hyperandrogenism (hirsutism and/or
		Imaging criteria for polycystic ovarian morphology	Hyperandrogenaemia)
Exclusion criteria:	Other causes of amenorrhoea and hyperandrogenism		
Reference	(Zawadski and Dunaif 1992)	(ESHRE/ASRM 2004)	(Azziz et al. 2006)

Table 7 Published ultrasound criteria for diagnosis of polycystic ovarian morphology

Source	Ultrasound modality	Number of follicles	Follicular diameter (mm)	Ovarian volume (cm^3)
Balen et al. 2003 (widely used in clinical practice)	Trans-vaginal	12 or more	2–9	> 10 Ovarian area acceptable surrogate marker
Jonard et al. 2003	Trans-vaginal	12 or more	2–9	
Adams et al. 1985	Trans-abdominal	10 or more	2–8	

hosted by the European Society for Reproduction and Embryology and the American Society for Reproductive Medicine ESHRE/ASRM (2004) require any two of the following three criteria: menstrual dysfunction, androgen excess or ultrasound features to be present. Using the Rotterdam criteria the diagnosis may be made in females with

- Normal ovulatory cycles, but polycystic ovaries on ultrasound and hyperandrogenism (Ovulatory PCOS)
- Irregular cycles and polycystic ovaries on ultrasound, but with no evidence of hyperandrogenism/ androgen excess
- Irregular cycles and hyperandrogenism/androgen excess

PCO morphology need only be demonstrated in a single ovary in order to fulfil the ultrasound criteria.

The Androgen Excess Society diagnostic criteria (Azziz et al. 2006) require the presence of androgen excess with menstrual dysfunction and/or ultrasound changes. All of these criteria assume that other causes of menstrual dysfunction and androgen excess have been excluded including nonclassical congenital adrenal hyperplasia (21-hydroxylase deficiency), virilising androgen-secreting ovarian or adrenal neoplasm, Cushing's syndrome, hyperprolactinaemia, prolactinoma, primary hypothyroidism, acromegaly and simple obesity with early postmenarchal physiologic anovulation.

Imaging in PCOS

Sonographic criteria for the diagnosis of polycystic ovary morphology (PCO) were established by Adams et al. (1985). PCO was defined on any single image plane as an ovary comprising of multiple cysts between 2 and 18 mm in diameter which are evenly distributed around the periphery accompanied by an increased quantity of ovarian stroma (Table 7) (Fig. 8). It should be noted that multifollicular ovaries can be a normal finding in adolescence (Fig 2).

Transvaginal ultrasound is a highly sensitive and specific tool for depicting PCO. Transvaginal ultrasound is not widely utilised in the adolescent population as most girls are virginal. Transabdominal ultrasound is limited by the inability to visualise one or both ovaries in up to 20% of patients. Transabdominal US performs poorly in obese patients.

The Rotterdam consensus criteria recognise PCOS is a functional disorder and that the presence or

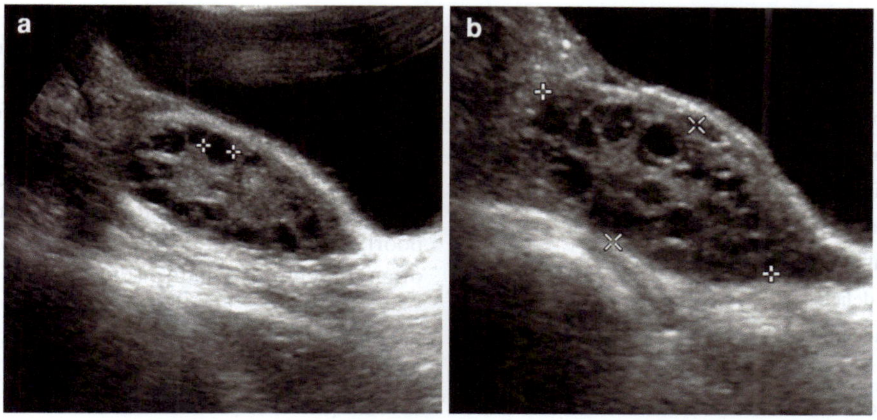

Fig. 8 Polycystic ovaries. **a** Longitudinal sonogram of an ovary demonstrating polycystic ovary (PCO) morphology. **b** PCO (between callipers) showing the classical peripheral 'necklace' distribution of small follicles. The presence of abundant stroma accounts for increased ovarian volume

absence of PCO alone does not establish or exclude a diagnosis of PCOS (Rotterdam ESHRE/ASRM 2004). Revised ultrasound criteria for the diagnosis of PCO were proposed in 2003 (summarised in Table 7) and are defined by the presence of one of the following: either 12 or more follicles measuring 2–9 mm in diameter or an increased ovarian volume (10 cm^3) (Balen et al. 2003). As ovarian size is calculated using a formula for a prolate ellipse the presence of a single follicle exceeding 10 mm in diameter should prompt a repeat scan at a time of ovarian quiescence in order to provide a more accurate calculation of volume and area, with area considered an adequate surrogate marker for volume (Balen et al. 2003). Alternative sonographic criteria for PCO have also been described and are summarised in Table 7.

The 'string of pearls' peripheral distribution of ovarian follicles, ovarian stromal hyperechogenicity and increased stromal volume are all specific markers of PCO but are not included in the Rotterdam consensus guideline statement on ultrasound imaging.

Controversies in Diagnosing PCOS in Adolescents

The diagnosis of PCOS in adolescence is particularly challenging. Although there are clearly developed consensus guidelines, the application of these to the adolescent girl is troublesome for the following reasons:

- There is a paucity of normative data describing androgen levels in perimenarchal and early postmenarchal girls.
- Physiologic anovulation commonly occurs in the first 2 years following menarche and it is difficult differentiate this from PCOS. Acne and hirsutism are common complaints in otherwise healthy adolescents.
- Reliance on the transabdominal ultrasound approach in most adolescents.

4.4.2 Premature Ovarian Failure/Primary Ovarian Insufficiency

Premature ovarian failure (POF) is a condition which affects women under the age of 40 years and is characterised by amenorrhoea of at least 4 months duration, hypooestrogenism and hypergonadotropinism (elevated FSH) (Rebar 2008). POF is a heterogeneous disorder which is also referred to as premature menopause, primary ovarian insufficiency (POI), hypergonadotropic amenorrhoea, hypergonadotropic hypogonadism and hypergonadotropic failure. The incidence of POF in women under 20 years is around 1 in 10,000.

POF results from either a reduction in the initial number of primordial ovarian follicles, an increase in germ cell apoptosis, premature ovarian follicular destruction or follicular dysfunction. POF may be associated with intermittent follicular development, ovulation and menstrual bleeding.

The cause of POF in most girls is rarely identified. Common causes which should be sought include X-chromosomal abnormalities, fragile X premutations and autoimmune causes (Welt 2008). The main causes of POF are summarised in Table 8.

Table 8 Causes of ovarian insufficiency and premature ovarian failure

Idiopathic
Familial (autosomal and X-linked dominant)
Infection—tuberculosis, mumps, cytomegalovirus, herpes
Gonadal dysgenesis
Turner syndrome 45,X and 45,X/46,XY mosaicism
46,XY gonadal dysgenesis (Swyer syndrome)
17-hydroxylase deficiency
Fragile X premutations
Trisomy X
Balanced X chromosome translocations
Gonadotropin receptor gene mutations
Autoimmune oophoritis
Polyglandular failure Type I (mucocutaneous candidiasis and hypoparathyroidism)/Polyglandular failure Type II (adrenal insufficiency and other autoimmune disease)
Chemotherapy
Pelvic irradiation
Surgery including gonadectomy
Ovarian torsion
DiGeorge syndrome
Galactosaemia
Thalassaemia
Rare syndromic causes
Congenital disorders of glycosylation
Blepharophimosis-ptosis-epicanthus inversus syndrome (BPES)
Pseudohypoparathyroidism Type Ia

Gonadal Dysgenesis

Gonadal dysgenesis refers to a range of conditions in individuals with a female phenotype and dysgenetic or 'streak' gonads. The Müllerian structures are intact. These disorders include Turner syndrome, 45,X/46,XY mixed gonadal dysgenesis and pure gonadal dysgenesis. The principal endocrine manifestation is pubertal delay. Occasionally presentations may be delayed with a clinical picture of primary amenorrhoea.

Turner Syndrome

Turner syndrome (Ullrich–Turner syndrome) occurs in females with an absent or structurally abnormal second X chromosome. Premature ovarian failure occurs commonly. Girls with Turner syndrome have a normal complement of primordial follicles in early fetal life which are typically depleted by the first decade of life due to accelerated apoptosis. Premature ovarian failure results in a hypooestrogenic state with elevated FSH levels. On ultrasound the uterus is immature and lacks a definable endometrial stripe. The ovaries are small, poorly vascularised, dysplastic, lack follicles and are often difficult to visualise (Fig. 9).

Fragile X Premutations

Fragile X syndrome is an X-linked, trinucleotide-CGG repeat disease. More than 200 triplet repeats of the Fragile X Mental Retardation-1 gene (FMR1 Xq27.3) results in the full syndrome with clinical features including developmental delay, autism and mental retardation. Female carriers of the FMR1 premutation (between 55 and 200 CGG repeats) are at increased risk of POF, with earlier menopause occurring in proportion to an increasing number of triplet repeats.

Chemotherapy and Radiotherapy

Acute ovarian failure and POF are recognised complications of ovarian exposure to radiation therapy and chemotherapy particularly alkylating agents (Sklar et al. 2006; Chemaitilly et al. 2006) (Fig. 10). The depletion of the non-renewable reserve of primordial ovarian follicles has been evaluated in a cohort of adult survivors of childhood cancer treated with radiotherapy and alkylating agents. Ovarian functional reserve in cancer survivors was compared to age matched controls (Larsen et al. 2003) using antral follicle counts and ovarian volumes obtained by ultrasound in the early follicular phase of the menstrual cycle (days 3–5). Cancer survivors had an advanced ovarian age with POI observed even in those with spontaneous menstrual cycles. Cranial irradiation above 30 GY is known to cause hypogonadotropic hypogonadism (Sklar 1999).

Autosomal Gene Mutations Causing Follicle Dysfunction

Gonadotropin receptor defects cause failure of normal ovarian follicle growth. Autosomal recessive FSH receptor gene mutations result in primary amenorrhoea, elevated FSH levels with small ovaries. Gene mutations resulting in LH receptor inactivation are a cause of primary amenorrhoea in girls.

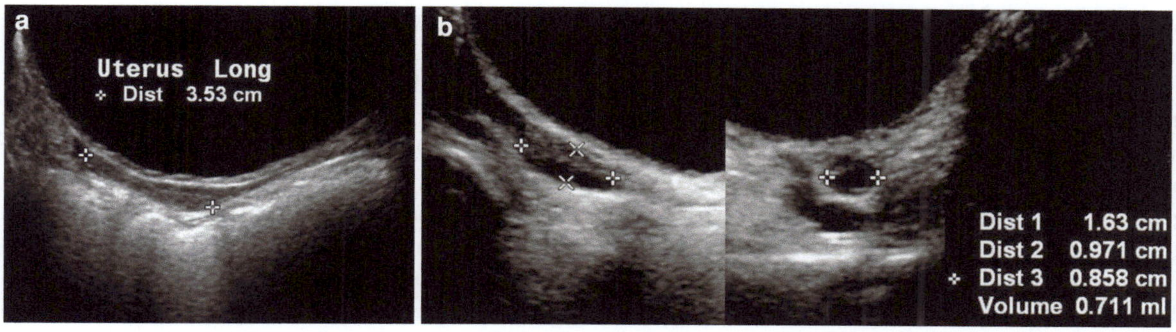

Fig. 9 Turner syndrome. **a** Longitudinal ultrasound scan in a 15-year-old 45,X0 girl with an infantile tubular uterus. **b** Composite ultrasound imaging for ovarian volume calculation. The ovaries are 'streak' and of small volume showing scant follicles

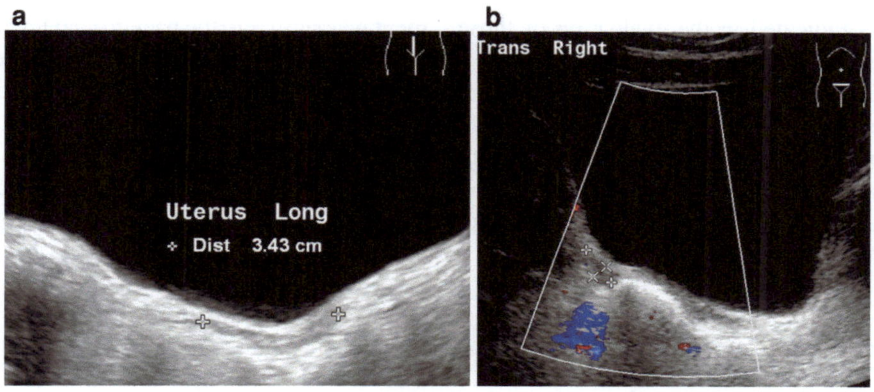

Fig. 10 Premature ovarian failure following prior busulphan chemotherapy for haematological malignancy. **a** Longitudinal ultrasound scan in a 16 year-old with an immature tubular uterus, a faint endometrial echo is just visible. **b** The right ovary is barely visible and of small volume showing no discernible follicle

Autoimmune Oophoritis

Up to 10% of cases POF are associated with autoimmunity or adrenal insufficiency related to an autoimmune oophoritis. Autoimmune ovarian failure resulting from premature follicle destruction may occur in both polyglandular syndrome type I and type II. Type I polyglandular syndrome presents in childhood with mucocutaneous candidiasis, hypoparathyroidism and Addison's disease and is accompanied by POI in 60% of cases. Polyglandular failure type II is characterised by adrenal insufficiency and hypothyroidism, occurring largely in adult women with POI occurring in only around 10% of cases (Hoek et al. 1997).

Beta-Thalassaemia Major

In a small prospective study of 31 adolescent females with beta-thalassemia major; a high proportion (42%) presented with delayed puberty. Hypothalamic ovarian pituitary axis dysfunction was found in 48 and 39% had hypogonadotropic hypogonadism. Ovarian failure occurred in 16% of patients. High levels of serum ferritin and pituitary iron overload was deemed to be the cause of ovarian failure (Al-Rimawi et al. 2005).

Clinical Investigation of Premature Ovarian Insufficiency

The diagnosis of POF is confirmed by serum FSH more than 40 mu/L on at least two occasions, at least 1 month apart. This disease may have a fluctuating course with high FSH levels returning to normal. Ovulatory function may be subsequently regained. LH levels are also elevated but FSH is usually disproportionately higher than LH. Serum oestradiol levels are typically low. Additional investigation should include karyotype, thyroid function, adrenal and thyroid autoantibody and FMR1 premutation screening.

Imaging Studies in Ovarian Insufficiency
In POI pelvic ultrasonography is useful to document ovarian morphology (streak gonad in gonadal dysgenesis) and to identify multifollicular ovaries suggesting a diagnosis of autoimmune oophoritis.

In secondary POI imaging should be focussed on the likely underlying cause. If thyroid dysfunction is suspected then investigation should begin with clinical and endocrine evaluation. Neck ultrasound and, if appropriate, thyroid scintigraphy should be considered. Cranial MRI to assess the pituitary fossa and hypothalamus is indicated in the evaluation of those with persisting headache which is unfortunately a rather non-specific and fairly common symptom but should be undertaken promptly if there is visual field defect, hyperprolactinaemia or amenorrhoea with unexplained marked oestrogen deficiency. Evaluation of bone mineral density in adolescents with POI is not established clinical practice.

4.5 Amenorrhoea of Adrenal Origin

4.5.1 Non-classical Congenital Adrenal Hyperplasia

Congenital adrenal hyperplasia (CAH) are a group of monogenic disorders, inherited as autosomal recessive traits in which the adrenocortical enzymes responsible for the production of cortisol from cholesterol are deficient. The most common enzymatic defect is deficiency of 21-hydroxylase due to a mutation of the CYP21A2 gene. This principally results in the classical form of CAH characterised by virilisation with or without salt wasting but in around 5–10% of cases a nonclassic form of congenital adrenal hyperplasia (NCAH) is present.

NCAH is seen in individuals with signs and symptoms of hyperandrogenism. Clinical features include advanced bone age, early pubic hair (premature adrenarche/pubarche), precocious puberty, initial accelerated growth velocity with premature growth arrest in childhood, cystic acne, hirsutism, male pattern alopecia, menstrual disorders (menstrual irregularity, primary or secondary amenorrhoea) and subfertility. NCAH can be asymptomatic. There is a higher incidence of females with NCAH giving birth to offspring with the classical form of CAH. Rapid onset or progressive hirsutism should alert to the possibility of Cushing's syndrome or a virilising tumour.

Sonography of the adrenal glands show diffuse enlargement without fat deposition or focal nodular changes. The role of imaging is to exclude virilising adrenal or gonadal tumours. Ovarian adrenal rest tumours are rare (Russo et al. 1998). On ultrasound adrenal rest tumours within the ovary may be difficult to differentiate from cystic ovarian tissue (Stikkelbroeck et al. 2003). Polycystic ovarian morphology (Fig. 8) has been described in CAH with wide variation in the reported prevalence. The prevalence in a small retrospective case series of CAH under treatment was similar to the background level in the general population of 15% (Stikkelbroeck et al. 2004). However, the highest reported prevalence of PCO was up to 85% (Hague et al. 1990) in adult CAH patients with 21-hydroxylase deficiency with a lower prevalence in younger patients. It is important to exclude NCAH in any individual with clinical and/or imaging features of PCOS.

4.5.2 Lipoid Congenital Adrenal Hyperplasia

Lipoid congenital adrenal hyperplasia (lipoid CAH) is a severe and extremely rare form of CAH in which adrenal and gonadal steroidogenesis is defective due to mutations of the steroidogenic acute regulatory (StAR) protein. The inheritance pattern is autosomal recessive. The condition is often fatal if undiagnosed in early life due to salt wasting.

Affected infants usually have a normal 46,XY male karyotype; however, the external genitalia are female in appearance due to impaired testosterone synthesis. Müllerian structures are absent due to the presence of anti-Müllerian hormone. Subsequently there is a conspicuous lack of pubertal development with primary amenorrhoea. 46,XX subjects with lipoid CAH develop Müllerian structures and undergo spontaneous feminisation with breast development and no delay in puberty. Cyclical vaginal bleeding coincides with the timing of puberty.

The diagnostic imaging features relate to the presence of fat accumulation within the adrenal glands. Fat accumulation on ultrasound may be difficult to visualise in infants and non-visualisation of the adrenal glands may be clue to the diagnosis. CT or preferably MRI will demonstrate preferential accumulation of fat in the enlarged adrenal cortices with normal medullary size and architecture. (Kohda et al. 2006). Polycystic ovarian morphology may be seen.

4.5.3 Adrenal Tumour

Adrenocortical tumours (ACT) are rare in children. The endocrine manifestations of ACT include virilisation and less commonly hypercortisolaemia (slow growth, obesity with centripetal fat distribution, acne, hirsutism, striae, amenorrhoea). Primary hyperaldosteronism (Conn's syndrome) is extremely rare in childhood and adolescence. The clinical features of virilisation vary but range from premature pubarche, prepubertal breast development, hypertrophy of the clitoris, acne, weight gain, deepening of the voice and accelerated growth velocity. Atypical congenital adrenal hyperplasia is a more common cause of virilisation in this age group and must be excluded. The investigation of the virilised girl is discussed in Delayed and precocious puberty. Oestrogen secretion occurs very rarely and also induces accelerated growth and skeletal maturity with breast development and vaginal bleeding in prepubertal girls. Approximately 40% of patients are hypertensive at diagnosis due to glucocorticoid or mineralocorticoid excess or compression of the renal artery (Michalkiewicz et al. 2004). Older girls are more likely to have non-functioning tumours and present more commonly with abdominal pain and weight loss.

The genetic associations of ACT include Li-Fraumeni syndrome and Beckwith-Wiedemann syndrome. Rare associations include multiple endocrine neoplasia type 1 (MEN 1) and Lynch familial neoplasia (Albaugh and Chen 2001). Referral to clinical genetics is mandatory in all patients.

Approximately 90% of ACT are malignant and they account for 0.2% of all paediatric solid malignancies. In the paediatric population patients present most commonly below the age of 5 years and girls are affected more commonly than boys. The distinction between cortical adenomas (benign) and carcinomas (malignant) can be very difficult in many cases. The tumour size and weight offer only a very rough indication of malignant potential. Tumour nodules less than 5 cm in diameter and weight less than 200 g are likely to be adenomas, whereas malignant tumours are larger and heavier.

In general US should be used to screen for a suspected adrenal mass. The adrenal gland becomes more difficult to visualise in the older child. A small case series of children with virilising adrenocortical tumour has shown low sensitivity for detecting small functioning adrenal tumours with US (Bonfig et al. 2003). CT is useful to depict calcification and vascular involvement but ultrasound has a specific role to evaluate for renal vein and IVC tumour extension. MRI is superior in lesion detection and characterisation. (Fig. 11). Optimal treatment involves complete tumour resection with appropriate hormone replacement therapy (Fig. 12).

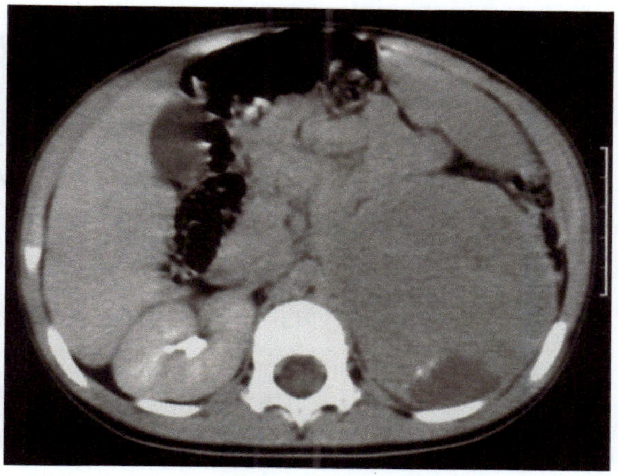

Fig. 11 Adrenocortical carcinoma. Axial contrast-enhanced CT of a large left adrenal tumour in a child with hypercortisolism with a single fleck of calcification. Neuroblastoma should always be considered in the differential of a paediatric adrenal mass

4.6 Disorders of the Genital Outflow Tract

Congenital abnormalities of the uterus and lower genital outflow tract are an important cause of primary amenorrhoea and should be suspected in girls with absence of menarche after full development of secondary sexual characteristics. Disorders may result from:

- Müllerian duct agenesis or hypoplasia (discussed in detail in Structural Abnormalities of the Female Reproductive Tract).
- Incomplete Müllerian duct canalisation (discussed in detail in Structural Abnormalities of the Female Reproductive Tract).
- Specific anatomical defects such as imperforate hymen and intact vaginal septum

The presence of stenosis or atresia of the genital tract allows defects to be classified as either obstructed or

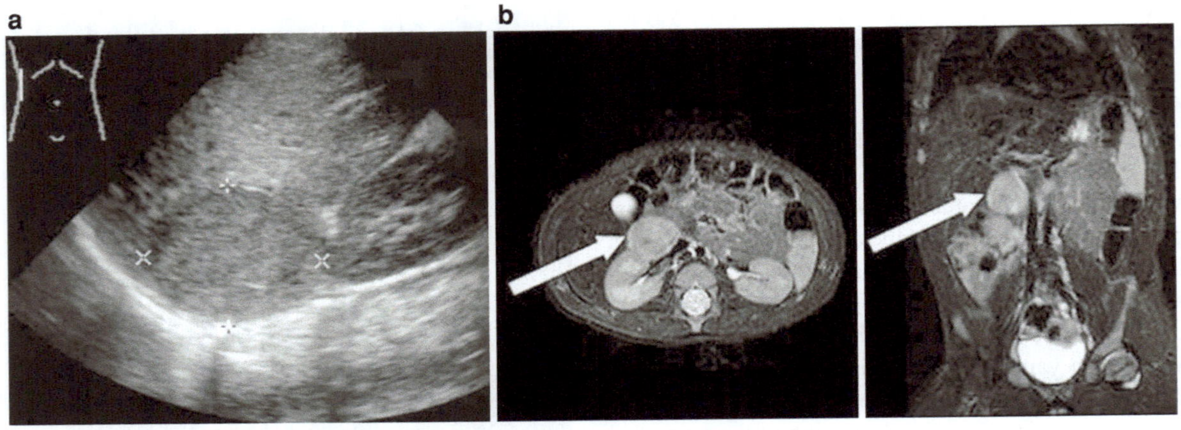

Fig. 12 Virilising adrenal tumour. **a** Longitudinal sonogram showing a homogenous adrenal tumour between callipers. **b** Axial and coronal T2-weighted MR images of the right adrenal tumour (*arrows*). *Images reproduced from* Bonfig et al. 2003 *with permission from Springer Publishers*

unobstructed. Obstruction of the genital tract prevents the egress of menstrual secretions resulting in retrograde menstruation and an increased risk of developing secondary endometriosis and pelvic adhesions.

Other causes of primary amenorrhoea with established secondary sexual characteristics include complete androgen insensitivity syndrome, late onset disturbance of the hypothalamic-pituitary-ovarian-uterine axis and any of the numerous causes of hypogonadotropic hypogonadism.

4.6.1 Müllerian Anomalies

A simplified classification of congenital Müllerian developmental anomalies include disorders of lateral Müllerian duct fusion (duplication defect with or without obstruction) and disorders of vertical fusion (canalisation defects with or without obstruction).

Müllerian Agenesis or Hypoplasia

The most extreme form of congenital Müllerian duct abnormalities are Müllerian duct aplasias resulting in segmental agenesis of the uterus and/or vagina with accompanying variable degrees of uterovaginal hypoplasia (Buttram and Gibbons 1979).

Mayer-Rokitansky–Küster–Hauser syndrome (MRKH) syndrome is defined by a range of vaginal anomalies consisting of agenesis of the proximal two-thirds to complete agenesis of the vagina and cervix to an almost normal appearance (Fig. 13). A rudimentary uterus is often present which occasionally may contain functioning endometrial tissue. This can lead to cyclical pain and endometriosis in the presence of vaginal agenesis.

MRKH patients show normal development of the female external genitalia with female karyotype (46,XX) and normal progression through thelarche and pubarche with primary amenorrhoea. Imaging with ultrasound and MRI demonstrates a septate rudimentary uterus which may occasionally contain functioning endometrial tissue, aplasia of the cervix and vagina with normal or hypoplastic adnexa. Associated abnormalities include renal dysplasia and cervical somite abnormalities (MURCS association: Müllerian duct aplasia, Renal dysplasia, Cervical Somite anomalies) (Duncan et al. 1979).

4.6.2 Imperforate Hymen

The hymen is a mucous membrane which occludes the external vaginal opening and is usually perforate at birth. Imperforate hymen results from an in utero defect of canalisation of the hymenal membrane at the vaginal orifice or rarely postnatally following scarring from previous infection. This is the most common genital obstructive defect and is usually not associated with any other Müllerian or urogenital defects.

Imperforate hymen typically presents as an interlabial swelling/bulging membrane at the introitus. The differential diagnosis of an interlabial swelling includes urethral prolapse, prolapsed ureterocele, perineal abscess, paraurethral cyst, Skene duct cyst or vaginal rhabdomyosarcoma (Nussbaum and Lebowitz 1983).

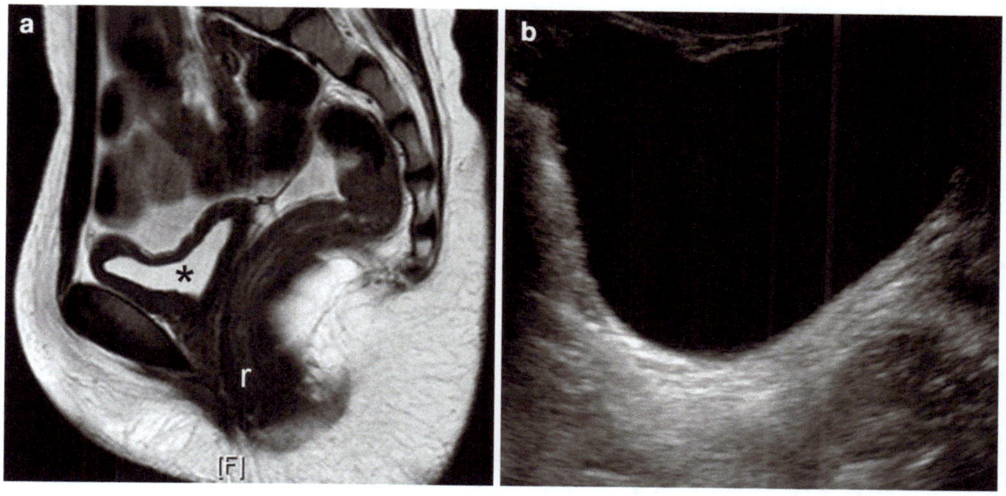

Fig. 13 Mayer-Rokitansky–Kuster–Hauser (MRKH) syndrome. **a** Sagittal T2 TSE image and, **b** longitudinal ultrasound scan showing absence of the uterus and vagina. Rectum (r) urinary bladder (*)

Imperforate hymen presenting in the neonatal period results from the build-up mucous secreted by the uterus under maternal and placental hormonal influence (mucocolpos). Symptoms in the adolescent include lower abdominal pain which is initially cyclical with a perceived delay in onset of menarche and a history of primary amenorrhoea with physical examination confirming the presence of secondary sexual characteristics. A pelvic mass results from the accumulation of vaginal and uterine secretions resulting in either haematocolpos or haematometrocolpos (Fig. 14). Ultrasound will typically show a fluid-distended vagina causing local mass effect. Fluid may also accumulate in the uterus and occasionally in the fallopian tubes. The fluid content may be anechoic or contain internal echoes depending on the amount of proteinacious material or blood products present. Imperforate hymen cannot be differentiated from a low transverse vaginal septum by ultrasound. MRI is not indicated unless additional abnormalities are demonstrated by ultrasound. Treatment involves surgical hymenectomy to establish a patent vagina.

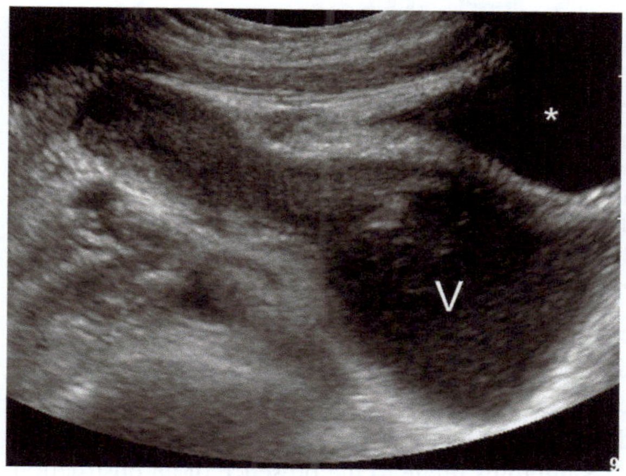

Fig. 14 Imperforate hymen. Longitudinal ultrasound showing a fluid-distended vagina (v) in a 12-year-old girl secondary to an imperforate hymen. (*) urinary bladder

4.6.3 Vaginal Septal Anomalies

Intact vaginal septae (see Structural Abnormalities of the Female Reproductive Tract) result from failure of canalisation of the vaginal plate which separates the evaginated caudal portion of the fused Müllerian ducts from the cranial aspect of the urogenital sinus. Presenting symptoms are similar to imperforate hymen.

Transverse Vaginal Septum

Transverse vaginal septae may occur in the upper, middle, or lower thirds of the vagina with most occurring in the upper and middle portions of the vagina (Fig. 15). Associated anomalies are rare. Imaging features are similar to imperforate hymen.

Longitudinal Vaginal Septum

A complete or partial longitudinal vaginal septum is usually associated with cases of uterus didelphys. Uterus didelphys is a disorder of lateral Müllerian duct fusion resulting in a duplication anomaly

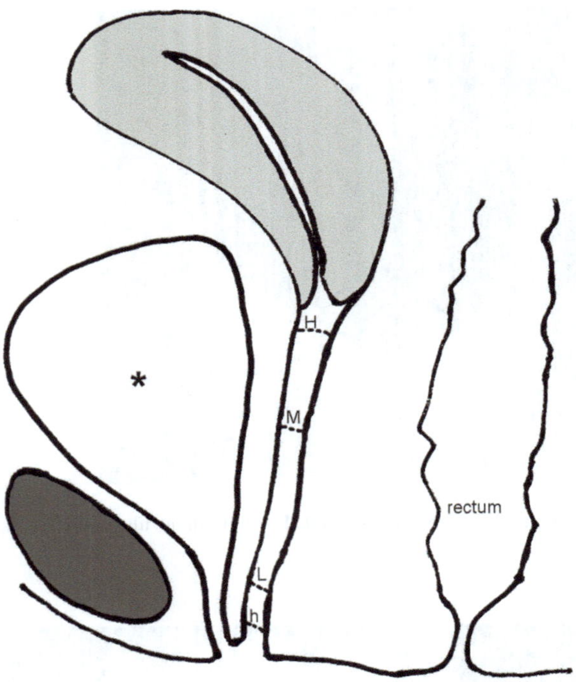

Fig. 15 Position of congenital membranes which can obstruct the vagina. Low transverse vaginal septae lie in close proximity to the expected position of an imperforate hymen which accounts for the difficulty in differentiation between these distinct entities on diagnostic imaging. High (H), middle (M) and low (L) transverse septae. Hymen (h) and bladder (*)

comprising of two completely separate uterine cavities each with preserved zonal anatomy and endocervical canals (Fig. 16). Neither, one or both didelphic cavities may be obstructive.

Symptoms relate to the presence of an obstruction. Uterus didelphys typically becomes symptomatic at menarche, with an obstructed hemivagina resulting in lower abdominal pain which is initially cyclical and coincides with menstrual bleeding from the unobstructed side. Non-obstructed uterus didelphys is often asymptomatic and usually detected incidentally on clinical examination or on ultrasound.

Routine ultrasound rarely demonstrates a vaginal septum convincingly, but its presence should be inferred in the setting of uterus didelphys. Hydrosonographic evaluation in the detection of intact vaginal septae has been reported (Caloia et al. 1998). T2 weighted MR imaging is ideally suited to evaluate uterus didelphys and the presence of a vaginal septum which is seen as thin uniform hypointense band at the level of the obstructed vagina. Associated anomalies include absent or hypoplastic kidney ipsilateral to the obstructed endocervical canal (Orazi et al. 2007) and rarely multicystic dysplastic kidney (Prada Arias et al. 2005).

4.6.4 Androgen Insensitivity Syndrome (AIS)

Complete androgen insensitivity syndrome (CAIS) (see Structural Abnormalities of the Female Reproductive Tract) is a rare disorder of sexual differentiation with a prevalence of approximately 1:10 000–1:40 000 live births. An affected individual will have female external genital phenotype with female gender identity in the presence of a male XY karyotype and male gonads. The diagnostic criteria for CAIS are summarised in Table 9.

CAIS develops in early fetal life due to mutational defects in intracellular androgen receptor function. Approximately 70% of androgen receptor mutations are inherited in an X-linked recessive fashion (Hughes and Deeb 2006). Complete and partial forms of androgen insensitivity are recognised including partial androgen insensitivity syndrome (PAIS) characterised by ambiguous or undermasculinised genitalia and mild androgen insensitivity syndrome (MAIS).

Patients with androgen insensitivity produce physiological or elevated levels of testosterone and dihydrotestosterone from the testes. Female external genitalia differentiate despite circulating testosterone. Neonates born with CAIS will appear as a female infant. Müllerian inhibitory substance is produced in the testes resulting in agenesis of the fallopian tubes, uterus and proximal vagina. The gonads may be located in the labia majora, inguinal ring or in the abdomen (Fig. 17). Up to 90% of premenarcheal girls with CAIS will present with inguinal hernias (Gans and Rubin 1962) and this diagnosis should be considered in girls with inguinal hernias. However, surveys of clinical practice report that few surgeons routinely request karyotyping, androgen levels or ultrasound of the pelvic organs in girls presenting in with inguinal hernias (Viner et al. 1997; Burge and Sugarman 2002).

In adolescent life young women with CAIS present with primary amenorrhoea greater than 2 years after the development of breast growth. Late presentation of CAIS is a rare but important cause of primary amenorrhoea. Clinical examination reveals a phenotypic female with normal breast development, height which

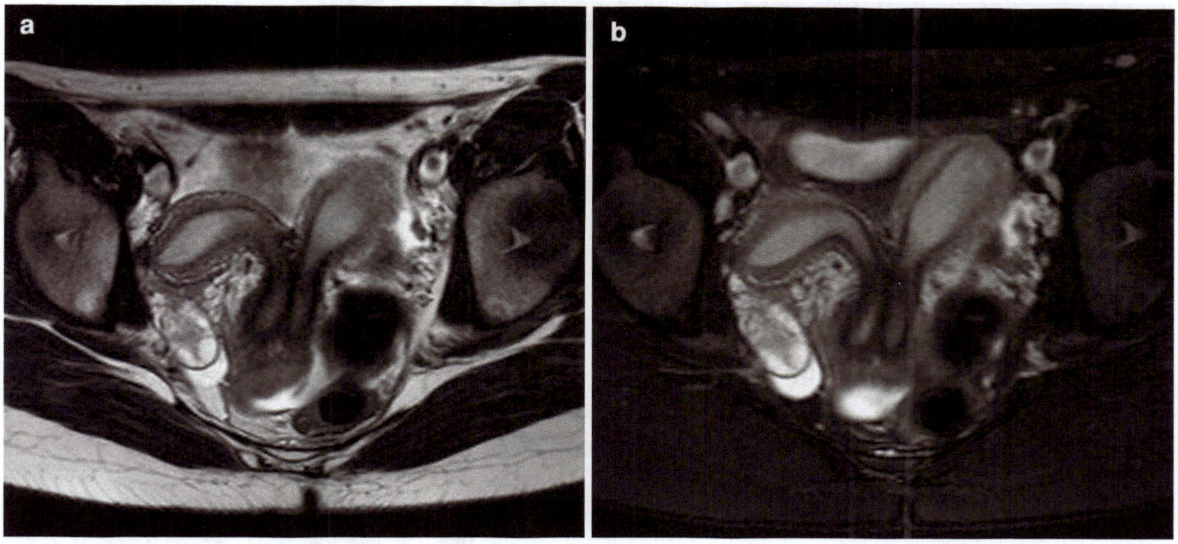

Fig. 16 Uterus didelphys. **a** Para-axial T2 TSE and **b** T2-weighted SPAIR images of the pelvis showing uterus didelphys noted incidentally on initial ultrasound of the renal tract for recurrent urinary tract infection. No associated hydrocolpos or renal agenesis was present

Table 9 Diagnostic criteria for complete androgen insensitivity syndrome

1. Normal female external genitalia in a 46,XY individual with testes
2. Absence of virilisation despite normal or high male levels of testosterone
3. Markedly decreased or absence of post-pubertal axillary and pubic hair growth
4. Demonstration of an androgen receptor (AR) gene mutation
5. Spontaneous feminisation at puberty with absence of menarche before gonadectomy
After (Wisniewski et al. 2000)

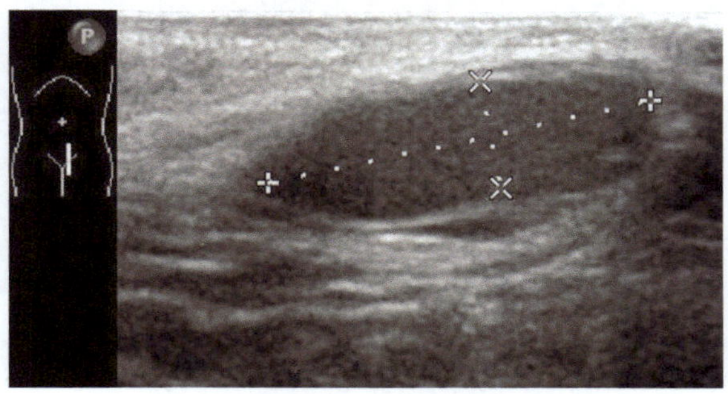

Fig. 17 Infant with Congenital androgen insensitivity syndrome (CAIS). 20-month-old CAIS patient with female external genitalia and two palpable lumps in the labial folds. High resolution ultrasound showing a labial gonad (between callipers)

is normal or slightly advanced in most cases and absent or minimal axillary and pubic hair (Oakes et al. 2008). Breast development results from endogenous aromatisation of testosterone to oestrogens. The external genitalia appear normal. A rudimentary blind ending vagina can be demonstrated by physical examination and imaging (Fig. 18a–b). The main differentials include Mayer-Rokitansky-Kuster-Hauser (MRKH) syndrome (Fig. 13) and Müllerian agenesis. In these conditions testosterone levels are normal. Transabdominal ultrasound will accurately document vaginal length (Sarpel 2005), Müllerian aplasia and the location and appearances of the gonads. Careful evaluation with a high resolution linear probe of the perineum and inguinal regions will depict extra-abdominal gonads (Fig. 18).

The incidences of dysgerminoma and gonadoblastoma have been reported to be 0.8% in CAIS and 5.5% in AIS (Rajpert-Demeyts 2006). Laparoscopic orchidectomy should be undertaken once final height is attained and breast development completed.

Bone mineral density in women with CAIS is reported to be decreased (Sobel et al. 2006). A small study of both pre and post-orchiectomy girls with CAIS has shown no significant difference in bone biochemical markers or fracture risk as assessed by

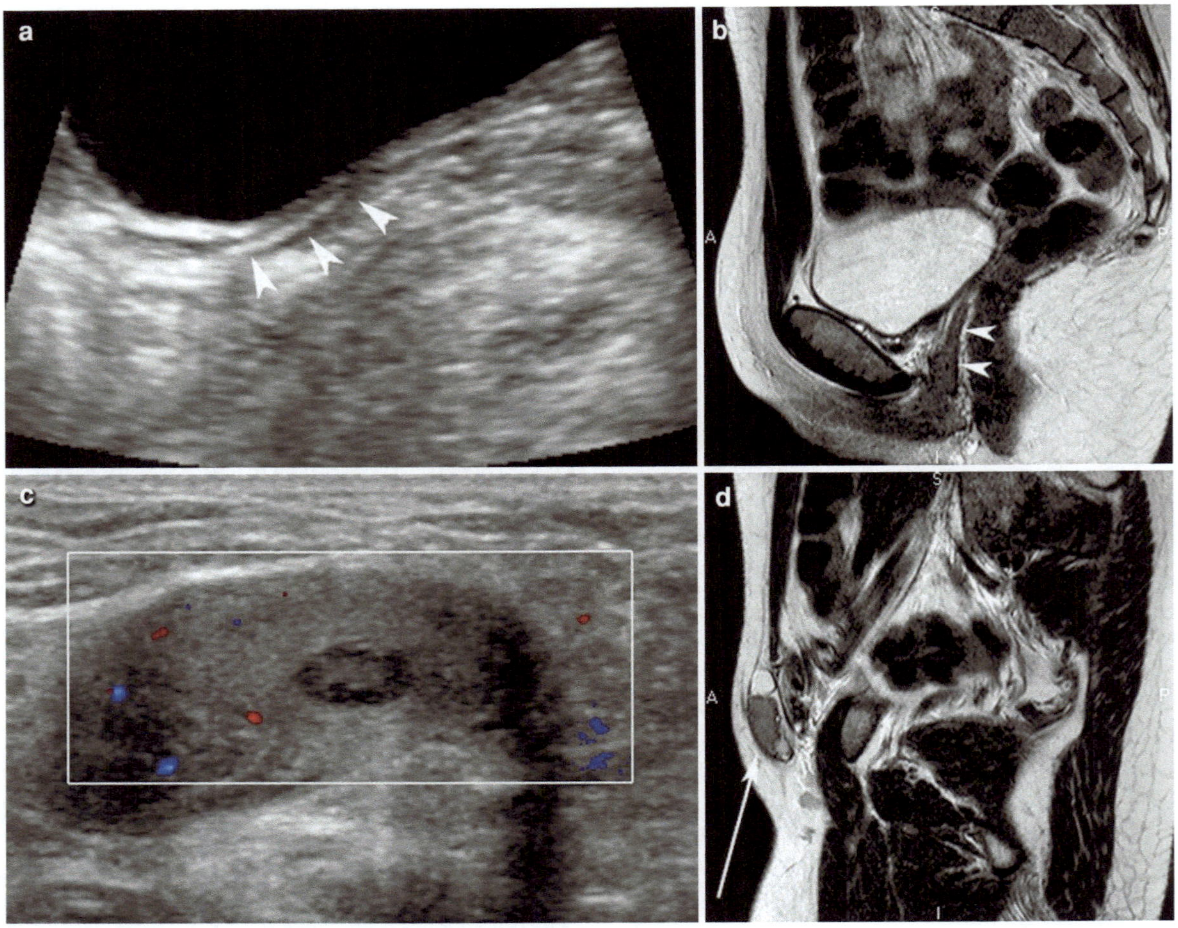

Fig. 18 Teenager with Congenital androgen insensitivity syndrome (CAIS). Selected images from a 16-year-old CAIS patient referred with primary amenorrhoea. **a** Longitudinal US and **b** sagittal T2-weighted MRI depicting absent Müllerian structures, the uterus and upper vagina are absent, a rudimentary 'short' vagina is present (*arrowheads*). **c** Colour Doppler US of the left groin crease confirms the presence of a mixed echotexture inguinal gonad with a focal internal nodule. **d** Sagital T2-weighted MRI of the inguinal gonad. This was removed and confirmed to be a dysgenetic gonad consisting of an immature testis with no germ cells and a Sertoli-cell adenoma (nodule on ultrasound)

DEXA scanning compared to controls (Bertelloni et al. 1998).

4.7 Vaginal Bleeding and Vaginal Discharge in Childhood

4.7.1 Neonates

Vaginal discharge (leucorrhoea) in the newborn female is not uncommon and almost always of no clinical significance. The neonatal vaginal mucosa can hypertrophy as a result of intrauterine exposure to maternal and placental oestrogens. This is seen on ultrasound as a transient prominent uniform echogenic midline endometrial stripe which is shed once oestrogen influence subsides (Fig. 19). Occasionally there may be a concomitant oestrogen withdrawal bleed. The yield of pathology from diagnostic imaging in this age group is very low. Pelvic ultrasound is not routinely indicated but may rarely be required to allay parental anxiety and should be performed if symptoms persist beyond 3 weeks.

4.7.2 Premenarchal Children

Vaginal bleeding in prepubertal child is abnormal and should be investigated. Beyond the neonatal period vaginal discharge should not be seen in a healthy prepubertal girl. There is a wide differential diagnosis

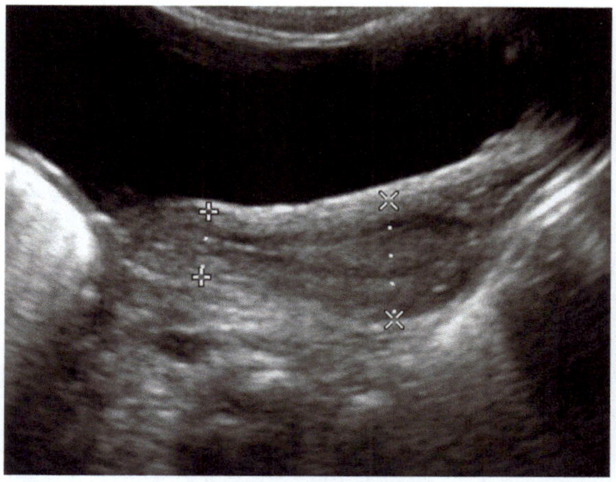

Fig. 19 Neonatal uterine stripe. Inverted pear-shaped uterus (between callipers) in a 4-week-old girl referred with leucorrhoea. The uterine strip is prominent but of uniform echotexture, the remainder of the study was normal. The overall appearances are reassuring and the symptoms should normally resolve

for prepubertal pelvic discharge and bleeding (Table 10). In most instances the underlying condition is benign and self-limiting. Poor perineal hygiene and chemical irritants are common causes. The prepubertal vagina is relatively short, has no innate immunoglobulin immunity and a pH which favours microbial colonisation. The labia are thin and vulvovaginal soft-tissues are sensitive. Pelvic swabs obtained for microbial culture yielding organisms related to sexually transmitted diseases should prompt consideration of sexual abuse.

Pelvic ultrasound is useful to exclude significant ovarian, adrenal or uterovaginal pathology such as a tumour or a retained vaginal foreign body.

Table 10 Differential diagnosis of per vaginal discharge and bleeding in childhood

Physiologic
Poor perineal hygiene
Chemical irritant
Trauma (accidental and non-accidental)
Dermatoses
Infection (sexually transmitted disease, pelvic abscess, atypical infections)
Blood dyscrasia
Precocious puberty
Foreign body
Factitious
Haemangioma
Rhabdomyosarcoma
Carcinoma
Urologic causes of apparent vaginal bleeding
Ectopic ureter
Urethral or ureterocele prolapse
Urethral polyp

4.8 Vaginal Foreign Body

Common vaginal foreign bodies include tissue paper in the young child and retained tampons in postmenarchal girls. A history recalling insertion of a foreign body is rarely forthcoming. Presenting symptoms may include persistent vaginal bleeding or blood stained offensive or serous discharge, abdominal pain and occasionally genital itching. Clinical examination should include inspection of the external genitalia.

Non-invasive diagnostic imaging may aid in the diagnosis of vaginal foreign body. Radiopaque objects may be visible on radiographs. Sonography is useful in demonstrating a foreign body particularly if characteristic indentation of the posterior bladder wall is noted (Fig. 20). (Caspi et al. 1994, 1995). Magnetic resonance imaging may depict non-ferrous foreign bodies that have migrated beyond the vaginal wall (Kihara et al. 2001). Non-invasive diagnostic imaging may not correctly identify all foreign bodies and where there is a high index of suspicion despite negative imaging direct visualisation via examination under anaesthesia and/or vaginoscopy should be performed and remains the diagnostic gold standard. Contrast vaginography may also be performed at this time to document long-term complications including vaginal stenosis and fistula formation.

4.9 Neoplasms

4.9.1 Rhabdomyosarcoma

Embryonal rhabdomyosarcoma although rare is the most common malignant neoplasm of the female genital tract in young girls. Peak incidence is bimodal, occurring around 2 years of age and later in the second decade of life. Presenting symptoms include vaginal discharge, intermittent vaginal bleeding with a prolapsing fleshy mass at the introitus with or without passage of polypoidal tumour from the

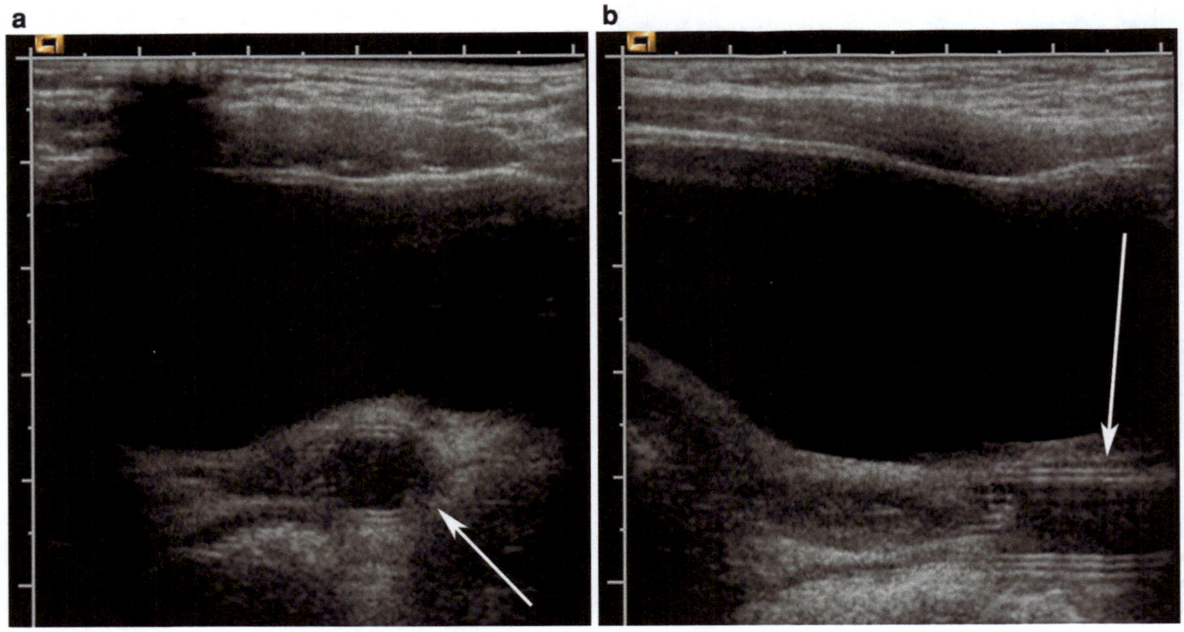

Fig. 20 Vaginal foreign body. Transabdominal high resolution ultrasound. **a** Transverse and **b** longitudinal images showing an intravaginal foreign body (biro pen) deeply embedded in the upper third of vagina. The foreign body is seen as a linear mass (*arrow*) which is of hexagonal cross-section Images courtesy of Dr. Paul Humphries Consultant Paediatric Radiologist MRCP FRCR, London, UK

vagina. The botryoid variant of rhabdomyosarcoma usually presents in infancy as a submucosal polypoidal mass, typically arising from the vagina or urinary bladder and rarely from the uterine cervix.

Outcome is dependent upon tumour size, local extent and the histological subtype; embryonal is the most common subtype with the most favourable prognosis. The botryoid variant is locally aggressive. Around one-third of cases are metastatic at diagnosis. Metastatic sites include the locoregional lymph nodes, lungs, liver, kidneys and pericardium. Vaginal lesions have a better prognosis than cervical lesions. The usual location is the anterior vaginal wall just below the cervix. The typical ultrasound appearances are of a polypoidal mass with a configuration resembling a cluster of grapes within a hollow structure (Agrons et al. 1997). Obstructing lesions can result in a build up of fluid in the uterine cavity. MRI is required for local staging (Fig. 21).

4.9.2 Endodermal Sinus Tumour

Endodermal sinus tumour is a rare aggressive type of malignant germ cell tumour associated with elevated serum alpha-fetoprotein levels. Tumour is typically located in the sacrococcygeal region or ovaries but can occasionally occur in the vagina in young children usually under 3 years old. Symptoms include vaginal bleeding or bloody vaginal discharge. Imaging cannot reliably differentiate from sarcoma botryoides and histopathologic confirmation is required. Prognosis is poor despite radical adjuvant therapy.

4.10 Vascular Malformations

Vascular malformations occasionally occur in the external genitalia or adjacent perineum.

4.10.1 Haemangioma

Infantile haemangioma is the most common type of genital or perineal vascular malformation. Imaging features are similar to those of any infantile haemangioma and the lesion will follow a typical course of proliferation, involution and involuted (Vogel et al. 2006). Complications include ulceration, bleeding and local mass effect. Ultrasound is usually diagnostic. MRI should be reserved for complex or atypical presentations or and when additional malformations must

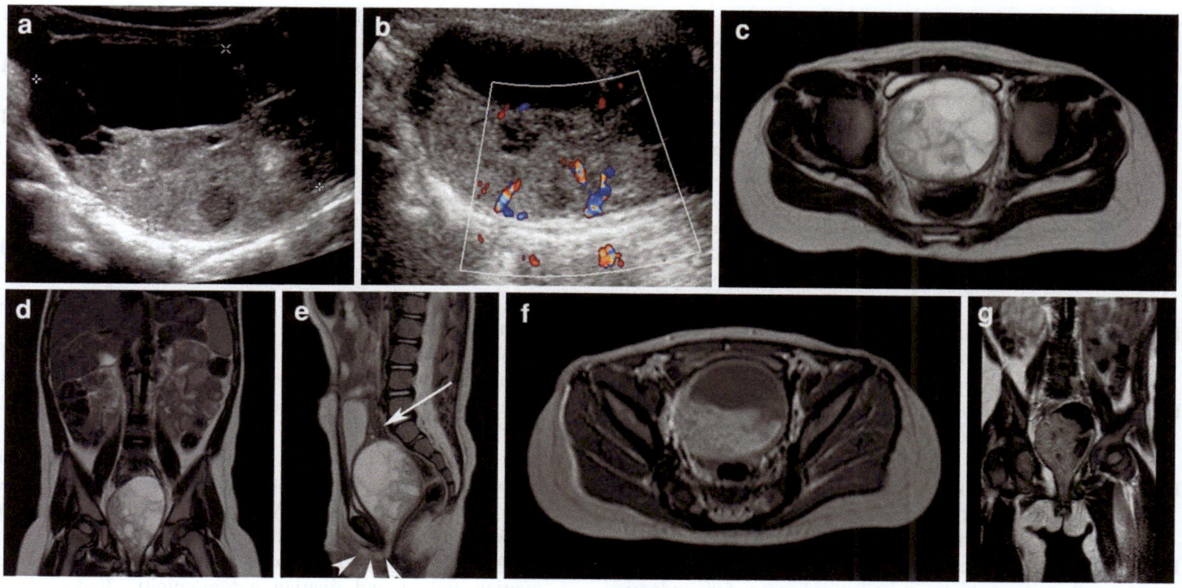

Fig. 21 Vaginal rhabdomyosarcoma. Twenty three-month-old girl presenting with vaginal bleeding. **a–b** Transverse sonograms showing **a** a complex pelvic mass lesion within a distended vagina **b** showing colour Doppler flow to the solid components. **c** Axial, **d** coronal and **e** Sagittal T2 TSE images showing a heterogenous mass lesion distending the vagina but not involving the uterus (*arrow*). Fleshy tissue was visible at the introitus (*arrowheads*). **f–g** T1 post intravenous-gadolinium axial and coronal images confirming an enhancing vaginal mass

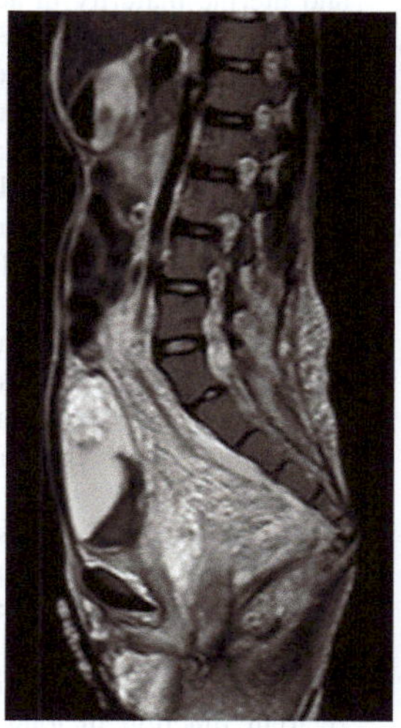

Fig. 22 Pelvic vascular malformation. Sagittal T2-weighted SPAIR image of a 13-year-old female with diffuse haemangiolymphangioma infiltrating the perineum, urinary bladder, pelvis and erector spinae muscle complex. The urinary bladder contains a blood product-urine fluid level

be excluded (Fig. 22). PELVIS (perineal haemangioma, external genitalia malformations, lipomyelomeningocele, vesicorenal abnormalities, imperforate anus, and skin tag) and SACRAL (spinal dysraphism, anogenital anomalies, cutaneous anomalies, and renal and urologic anomalies associated with angioma of lumbosacral localisation) syndromes have recently been reported describing the association of perineal haemangioma with pelvic malformations (Girard et al. 2006; Stockman et al. 2007). Treatment of vascular malformations should involve an expert multidisciplinary team.

Complex locally aggressive and infiltrative haemangiomata include disorders such as kaposiform hemangioendothelioma and kaposiform lymphangioendothelioma. Disease extent in these cases is best evaluated with MRI. Treatment includes a combination of sclerotherapy, selective embolisation and surgery.

References

Adams J, Polson DW, Abdulwahid N et al (1985) Multifollicular ovaries: clinical and endocrine features and response to pulsatile gonadotrophin releasing hormone. Lancet 2: 1375–1399

Agrons GA, Wagner BJ, Lonergan GJ et al (1997) From the archives of the AFIP. Genitourinary rhabdomyosarcoma in children: radiologic-pathologic correlation. Radiographics 17:919–937

Albaugh G, Chen M (2001) Adrenocortical carcinoma in two female children. Pediatr Surg Int 17:71–74

Al-Rimawi HS, Jallad MF, Amarin ZO et al (2005) Hypothalamic-pituitary-gonadal function in adolescent females with beta-thalassemia major. Int J Gynaecol Obstet 90:44–47

Apter D, Viinikka L, Vihko R (1978) Hormonal patterns of adolescent menstrual cycles. J Clin Endocrinol Metab 47:944–954

Azziz R, Carmina E, Dewailly D et al (2006) Position statement: criteria for defining polycystic ovary syndrome as a predominantly hyperandrogenic syndrome: an androgen excess society guideline. J Clin Endo Metab 91: 4237–4245

Bakos O, Lundkvist E, Bergh T (1993) Transvaginal sonographic evaluation of endometrial growth and texture in spontaneous ovulatory cycles—a descriptive study. Hum Reprod 83:799–806

Balen AH, Laven JS, Tan SL et al (2003) Ultrasound assessment of the polycystic ovary: international consensus definitions. Hum Reprod Update 9:505–514

Benvenga S, Campenní A, Ruggeri RM, Trimarchi F (2000) Hypopituitarism secondary to head trauma. J Clin Endocrinol Metab 85:1353–1361

Bertelloni S, Baroncelli GI, Federico G et al (1998) Altered bone mineral density in patients with complete androgen insensitivity syndrome. Horm Res 50:309–314

Blair JC (2010) Prevalence, natural history and consequences of posttraumatic hypopituitarism: a case for endocrine surveillance. Br J Neurosurg 24:10–17

Blendonohy PM, Philip PA (1991) Precocious puberty in children after traumatic brain injury. Brain Inj 5:63–68

Bonfig W, Bittmann I, Bechtold S et al (2003) Virilising adrenocortical tumours in children. Eur J Pediatr 162: 623–628

Bonneville F, Cattin F, Marsot-Dupuch K et al (2006) T1 signal hyperintensity in the sellar region: spectrum of findings. Radiographics 26:93–113

Burge DM, Sugarman IS (2002) Exclusion of androgen insensitivity syndrome in girls with inguinal hernias: current surgical practice. Pediatr Int Surg 18:701–703

Buttram VC, Gibbons WE (1979) Müllerian anomalies: a proposed classification—an analysis of 144 cases. Fertil Steril 32:40–46

Buzi F, Pilotta A, Dordoni D et al (1999) Pelvic ultrasonography in normal girls and in girls with pubertal precocity. Acta Paediatr 88:246–247

Caloia DV, Morris H, Rahmani MR (1998) Congenital transverse vaginal septum: vaginal hydrosonographic diagnosis. J Ultrasound Med 17:261–264

Caspi B, Zalel Y, Elchalal U et al (1994) Sonographic detection of vaginal foreign bodies. J Ultrasound Med 13: 236–237

Caspi B, Zalel Y, Katz Z et al (1995) The role of sonography in the detection of vaginal foreign bodies in young girls: the bladder indentation sign. Pediatr Radiol 25:S60–S61

Ceballos R (1966) Pituitary changes in head trauma. Analysis of 102 consecutive cases of head injury. Ala J Med Sci 3:185–198

Chemaitilly W, Mertens AC, Mitby P et al (2006) Acute ovarian failure in the childhood cancer survivor study. J Clin Endocrinol Metab 91:1723–1728

Cytowic RE, Smith A, Stump DA (1986) Transient amenorrhea after closed head trauma. N Engl J Med 314:715

Duncan PA, Shapiro LR, Stangel JJ et al (1979) The MURCS association: Müllerian duct aplasia, renal aplasia, and cervicothoracic somite dysplasia. J Pediatr 95:399–402

Ehrmann DA (2005) Polycystic ovary syndrome. N Engl J Med 352:1223–1236

Franks S (1995) Polycystic ovary syndrome. N Engl J Med 333:853–861

Gans S, Rubin CL (1962) Apparent females with hernias and testes. Am J Dis Child 104:82–86

Garden AS (1998) Problems with menstruation. In: Garden AS (ed) Paediatric and adolescent gynaecology. Hodder Arnold, London, pp 127–154

Gillam MP, Molitch ME, Lombardi G et al (2006) Advances in the treatment of prolactinomas. Endocr Rev 27:485–534

Girard C, Bigorre M, Guillot B et al (2006) PELVIS syndrome. Arch Dermatol 142:884–888

Hague WM, Adams J, Rodda C et al (1990) The prevalence of polycystic ovaries in patients with congenital adrenal hyperplasia and their close relatives. Clin Endocrinol (Oxf) 33:501–510

Herman-Giddens M, Slora J, Wasserman R et al (1997) Secondary sexual characteristics and menses in young girls seen in office practice: a study from the pediatric research in office settings network. Pediatrics 99:505–512

Hoek A, Schoemaker J, Drexhage HA (1997) Premature ovarian failure and ovarian autoimmunity. Endocr Rev 18:107–134

Hughes I, Deeb A (2006) Androgen resistance. Best Pract Res Clin Endocrinol Metab 20:577–598

Jonard S, Robert Y, Corter-Rudelli C et al (2003) Ultrasound examination of polycystic ovaries: is it worth counting the follicles? Hum Reprod 18:598–603

Key A, Mason H, Allan R et al (2002) Restoration of ovarian and uterine maturity in adolescents with anorexia nervosa. Int J Eat Disord 32:319–325

Khadr SN, Crofton PM, Jones PA et al (2010) Evaluation of pituitary function after traumatic brain injury in childhood. Clin Endocrinol (Oxf) 73:637–643

Kihara M, Sato N, Kimura H et al (2001) Magnetic resonance imaging in the evaluation of vaginal foreign bodies in a young girl. Arch Gynecol Obstet 265:221–222

Koff E, Rierdan J (1996) Premenarcheal expectations and postmenarcheal experiences of positive and negative menstrual related changes. J Adolesc Health 18:286–291

Kohda E, Yamazaki H, Hisazumi H et al (2006) Imaging of congenital lipoid adrenal hyperplasia. Radiat Med 24: 217–219

Lai KY, de Bruyn R, Lask B et al (1994) Use of pelvic ultrasound to monitor ovarian and uterine maturity in childhood onset anorexia nervosa. Arch Dis Child 71: 228–231

Larsen EC, Muller J, Schmiegelow K et al (2003) Reduced ovarian function in long-term survivors of radiation- and chemotherapy-treated childhood cancer. J Clin Endocrinol Metab 88:5307–5314

Legro RS, Lin HM, Demers LM et al (2000) Rapid maturation of the reproductive axis during perimenarche independent of body composition. J Clin Endocrinol Metab 85:1021–1025

Mason HD, Key A, Allan R et al (2007) Pelvic ultrasonography in anorexia nervosa: what the clinician should ask the radiologist and how to use the information provided. Eur Eat Disord Rev 15:35–41

Michalkiewicz E, Sandrini R, Figueiredo B et al (2004) Clinical and outcome characteristics of children with adrenocortical

tumors: a report from the International Pediatric Adrenocortical Tumor Registry. J Clin Oncol 22:838–845
Moon RJ, Sutton T, Wilson PM et al (2010) Pituitary function at long-term follow-up of childhood traumatic brain injury. J Neurotrauma 27:1827–1835
Nussbaum AR, Lebowitz RL (1983) Interlabial masses in little girls: review of imaging and recommendations. AJR Am J Roentgenol 141:65–71
Oakes MB, Eyvazzadeh AD, Quint E et al (2008) Complete androgen insensitivity syndrome-a review. J Pediatr Adolesc Gynecol 21:305–310
Orazi C, Lucchetti MC, Schingo PM et al (2007) Herlyn-Werner-Wunderlich syndrome: uterus didelphys, blind hemivagina and ipsilateral renal agenesis. Sonographic and MR findings in 11 cases. Pediatr Radiol 37:657–665
Ostrov SG, Quencer RM, Hoffman JC et al (1989) Hemorrhage within pituitary adenomas: how often associated with pituitary apoplexy syndrome? AJR Am J Roentgenol 153:153–160
Piotin M, Tampieri D, Rufenacht DA et al (1990) The various MRI patterns of pituitary apoplexy. Eur Radiol 9:918–923
Prada Arias M, Muguerza Vellibre R, Montero Sanchez M et al (2005) Uterus didelphys with obstructed hemivagina and multicystic dysplastic kidney. Eur J Pediatr Surg 15: 441–445
Rajpert-DeMeyts M (2006) Developmental model for the pathogenesis of testicular carcinoma in situ: genetic and environmental aspects. Hum Reprod Update 12:303–323
Rebar RW (2008) Premature ovarian "failure" in the adolescent. Ann N Y Acad Sci 1135:138–145
Rogg JM, Tung GA, Anderson G et al (2002) Pituitary apoplexy: early detection with diffusion-weighted MR imaging. AJNR 23:1240–1245
Russo G, Paesano P, Taccagni G et al (1998) Ovarian adrenal-like tissue in congenital adrenal hyperplasia. N Engl J Med 339:853–854
Sarpel U (2005) The incidence of complete androgen insensitivity in girls with inguinal hernias and assessment of screening by vaginal length measurement. J Pediatric Surg 40:133–136
Shulman A, Shulman N, Weissenglass L et al (1989) Ultrasonic assessment of the endometrium as a predictor of oestrogen status in amenorrhoeic patients. Hum Reprod 4:616–619
Sklar CA (1999) Reproductive physiology and treatment related loss of sex hormone production. Med Pediatr Oncol 33:2–8
Sklar CA, Mertens AC, Mitby P et al (2006) Premature menopause in survivors of childhood cancer: a report from the childhood cancer survivor study. J Natl Cancer Inst 98:890–896
Sobel V, Schwartz B, Zhu YS et al (2006) Bone mineral density in the complete androgen insensitivity and 5-alpha reductase deficiency syndromes. J Clin Endocrinol Metab 91:3017–3023
Steele CA, MacFarlane IA, Blair J et al (2010) Pituitary adenomas in childhood, adolescence and young adulthood: presentation, management, endocrine and metabolic outcomes. Eur J Endocrinol 163:515–522
Stikkelbroeck NM, Hermus AR, Braat DD et al (2003) Fertility in women with congenital adrenal hyperplasia due to 21-hydroxylase deficiency. Obstet Gynecol Surv 58:275–284
Stikkelbroeck NM, Hermus AR, Schouten D et al (2004) Prevalence of ovarian adrenal rest tumours and polycystic ovaries in females with congenital adrenal hyperplasia: results of ultrasonography and MR imaging. Eur Radiol 14:1802–1806
Stockman A, Boralevi F, Taieb A et al (2007) SACRAL syndrome: spinal dysraphism, anogenital, cutaneous, renal and urologic anomalies, associated with angioma of lumbosacral localization. Dermatology 214:40–45
Tanriverdi F, Senyurek H, Unluhizarci K et al (2006) High risk of hypopituitarism after traumatic brain injury: a prospective investigation of anterior pituitary function in the acute phase and 12 months after trauma. J Clin Endocrinol Metab 91:2105–21011
The Rotterdam ESHRE/ASRM-Sponsored PCOS Consensus Workshop Group (2004) Revised 2003 consensus on diagnostic criteria and long-term health risks related to polycystic ovary syndrome. Fertil Steril 81:19–25
Treasure JI, King EA, Gordon PAL et al (1985) Cystic ovaries: A phase of anorexia nervosa. Lancet 1379-1382
Treasure JL, Wheeler M, King EA et al (1988) Weight gain and reproductive function: ultrasonographic and endocrine features in anorexia nervosa. Clin Endocrinol 29:607–616
Viner RM, Teoh Y, Williams DM et al (1997) Androgen insensitivity syndrome: a survey of diagnostic procedures and management in the UK. Arch Dis Child 77:305–309
Vogel A, Alesbury J, Burrows P et al (2006) Vascular anomalies of the female external genitalia. J Pediatr Surg 41:993–999
Welt CK (2008) Primary ovarian insufficiency: a more accurate term for premature ovarian failure. Clin Endocrinol 68:499–509
Wisniewski AB, Migeon CJ, Meyer-Bahlburg HFL (2000) Complete androgen insensitivity syndrome: long-term medical, surgical, and psychosexual outcome. J Clin Endocrinol Metab 85:2664–2669
Zawadski JK, Dunaif A (1992) Diagnostic criteria for polycystic ovary syndrome: towards a rational approach. In: Dunaif A, Givens JR, Haseltine FP, Merriam GE (eds) Polycystic Ovary Syndrome. Current Issues in Endocrinology and Metabolism. Blackwell Scientific Publications, Boston

Gynaecological Causes of Pelvic Pain

Gurdeep S. Mann, Angela T. Byrne, and Anne S. Garden

Contents

1 **Introduction** 174
2 **Definition and Causes of Acute and Chronic Pelvic Pain** 174
3 **Clinical Evaluation** 176
4 **Pain Related to Periods** 176
4.1 Dysmenorrhoea 176
4.2 Cyclical Pain 176
4.3 Chronic Pain 176
4.4 Pain Unrelated to Periods 176
4.5 Imaging 177
5 **Ovarian Cysts** 177
5.1 Childhood Ovarian Cyst 177
5.2 Adolescent Ovarian Cysts 179
5.3 Haemorrhagic Ovarian Cyst 181
5.4 Cystic Corpus Luteum 184
6 **Obstruction of the Gynaecological Tract** 185
7 **Teratomas** 188
8 **Ovarian/Adnexal Torsion** 190
8.1 Massive Ovarian Oedema 193
8.2 Isolated Fallopian Tube Torsion 193
9 **Peritoneal Inclusion Cyst (PIC)** 195
10 **Paraovarian/Paratubal Cysts** 195
11 **Hydrosalpinx** 195
12 **Pelvic Inflammatory Disease** 198
13 **Pregnancy** 199
13.1 Ectopic Pregnancy 200
13.2 Gestational Trophoblastic Neoplasia 201
14 **Endometriosis** 202
15 **Adenomyosis** 205
16 **Uterine Leiomyoma** 205
17 **Pelvic Free Fluid** 205
18 **Conclusion** 206
References 206

G. S. Mann (✉)
Department of Radiology, Alder Hey Children's Hospital NHS Foundation Trust, Liverpool, UK
e-mail: gurdeep.mann@alderhey.nhs.uk

G. S. Mann
Department of Radiology,
Liverpool Women's Hospital NHS Foundation Trust,
Liverpool, UK

A. T. Byrne
Department of Radiology,
British Columbia Children's Hospital,
University of British Columbia,
Vancouver, BC, Canada

A. S. Garden
Division of Medicine, School of Health and Medicine,
Lancaster University, Lancaster, Lancashire, UK

A. S. Garden
University Hospitals of Morecambe Bay NHS Trust,
Kendal, Cumbria/Lancashire, UK

A. S. Garden
Alder Hey Children's Hospital NHS Foundation Trust,
Liverpool, UK

Abstract

Pelvic pain in girls is a common clinical complaint in childhood and throughout adolescence and an important cause of morbidity particularly in the postmenarchal female. Clinical evaluation in these patients is challenging. Abdominopelvic pain in the absence of a history of cyclical pain related to the menstrual cycle is a very non-specific symptom, with a range of

G. Mann et al. (eds.), *Imaging of Gynecological Disorders in Infants and Children*, Medical Radiology. Diagnostic Imaging, DOI: 10.1007/174_2011_436, © Springer-Verlag Berlin Heidelberg 2012

gynaecological and non-gynaecological causes. Non-gynaecological aetiologies of pain include gastrointestinal, urological, musculoskeletal and psychosomatic disorders. Gynaecological causes of pelvic pain include complications related to ovarian cysts (cyst rupture, haemorrhage or torsion), torsion of adnexal masses or normal ovaries, and fallopian tube pathology including torsion and pelvic inflammatory disease. Other causes of pain more specific to reproductively mature adolescents include ovulatory Mittelschmerz (mid-cycle) pain, endometriosis and complications of pregnancy. Exclusion of pregnancy in this age group is an important initial step in clinical management. This chapter concentrates on the imaging of the common and important causes of acute abdominal or pelvic pain with a gynaecologic aetiology. A brief discussion of the ultrasound imaging of pregnancy is included. The role of imaging in gynaecologic conditions resulting in chronic pelvic pain syndromes is also considered.

Abbreviations

PID	Pelvic inflammatory disease
CT	Computed tomography
MRI	Magnetic resonance imaging
US	Ultrasound
STIR	Short-tau inversion recovery
HOC	Haemorrhagic ovarian cyst
PIC	Peritoneal inclusion cyst
β-hCG	Beta human chorionic gonadotropin
HU	Hounsfield unit
SI	Signal intensity
AFP	Alpha fetoprotein
WI	Weighted-image
TSE	Turbo spin echo
HASTE	Half fourier acquisition single shot turbo spin echo
SPAIR	Spectral adiabatic inversion recovery
AVR	Adnexal volume ratio
PPV	Positive predictive value
NPV	Negative predictive value
3D	Three-dimensional
ADC	Apparent diffusion coefficient
DWI	Diffusion-weighted imaging
MOO	Massive ovarian oedema
PIC	Peritoneal inclusion cyst
IFTT	Isolated fallopian tube torsion
ESR	Erythrocyte sedimentation rate
TOA	Tubo-ovarian abscess
IU	International units
GTN	Gestational trophoblastic disease
PHM	Partial hydatiform mole
CHM	Complete hydatiform mole
PSTT	Placental site trophoblastic tumour
ETT	Epitheliod trophoblastic tumour
FIGO	International federation of gynaecology
AFS	American fertility society
IV	Intravenous
JZ	Junctional zone

1 Introduction

Abdominal and pelvic pain is a common problem in childhood and adolescence with up to 12.3% of girls reporting recurrent pain (Apley and Naish 1958). Gynaecological causes for such pain are relatively unusual and whilst this chapter will concentrate on the gynaecological causes, it is important that other causes are considered (Tables 1 and 2). Gynaecological causes of pelvic pain include complications related to ovarian cysts (cyst rupture, haemorrhage or torsion), torsion of adnexal masses or normal ovaries and fallopian tube pathology including torsion and pelvic inflammatory disease (PID). Other causes of pain more specific to the reproductively mature adolescent include ovulatory mittelschmertz (mid-cycle) pain, endometriosis and rarely complications of pregnancy. Exclusion of pregnancy in this age group is an important initial step in clinical management.

2 Definition and Causes of Acute and Chronic Pelvic Pain

Acute pelvic pain can be defined as noncyclical pelvic pain of less than three months duration (Cicchiello et al. 2011). In practical terms this definition is not that clinically useful and includes those with serious or life-threatening pathology which requires immediate resuscitation, diagnosis and definitive surgical management as well less serious conditions which only require conservative management. Associated symptoms may

Table 1 Differential diagnosis of acute pelvic pain in the adolescent and child

Gynaecological	*Non-pregnancy-related*
	Ovarian cyst (rupture, haemorrhage)
	Ovarian torsion
	Adnexal torsion
	Pelvic inflammatory disease
	Tubo-ovarian abscess
	Corpus luteum cyst haemorrhage
	Trauma (accidental/non-accidental)
	Tumour
	Foreign body
	Pregnancy-related
	Normal pregnancy
	Ectopic pregnancy
	Threatened miscarriage
	Retained products of conception (post-abortion endometritis)
Gastrointestinal	Appendicitis
	Perforation
	Bowel obstruction
	Volvulus
	Hernia
	Gastroenteritis
	Inflammatory bowel disease
	Abscess (perirectal, psoas)
	Mesenteric ischaemia
	Mesenteric lymphadenitis
Urological	Urolithiasis
	Acute Pyelonephritis
	Renal abscess
	Cystitis
	Urethritis
	Tumour
Musculoskeletal	Acute trauma
	Myofascial pain syndrome
Psychogenic	

include, fever, nausea and vomiting. A history of pelvic discharge or bleeding should alert to a gynaecological cause. Cyclical pain with or without other menstrual symptoms is more suggestive of gynaecological pain. The common gynaecologic and non-gynaecologic causes of acute pelvic pain are summarised in Table 1.

Table 2 Differential diagnosis of chronic pelvic pain in the adolescent and child

Gynaecological	Endometriosis
	Pelvic inflammatory disease
	Adhesions
	Congenital malformations of the genital tract
	Mittelschmerz
	Adenomyosis (rare)
Gastrointestinal	Constipation
	Irritable bowel syndrome
	Inflammatory bowel disease
	Celiac disease
Urological	Urolithiasis
	Chronic Pyelonephritis
	Chronic Cystitis
	Urethritis
Musculoskeletal	Scoliosis/kyphosis
	Spondylosis
	Spondylolisthesis
	Congenital anomaly
	Myofascial pain syndrome
Psychosocial	
Others	Porphyria

Acute pelvic pain of sudden onset is a common clinical presentation to the emergency department and frequently generates a request for diagnostic imaging. Ultrasound is the first-line imaging modality. Cross-sectional imaging is second line imaging unless part of a trauma series work-up where CT is indicated. In most other circumstances MRI is often preferable but contrast-enhanced CT is usually undertaken as it is more widely available in the acute setting. Radiographs have a very limited role in evaluating for non-gynaecological and gynaecological causes of acute pelvic pain.

Chronic pelvic pain is generally defined as recurrent or constant pain of at least 3 month's duration, or cyclical pain of 6 month's duration, which is sufficient to interfere with normal activities (Forcier 2009). Chronic pelvic pain which is cyclical is almost always gynaecologic in origin, whereas noncyclical chronic pelvic pain can have a host of other causes. The common gynaecologic and non-gynaecologic causes of chronic pelvic pain are summarised in Table 2. The role of diagnostic imaging in chronic pelvic pain is limited but can provide reassurance to exclude serious pathology. Again ultrasound is the first-line imaging modality of choice. A study of chronic pelvic pain in adolescents, investigated by laparoscopy, found no abnormality in 60%, endometriosis in 25%, ovarian cysts in 7%, paraovarian cysts in 3%, PID in 3% and adhesions in 2%. (Kontoravdis et al. 1999).

3 Clinical Evaluation

The first step in clinical assessment should include obtaining a clinical history which enables differentiation between acute and chronic pelvic pain and where relevant the timing of the pain in relation to the menstrual cycle. Whilst it is often difficult to get a clear history or periodicity in this age group, especially in girls whose periods are irregular, it is helpful to consider gynaecological pain as

- Pain related to periods
- Cyclical pain
- Pain unrelated to periods.

4 Pain Related to Periods

4.1 Dysmenorrhoea

Dysmenorrhoea (painful menstrual periods) is common, occurs in around 43% of teenagers (Svanberg and Ulmsten 1981) although one study reports an incidence of 80% (Hillen et al. 1999) and is the most common cause of short-term school absence in this age group (French 2008). It is caused by endometrial production of prostaglandins causing uterine contractions and myometrial ischaemia. The pain of dysmenorrhoea is typically lower abdominal, suprapubic and pelvic, although it also frequently radiates through to the back and down the anterior aspects of the thighs. It usually begins one to two days premenstrually, is worst on the first or second day of the period, the later days of the period usually being pain free. It occurs in ovulatory cycles, the first periods after the onset of menarche usually being painless. Pain associated with periods which last throughout the period, being just as painful at the end as on Day one, is more likely to have an underlying cause (see Table 3). Around 10% of adolescents reporting severe dysmenorrhoea will be found to have underlying pathology (Harel 2008).

Table 3 The main causes of persistent dysmenorrhoea in the adolescent population

Endometriosis
Genital outflow tract anomalies
Pelvic inflammatory disease
Abdominopelvic adhesions
Adenomyosis (rare)

Dysmenorrhoea responds well to non-steroidal anti-inflammatory preparations or the combined oral contraceptive pill. Pelvic imaging is not required in those who respond to medical therapy.

4.2 Cyclical Pain

Cyclical pain may be due to ovulation. Ovulation occurs 14 days prior to the period and diagnosis may be delayed in girls with an irregular menstrual cycle. While ultrasound may suggest the diagnosis through the findings of a collapsed follicle and free fluid in the pelvis, diagnosis is most usually made by suppression of ovulation by using the combined oral contraceptive pill which will result in abolition of the pain.

4.3 Chronic Pain

Chronic, intermittent pain may be due to a large ovarian cyst such as a teratoma. Smaller ovarian cysts—those 5 cm or less, particularly those with an anechoic appearance and without solid areas or septa, are normal physiologic cysts associated with follicular or corpus luteum development. Such ‘cysts’ do not cause pain, but can be a cause of unnecessary concern for a patient/parent, or a source of irritation for the gynaecologist—if they are reported as such! A repeat scan to ensure the ‘cyst’ has resolved is all that is required.

4.4 Pain Unrelated to Periods

Acute pain unrelated to periods provides the greatest diagnostic dilemma and may be due to ovarian cyst problems, ectopic pregnancy or PID. Chronic pain may be related to large ovarian ‘cysts’.

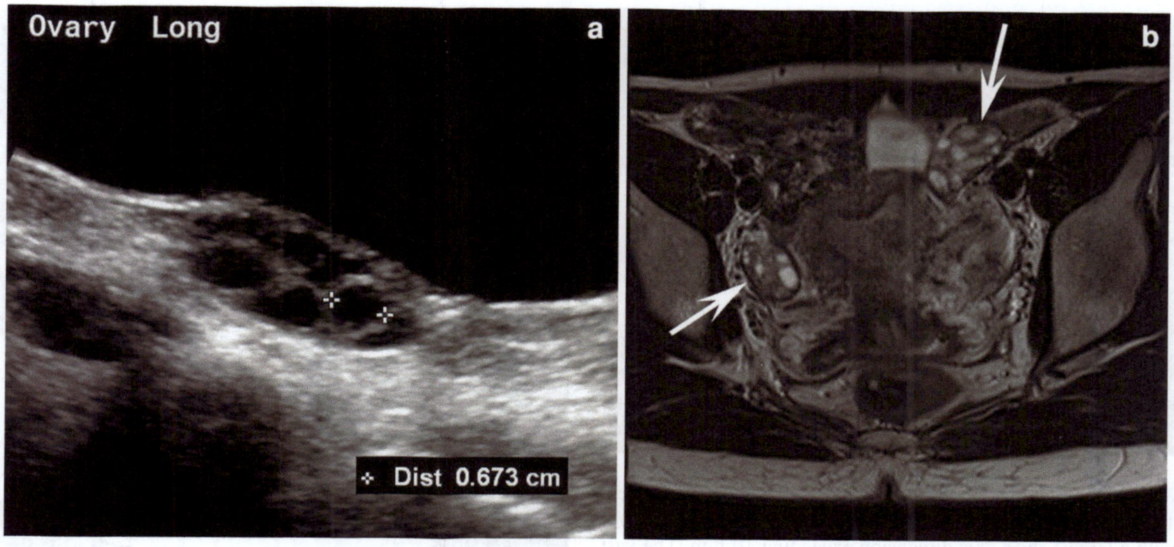

Fig. 1 **a** Typical sonographic appears of a multifollicular ovary containing several non-ovulatory follicles measuring no more than 9 mm in diameter. **b** Axial T2-weighted MRI of normal multifollicular ovaries (*arrows*)

4.5 Imaging

Imaging, particularly ultrasound, is important in the investigation of gynaecological pain in the paediatric and adolescent age group as bimanual examination should never be performed in a pre-pubertal girl without anaesthesia. Such clinical examination can be unhelpful even in an sexually active adolescent as they often find such an examination embarrassing and unpleasant and so find it difficult to relax—even when time is spent trying to reassure them prior to examination. For that reason, transvaginal ultrasound examination is rarely an option, and not typically offered in dedicated paediatric care facilities; trans-abdominal ultrasound in all cases should replace bimanual examination in this age group.

5 Ovarian Cysts

An ovarian cyst is defined by its size and sonographic appearances. The maximal diameter of an ovarian follicle (microcyst) is 10 mm (Fig. 1). Ovarian follicles are a normal finding and seen throughout childhood. An ovarian macrocyst, also referred to as 'ovarian cyst' is defined by a diameter exceeding 10 mm (Fig. 2). In postmenarcheal girls a dominant follicle will exceed 10 mm in diameter and should be considered a normal finding if appropriate to the stage of the menstrual cycle (Fig. 3). A simple cyst has barely perceptible thin-walls, uniformly anechoic content and no calcifications, associated mass or demonstrable vascularity on Doppler imaging. A single thin-walled septa (Fig. 4) or daughter cyst (Fig. 5) should not be considered indicative of a complex cyst.

Ovarian cysts are common in adolescence reflecting the cyclical hormonal changes related to menstruation which drives follicular maturation and involution. Simple ovarian cysts in childhood are follicular in origin. In postmenarchal girls ovarian cysts are usually follicular in origin but may be luteal or rarely thecal. Most ovarian cysts, typically measuring less than 5 cm in diameter, are entirely asymptomatic and will resolve spontaneously but do merit follow-up imaging to confirm resolution. Pain related to an ovarian cyst can result from cyst rupture, intracystic haemorrhage or where the cyst acts as fulcrum for adnexal torsion. Mittelschmerz occurs in the middle of the menstrual cycle and is a sharp pain related to ovarian follicle rupture during ovulation.

5.1 Childhood Ovarian Cyst

The ovaries show relatively slow growth in childhood and, on imaging appear fairly quiescent. The incidence

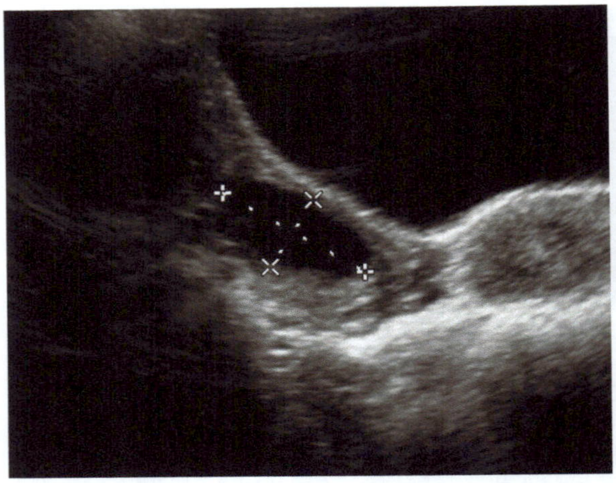

Fig. 2 Simple ovarian cyst. US image of a premenarcheal 11-year old with an anechoic follicular cyst (*between callipers*) with a largest short axis dimension exceeding 10 mm. The vast majority of ovarian cysts are asymptomatic and often detected as an incidental finding and will resolve on follow-up imaging

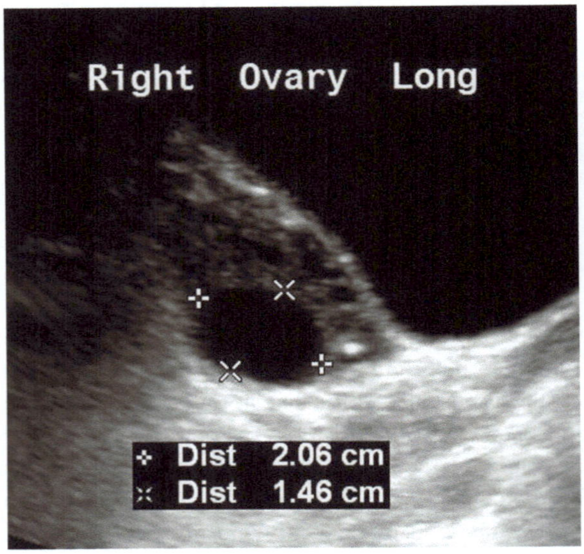

Fig. 3 US image of a postmenarcheal 16-year old with an anechoic dominant ovarian follicle (*between callipers*)

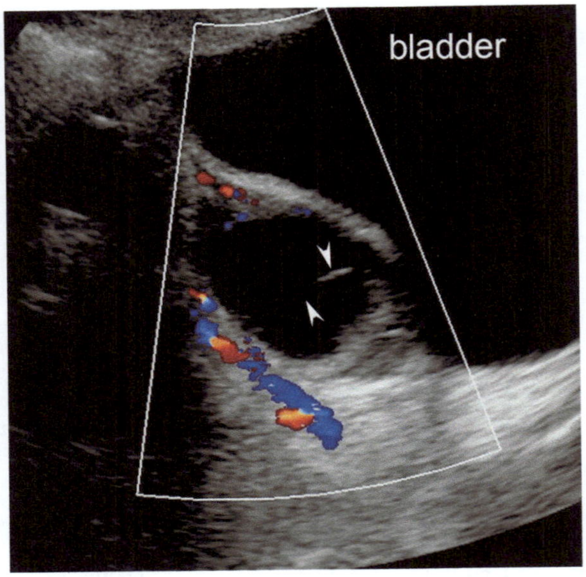

Fig. 4 Oblique colour Doppler US image of an ovarian cyst containing a thin uniform internal septum (*arrowheads*). No solid component, calcification or abnormal flow was demonstrated. This resolved on follow-up imaging

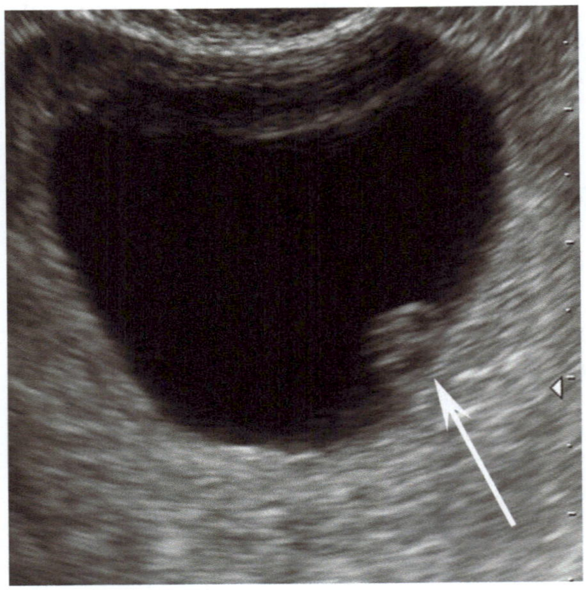

Fig. 5 Axial US image showing two small daughter cysts (*arrow*) lining the internal wall of an ovarian cyst

of ovarian cysts is lower in early childhood than in neonates and postmenarchal girls, corresponding with low-levels of gonadotropins and oestradiol production. Despite this, follicular maturation and involution is ongoing throughout childhood. Ovarian cysts in children generally result from disordered folliculogenesis and failure of cyst involution (Brandt and Helmrath 2005). The imaging appearances of ovarian cysts in this age group are similar to neonatal ovarian cysts. Asymptomatic cysts are typically documented on pelvic US for non-gynaecological indications. Small simple cysts which are anechoic and thin-walled can be monitored with surveillance US until resolution.

Table 4 Causes of benign ovarian tumours in children and adolescents

Benign epithelial tumours
Serous
Mucinous
Endometrioid
Borderline tumours
Serous
Mucinous
Germ cell tumours
Mature cystic teratoma
Functional teratomas
Gonadoblastoma
Sex cord stromal tumours
Thecoma
Fibroma
After Templeman and Fallat (2005)

Currently there is no consensus as to the management of ovarian cysts in this age group. The vast majority of cysts are follicular and functional in nature and most will resolve spontaneously. Management is based on cyst size, US characteristics, growth, persistence and symptoms. The aim of clinical management of ovarian cystic masses in children is where possible, to resolve symptoms whilst preserving functioning ovarian tissue and long-term fertility. There is a reasonable expectation that for the vast majority of children with ovarian lesions clinical management will be expectant and conservative. Ovarian malignancy is rare but not exceptional in this age group; most ovarian tumours will be benign (Islam et al. 2008). The subtypes of benign ovarian neoplasm encountered in paediatric practice are summarised in Table 4. Large ovarian cysts in this age group can be functional and associated with pseudo-precocious (gonadotropin-independent) puberty. The uterus should be evaluated with US to look for evidence of oestrogenisation with the length of the uterus and depth and quality of the endometrium documented. Autonomously hormonally active cysts are seen in McCune–Albright syndrome and occasionally in ovarian malignancy (see "Delayed and Precocious Puberty"). Helmrath et al. (1998) have reported ovarian neoplasms in the resection of three cases of apparently simple cysts which failed to involute on surveillance imaging.

Persisting, large, symptomatic or complex cysts merit surgical evaluation. Risk-stratification for these lesions should include pre-operative imaging initially with US and correlation with tumour markers. Timely involvement of a paediatric gynaecologist is important to plan appropriate surgical management and to prevent unnecessary ovarian biopsy, oophorectomy or salpingo-oophorectomy (Hernon et al. 2010).

5.2 Adolescent Ovarian Cysts

Ovarian cysts in the adolescent are very common. Most result from dysfunctional ovulation and persistence of the follicle. Other cysts include corpus luteum cysts and theca lutein cysts. The risk of ovarian malignancy is broadly inversely related to age and whilst rare, ovarian neoplasms are more common in this age group than any other encountered in paediatric practice.

Follicular ovarian cysts are typically 2–3 cm in diameter, simple, thin-walled, anechoic fluid-filled structures that develop in the first half of the menstrual cycle. These typically involute during the remainder of the menstrual cycle. In the absence of ovulation the cyst can grow larger (Fig. 6) but typically will resolve on imaging follow-up. A very large cyst may become symptomatic due to mass effect and are often referred to as a giant ovarian cyst. Abdominal pain and menstrual irregularity are common albeit non-specific associated symptoms. Most cysts will resolve over the next 2–3 menstrual cycles. Initial follow-up of US should be based on menstrual cycle length. We typically offer an initial 6-week follow-up US appointment in an asymptomatic girl with a simple adnexal cyst in whom the menstrual cycle length is around 4 weeks duration. Ultrasound examination of a girl with a ruptured ovarian cyst will reveal the collapsed sac with a large amount of free fluid in the Pouch of Douglas. While simple cysts show anechoic content on US, proteinaceous material will vary in echotexture but will show more echogenic content. On MRI a simple cyst is thin-walled with content of similar signal-intensity to urine or cerebrospinal fluid (Fig. 7). A proteinaceous cyst is bright on T1 W spin-echo imaging and will suppress on STIR or T2 W fat-saturated imaging (Fig. 8).

An adnexal cyst which does not resolve or continue to increase in size or complexity merits further evaluation. The differential diagnosis of an adnexal

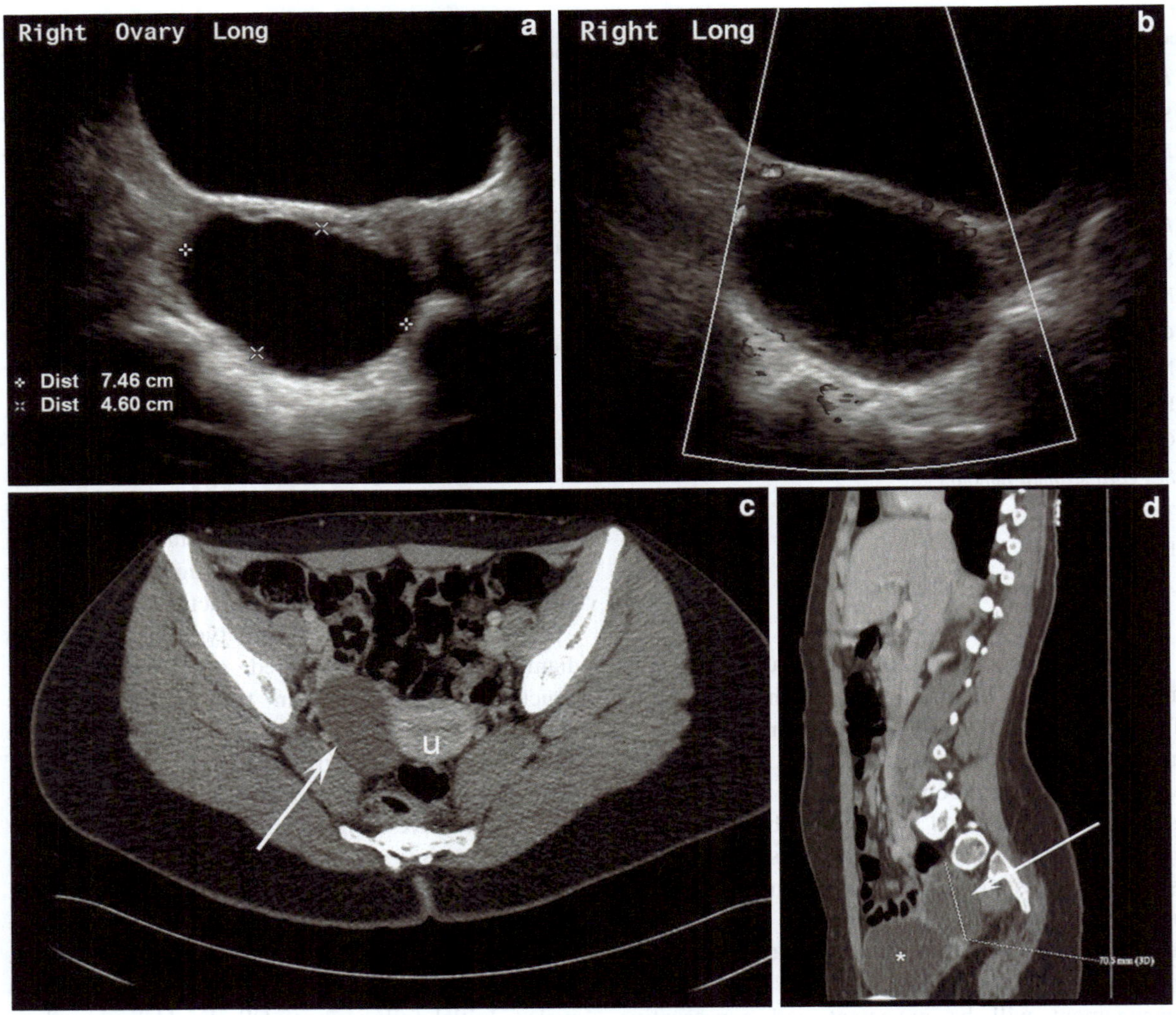

Fig. 6 **a** Gray-scale and **b** colour Doppler longitudinal US images of a large simple ovarian cyst. **c** Corresponding axial contrast-enhanced CT image and **d** sagittal reformatted image showing the hypoattenuating thin-walled ovarian cyst (*arrow*), (u) uterus (*) urinary bladder. The soft tissue contrast of CT is poor compared to that of US or MRI

cyst in the adolescent postmenarchal girl is summarised in Table 5 and includes peritoneal inclusion cyst (PIC), hydrosalpinx, tubo-ovarian abscess, paraurethral cyst (Fig. 9), paraovarian cyst, congenital uterine or tubal anomalies, ectopic pregnancy, endometriosis and ovarian tumour. In general before surgical removal of an adnexal cystic mass is undertaken correlation with serial imaging (US and where available MRI), tumour markers and discussion with a gynaecologist is indicated in order to prevent unnecessary oophorectomy.

Acute pain may result from bleeding into an ovarian cyst. Risk factors for bleeding include blood dyscrasias, anticoagulation and trauma. Most complex cysts in adolescents result from bleeding into a functional cyst. Bleeding typically occurs in the first 3 weeks of the menstrual cycle in a functional cyst and later in the cycle in a corpus luteum cyst. Differentiation between a haemorrhagic ovarian cyst (HOC) and other causes of a complex adnexal mass such as tumour may not be possible on diagnostic imaging. Complex cysts which do not resolve or continue to grow mandate a gynaecological or surgical opinion. The indications for surgical resection of a postpubertal ovarian cyst are summarised in Table 6.

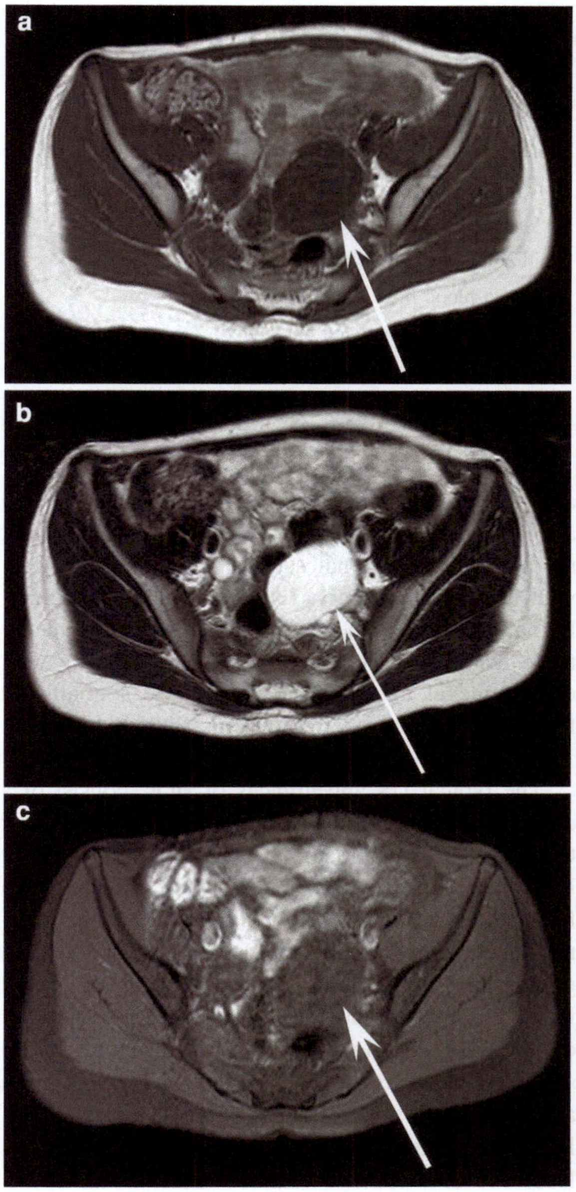

Fig. 7 MRI signal characteristics of a simple ovarian cyst (*arrow*). Axial **a** T1-weighted, **b** T2-weighted and **c** T2-weighted fat-suppressed imaging showing a left ovarian cyst which is isointense to fluid on all sequences. Comparison is typically made with the signal intensity of cerebrospinal fluid or urine

5.3 Haemorrhagic Ovarian Cyst

Bleeding into a follicular cyst or corpus luteum cyst can result in acute abdominopelvic pain. Rupture of a HOC is a cause of an acute abdomen. The gray-scale US appearances of a haemorrhagic follicular cyst and

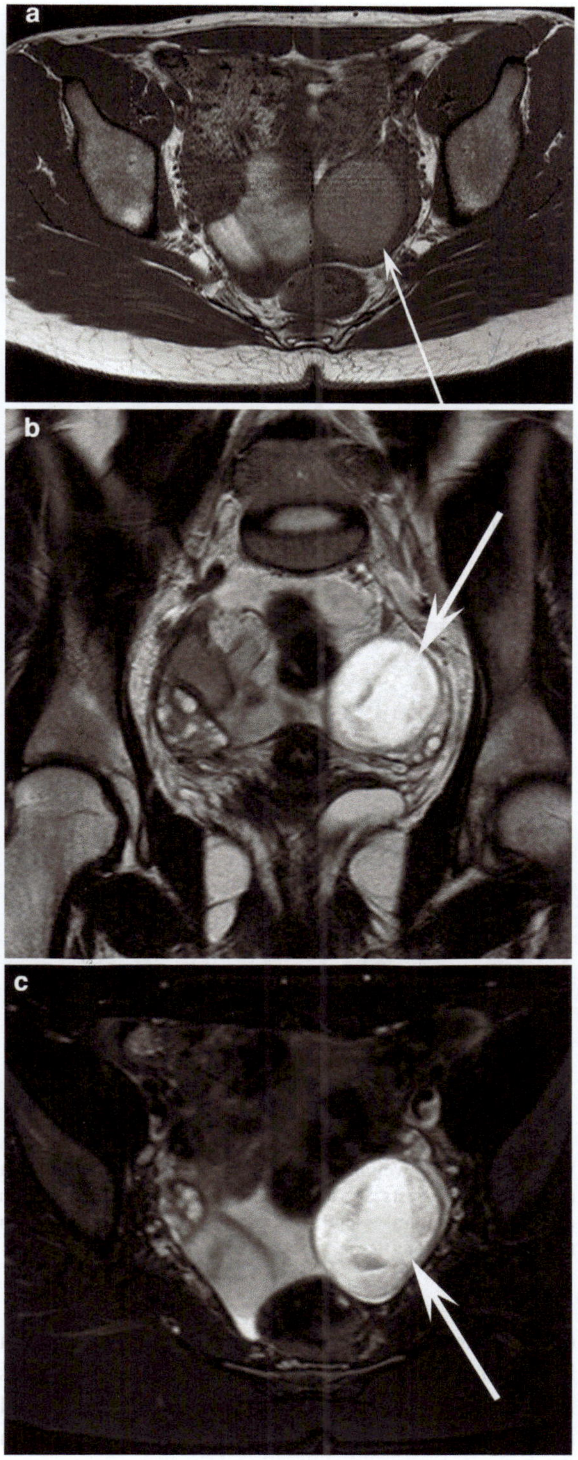

Fig. 8 MRI signal characteristics of a proteinaceous ovarian cyst (*arrow*). **a** Axial T1-weighted, **b** coronal T2-weighted and **c** axial T2-weighted fat-suppressed imaging showing a left ovarian cyst which is bright on T2-weighted imaging and of intermediate bright signal on T1. Pelvic free fluid is present

Table 5 Gynaecological causes of adnexal masses

Ovarian masses
Cyst
Benign tumour
Malignant tumour
Massive ovarian oedema
Peritoneal inclusion cyst
Tubo-ovarian torsion
Hydrosalpinx
Paratubal/paraovarian cyst
Paraurethral cyst
Ectopic pregnancy
Tubo-ovarian abscess
Endometrioma
Müllerian duct anomaly

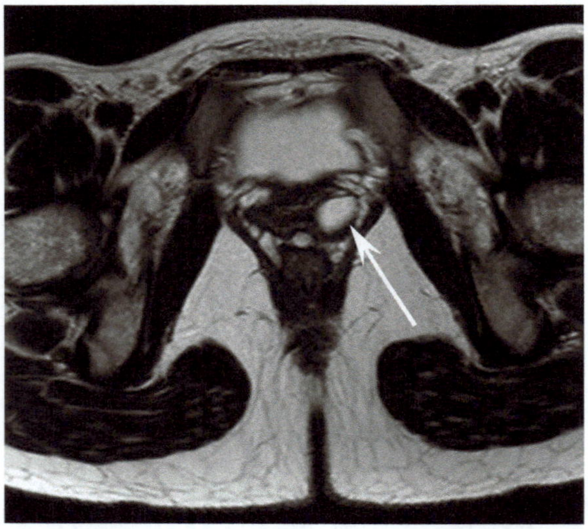

Fig. 9 Axial T2-weighted MR image of a paraurethral cyst (*arrow*). These cysts are uncommon and develop either from chronic paraurethral gland obstruction or are derived from remnant embryonic tissue

corpus luteum cyst are similar. The diagnosis of a haemorrhagic corpus luteum cyst (discussed below) is favoured when the cyst coincides with the luteal phase of the menstrual cycle or a positive serum β-hCG level.

The US appearances of a HOC depend on the age of the blood and the degree of clot formation or retraction. Fresh bleeding may initially appear

Table 6 Indications for considering surgical resection in the management of postpubertal ovarian cysts

Significant symptoms
Failure of cyst to involute on serial diagnostic imaging
Concern for torsion (even where imaging shows no lead point)
Concern for malignancy
Elevated AFP and β-hCG
Solid components or papillary projections
Increased blood flow
Complex or multiloculated mass
Where possible viable ovarian tissue should be conserved.
(After Brandt and Helmrath 2005)

anechoic to moderately echoic. Subacutely blood appears of mixed echotexture progressively becoming more complex. Internal septa may be present. Cyst wall thickness can vary. Eventually with clot dissolution, cyst content becomes anechoic. Unfortunately these features are nonspecific and may be seen with other adnexal masses. HOC may have sonographic features identical to dermoid cysts (Baltarowich et al. 1987).

The typical US appearances of HOC consist of a complex adnexal mass with variable posterior through transmission (Fig. 10). A HOC is defined by low-level echoes. In the first 24 h, the presence of a fine, reticular 'lacelike' pattern (Fig. 11) is diagnostically specific (Jain 2002). Curvilinear or triangular echogenic regions at the cyst wall may result from clot lysis. Internal fluid-debris levels can develop with clot liquefaction. The presence of fibrin strands and a retracting clot are key observations in allowing high confidence in the diagnosis of HOC. Approximately 90% of HOCs will exhibit at least one of these two features (Patel et al. 2005). Fluid–fluid levels and haemoperitoneum may be observed after cyst rupture.

Intact HOC typically appear unilocular on CT images, with an internal attenuation of 25–100 HU (Potter and Chandrasekhar 2008). Haemorrhagic cysts tend to display high signal intensity (SI) on T1-WI and intermediate to low signal on T2-WI (Fig. 12). Blood products may result in a crenulated cyst wall. The signal intensity of a haemorrhagic cyst should not differ with and without fat suppression which is helpful in differentiation from a dermoid. HOC demonstrated on cross-sectional imaging do not

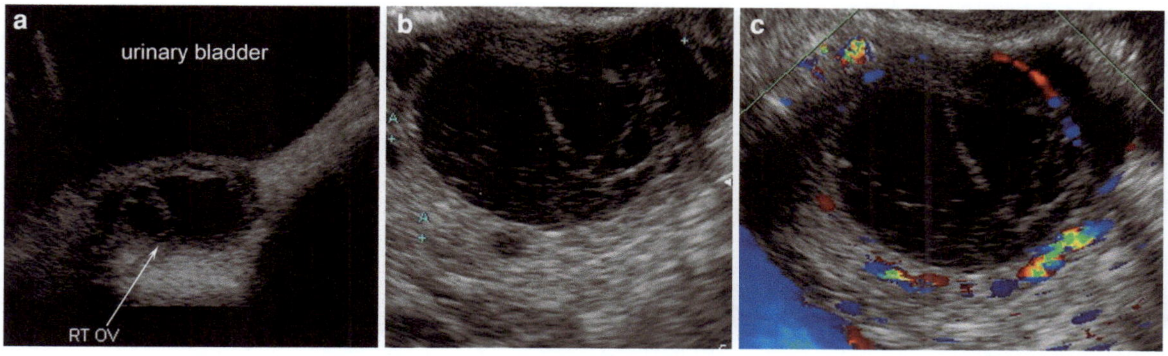

Fig. 10 Haemorrhagic ovarian cyst (HOC). **a** Transabdominal US showing an enlarged solid adnexal mass (*arrow*) with no discernible normal ovarian parenchyma. **b** Corresponding higher-resolution imaging and **c** colour Doppler US of the same lesion. Internal clot retraction is demonstrated and can give rise to highly variable internal appearances including avascular regions of solid appearing tissue. These appearances can be difficult to distinguish from adnexal torsion or cystic teratoma. HOC should regress and involute on follow-up imaging

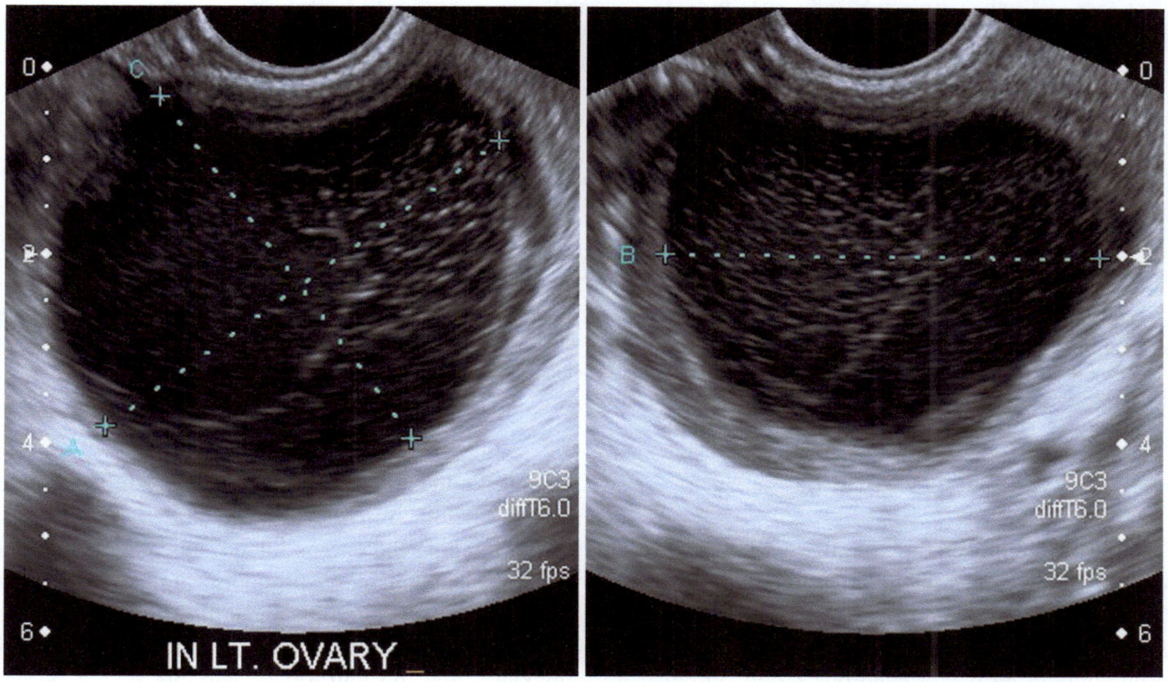

Fig. 11 Transvaginal US imaging showing a complex HOC with diffuse low-level echoes interspersed with a characteristic 'reticular' or 'lacelike' pattern due to fibrin strands which form as blood clots and retracts. HOC develop in follicular or corpus luteum cysts

require immediate ultrasound correlation unless there is significant associated haemoperitoneum. Follow-up imaging with US is mandated. Haemorrhagic cysts including corpus luteum cysts should decrease in size over the next menstrual cycle and resolve over 2–3 menstrual cycles. An endometrioma should be suspected and evaluated with MRI if a haemorrhagic cyst is unchanged in appearance over time in a postmenarchal girl. Cross-sectional imaging cannot reliably discriminate between a haemorrhagic cyst and a neoplasm which has bled. Laparoscopy and surgical resection should be considered for lesions which are stable but indeterminate and is indicated in growing lesions.

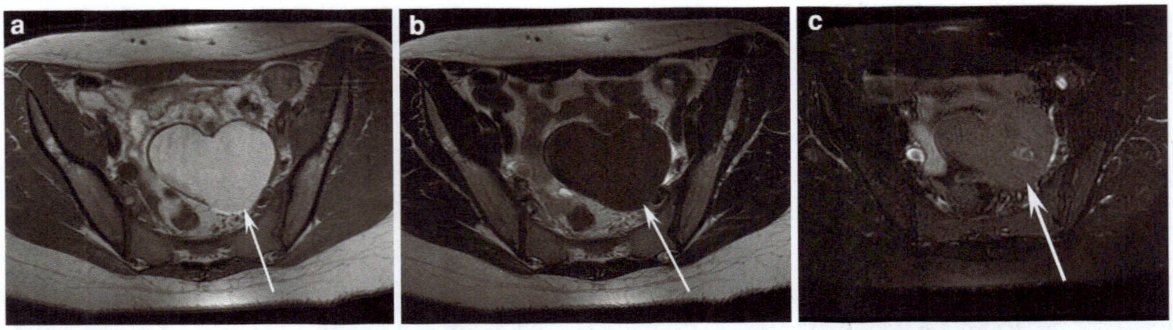

Fig. 12 MRI signal characteristics of a haemorrhagic ovarian cyst (*arrow*). Axial **a** T1-weighted, **b** T2-weighted and **c** T2-weighted fat-suppressed imaging showing a left ovarian cyst which is bright on T1, hypointense to fluid on T2 and of intermediate signal brighter than fat on fat-suppressed imaging. The differential would include haematosalpinx, if the appearances persist an endometrioma is more likely

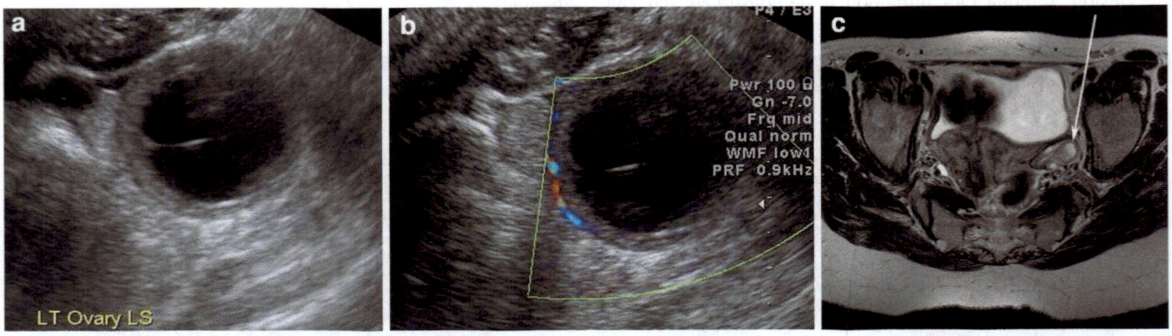

Fig. 13 Corpus luteum cyst. **a–b** Transvaginal US **a** showing the thick walls of a newly formed corpus luteum and **b** the typical increased peripheral vascularity of the luteal cyst wall. The presence of adjacent free fluid or more specifically haemoperitoneum is suggestive of luteal cyst rupture. **c** Axial T2-weighted MR image showing an involuting thick-walled luteal cyst (*arrow*)

5.4 Cystic Corpus Luteum

The corpus luteum is a functioning ovarian cyst which develops under the influence of luteinizing hormone following ovulation and implantation during the early luteal phase of the menstrual cycle. The wall of the corpus luteum derives a generous blood supply from neoangiogenesis which is essential in maintaining maternal progesterone levels. The corpus luteum itself is sustained by circulating maternal β-hCG.

Occasionally the corpus luteum may persist following ovulation in a non-pregnant female and is referred to as a corpus luteum cyst. This typically occurs in the late luteal phase of the menstrual cycle (within 14 days of ovulation). Corpus luteum cysts are usually solitary and measure 2.5–6.0 cm in maximal diameter. Pain may result from internal haemorrhage within the cyst, cyst rupture resulting in localised adnexal or pelvic free fluid, or failure of the corpus luteum to involute.

On imaging the corpus luteum cyst is thick-walled and may contain blood products (Fig. 13). The cyst content can vary from anechoic fluid, isoechoic echoes or contain debris from clot. The cyst wall thickness may be uniform or variable if clot retraction, adherent clot or cyst wall rupture are present. Sonographic through transmission is indicative of an underlying cyst (Jain 2002). Colour Doppler US of the luteinised cyst wall epithelium often results in increased peripheral flow. Cross-sectional imaging appearances are comparable with ultrasound findings. On CT the cyst is thick-walled, shows distinct wall enhancement and may contain blood products (Borders et al. 2004). Like haemorrhagic cysts, corpus luteum cysts tend to display high SI on T1-WI and intermediate to high signal on T2-WI. Blood products

Table 7 Simplified classification of congenital obstructive uterovaginal anomalies

Müllerian Organogenesis	Inadequate development of one or more Müllerian ducts	Uterine agenesis
		Uterine hypoplasia
		MRKH
Fusion	• Lateral fusion	Bicornuate uterus
	• Vertical fusion	Uterus didelphys
		Unicornuate uterus with a rudimentary horn
		Cervical atresia
		Vaginal septa
		Imperforate hymen
Septal resorption	Failure of resorption	Septate uterus

Table 8 Terminology used to describe gynaecological tract obstruction and accumulation of genital secretions

Prefix	Suffix
Haemato—blood	colpos—vaginal distension
Hydro[a]—serous fluid	metrocolpos—uterine & vaginal
Muco[a]—mucous	distension
Pyo—pus	metra—uterine distension
Aero—air or other gas	salpinx—fallopian tube distension
Uro[b]—urine	

[a] Mucous and serous fluid often referred to by the common prefix of 'hydro'
[b] Urine may accumulate in the presence of urogenital sinus

may result in a crenulated cyst wall. On MR the luteinised wall shows avid enhancement unlike typical follicular cysts. The corpus luteum eventually involutes to form the corpus albicans which is not visible on diagnostic imaging.

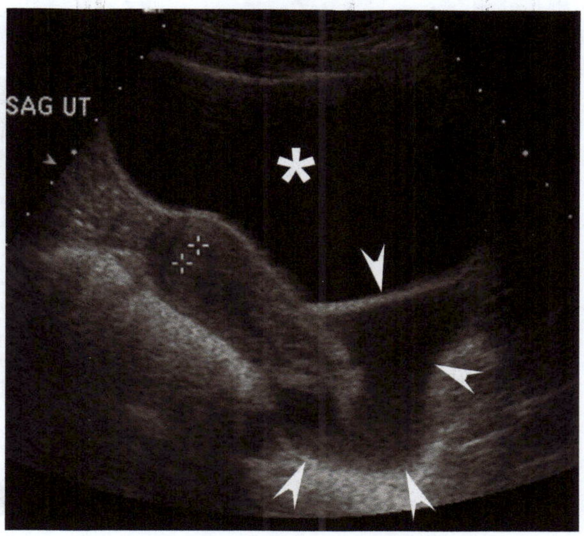

Fig. 14 Haemotocolpos secondary to an imperforate hymen. Longitudinal US image showing diffuse fine echoes distending the vagina (*arrowheads*). Uterine endometrium (*between callipers*), (*) Urinary bladder

6 Obstruction of the Gynaecological Tract

Obstruction of menstruation in the genital tract can be difficult to diagnose. Obstructed congenital uterovaginal anomalies typically present at menarche with the accumulation of blood in the genital tract proximal to the level of obstruction. The diagnosis of cryptomenorrhoea (hidden menstruation) may not be made initially, and the girl may well present several times to the emergency services, and even be admitted, before the diagnosis is made. This is particularly true in girls who have not yet developed a regular menstrual cycle and so the association with menstruation is missed. The underlying causes include imperforate hymen, vaginal septa, genital tract atresia and stenosis. A simplified classification of the causes and mechanisms of congenital obstructive uterovaginal anomalies are summarised in Table 7.

The most common causes of obstruction include a transverse vaginal septum or imperforate hymen. In girls with an imperforate hymen, clinical examination will show a central mass arising out-of the pelvis and separation of the labia will usually show the classical appearances of a 'blue bulge' at the introitus. Higher or thicker septa will not show the blue bulge appearance. Imaging with US cannot reliably

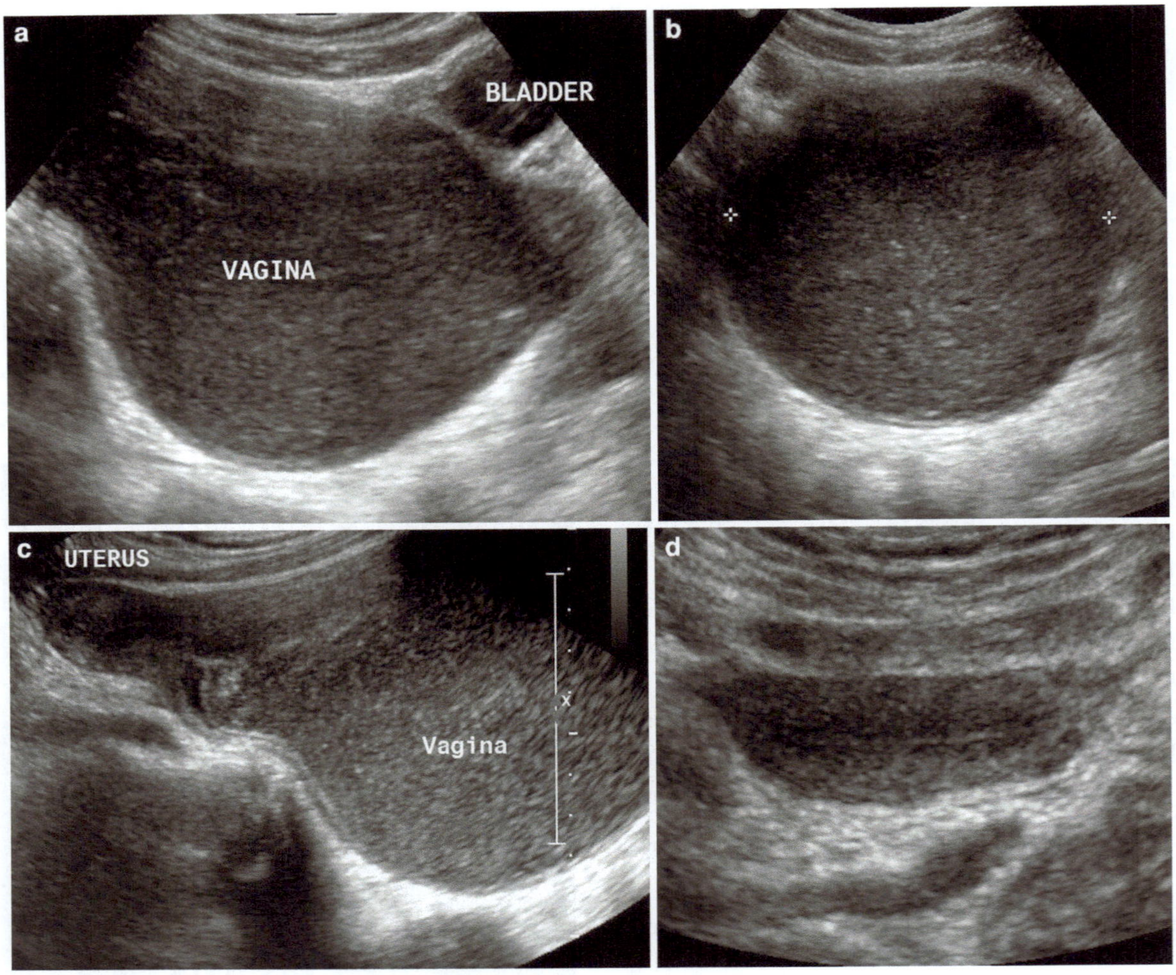

Fig. 15 Haematocolpos secondary to a transverse vaginal membrane. **a** Longitudinal and **b** transverse US imaging showing menstrual blood products distending the vagina. **c** Longitudinal and **d** transverse US imaging of the uterus

differentiate between high and low septa. MRI is useful in pre-operative planning by delineating the thickness of an obstructing membrane or septum, its position can be inferred by the level at which genital tract secretions accumulate (Olpin and Heilbrun 2009).

Presenting symptoms in the adolescent include delayed onset of menarche, primary amenorrhoea, dysmenorrhoea or cyclical pelvic pain. As blood accumulates with each menstrual cycle a palpable pelvic mass can result from haematocolpos or haematometrocolpos, the latter is a very rare entity. This may rarely result in urinary retention or an interlabial mass (Blask et al. 1991). Obstructive Müllerian anomalies preclude the outflow of menstruation increasing the likelihood of retrograde menstruation. A high incidence of decreased fertility and obstetric complications is common in later life. Genital tract obstruction can also present in the neonate or infant (see "Gynaecological Disorders in the Neonate and Young Child"). In children between these age groups serous fluid may accumulate from secretions by mucous glands in the cervix and vagina. Obstruction may occur at any level resulting in proximal accumulation of secretions. The nomenclature describing the level of obstruction and fluid type contained within the obstructed viscous are summarised in Table 8.

Ultrasound examination reveals a fluid-filled distended vagina. Fluid may also distend the uterus. Anechoic content is consistent with serous fluid

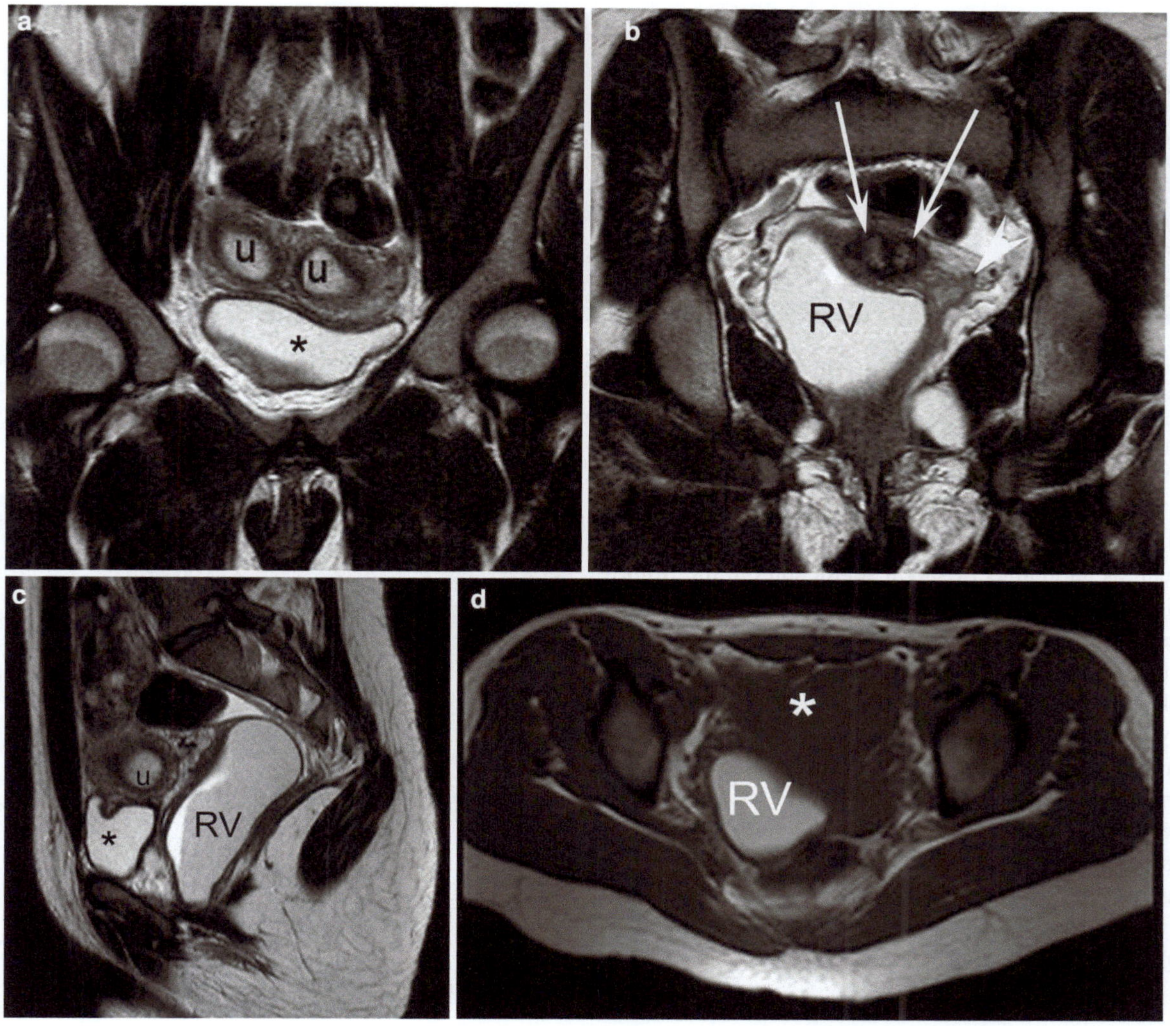

Fig. 16 Characteristic MR-imaging features of uterus didelphys. **a–b** Coronal T2-weighted-TSE imaging showing **a** failed Müllerian ductal fusion, with two widely divergent symmetric uterine horns (u) *above* the urinary bladder (*); and, **b** two cervixes (*arrows*). The *right* vagina (RV) is obstructed, the *left* vagina (*arrowhead*) is non-obstructed and the patient is still having cyclical menstrual bleeding. **c** High signal content is seen within the *right* vagina (RV) on sagittal T2 imaging and **d** axial T1-weighted-TSE imaging indicating the presence of blood. Unilateral hematocolpos implies the presence of an obstructing unilateral vaginal septum. Didelphic uteri account for approximately 10% of Müllerian duct anomalies. A longitudinal vaginal septum is present in around 75% of cases. Unilateral renal agenesis was not present in this case

(Fig. 14). If the fluid contains internal echoes this usually represents blood rather than pus (Fig. 15). Fluid which is of similar echotexture to the content of an endometrioma is compatible with degraded blood products. Obstruction of menstruation may also be associated with an obstructed rudimentary horn. Diagnosis may be delayed as these girls will menstruate normally from the unobstructed horn. Ultrasound will show the distended horn alongside the normal horn, which may well be mistaken for an adnexal cyst. On MRI serous fluid is hypointense on T1-WI and of high signal intensity on fat-suppressed and T2-WI. Increased T1 signal is seen with proteinaceous material (Fig. 16). Fluid levels are not uncommon. The appearances of blood breakdown products follow a predictable temporal sequence on MRI. Blood is typically hyperintense on T1-WI and low or variable signal on T2-WI and is not affected by fat suppression.

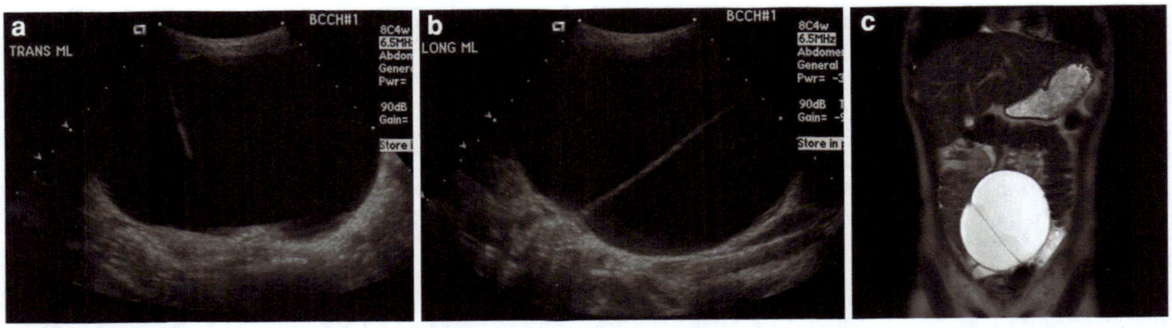

Fig. 17 Mature cystic teratoma. **a** Transverse and **b** longitudinal US images, **c** corresponding coronal T2-weighted HASTE image of a multicystic lesion surgically confirmed to be a mature teratoma arising from the left ovary. On US the inferior margin of the lesion was difficult to ascribe suggesting that this was a pelvic mass. The organ of origin of large lesions can be difficult to ascertain on US

MRI is useful in documenting the level of obstruction and presence of any associated malformations such as anomalies of sacral segmentation, the Müllerian ducts and renal upper tracts. Imperforate hymen is usually not associated with any other Müllerian abnormality and occurs as a result of incomplete canalisation of the urogenital sinus with the Müllerian duct system. Imperforate hymen cannot be differentiated from a low transverse vaginal septum by diagnostic imaging. Transverse vaginal septum is not associated with other urological or Müllerian anomalies. Longitudinal vaginal septum is usually associated with uterus didelphys, ipsilateral renal hypoplasia or agenesis (Orazi et al. 2007) and rarely multicystic dysplastic kidney (Prada Arias et al. 2005).

7 Teratomas

An important differential for a painful adnexal mass with complex imaging appearances is an ovarian tumour. Ovarian tumours in childhood are more commonly benign than malignant (Panteli et al. 2009). By far the most common lesions are germ cell tumours. The most common subtype is a mature cystic teratoma. Almost all mature teratomas contain a cystic component and are benign. Immature teratomas are potentially malignant and typically contain primitive neuroepithelium (Harms et al. 2006). Imaging alone cannot reliably differentiate between a benign and malignant teratoma. Serum tumour markers should be obtained. The surgical management of ovarian tumours is discussed further in Chap. "Gynaecological Neoplasia".

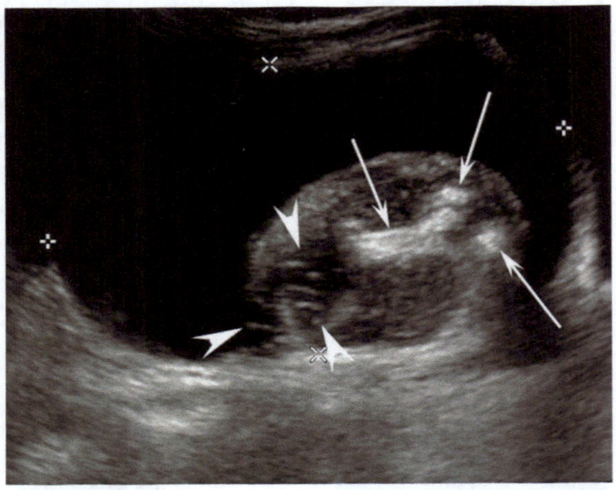

Fig. 18 Dermoid cyst. Transverse US showing a large well-defined cyst containing a complex rounded solid component of variable echotexture. The central echogenic component is predominately fat (*arrows*). Hair is present with a small area showing the characteristic multiple hyperechoic interfaces typical of the 'dermoid mesh' sign (*arrowheads*)

Teratomas contain derivatives from all three germ layers and are lined by squamous epithelium. In approximately 15–20% of cases disease is bilateral and over 15% of cases may be associated with torsion (Talerman 2003). Mature cystic teratomas contain elements of at least two of the three germ layers: endoderm, mesoderm and ectoderm. As ectodermal elements predominate, these lesions are also commonly referred to as 'dermoid cysts'.

The sonographic appearances of teratomas are highly variable and dependent on the overall composition of hypoechoic cyst fluid content (Fig. 17), as

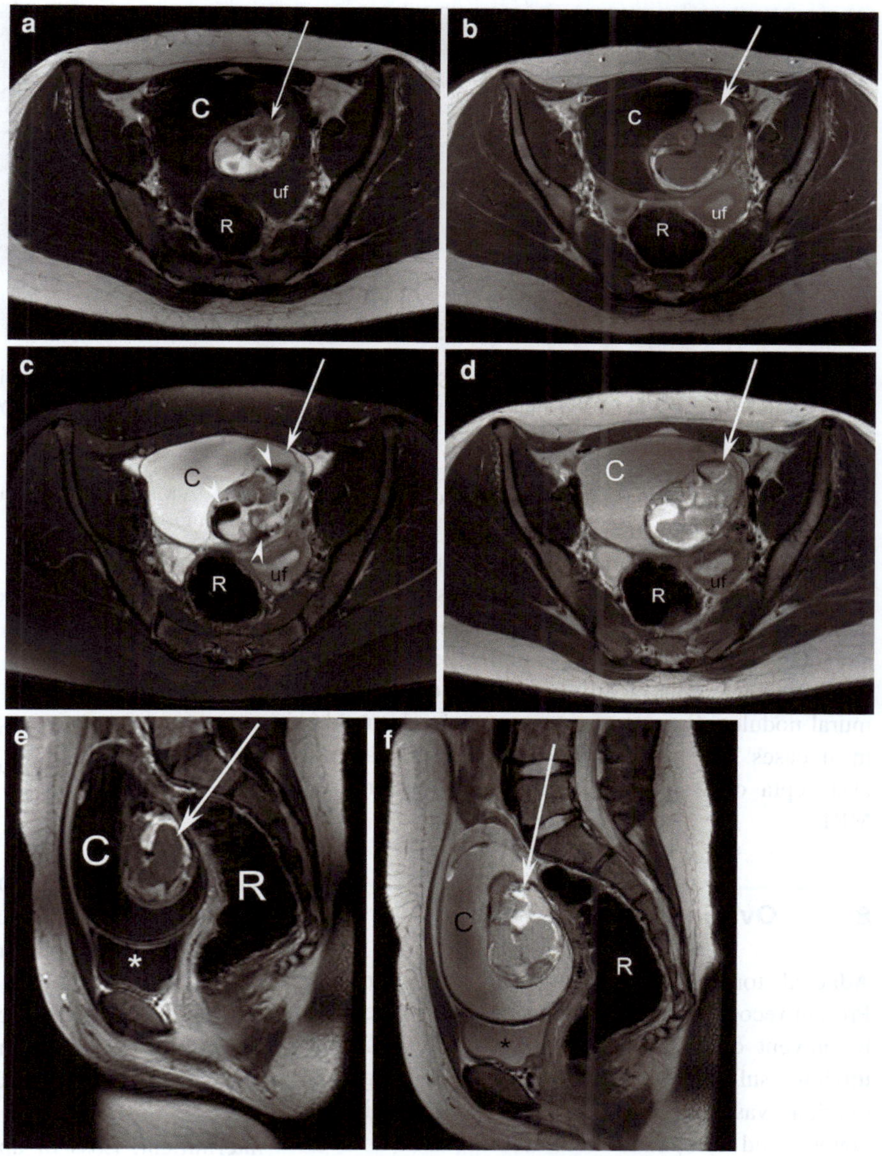

Fig. 19 Dermoid cyst. MRI imaging of the same lesion as Fig. 18 with a large macrocyst (C) and associated solid component (*arrow*). **a** Axial T1-weighted TSE showing scattered bright fatty tissue in the solid component, **b** axial T1-weighted TSE post gadolinium showing enhancing tissue within the centre of the solid component which is isointense to the uterine myometrium, **c** T2-weighted fat-suppressed SPAIR showing suppression of the fatty components (*arrowheads*), **d** axial-T2-weighted TSE and **e–f** sagittal T1 & T2-weighted TSE imaging showing the large cystic component. Urinary bladder (*), uterine fundus (uf), rectum (R)

well as the differing amounts and distribution of hyperechoic fat, teeth or hair.

Various specific sonographic findings characteristic of a cystic teratoma have been reported including the tip of the iceberg sign, fat-fluid levels, fat-hair levels, dermoid mesh sign (Fig. 18), dermoid plug sign (Rokitansky's protuberance) and echogenic intracystic fat balls (Beller 1998; Hutton and Rankin 1979; Kawamoto et al. 2001; Malde et al. 1992; Quinn et al. 1985). The tip of the iceberg sign refers to the interface of hair and sebum producing echogenic foci in the near field which result in obscuration of all but the most anterior portion of the cyst. The dermoid mesh sign is attributed to hair floating within the cyst yielding multiple linear echogenic interfaces (Fig. 18). The dermoid plug sign is an outgrowth of hair and other tissues from the inner surface of a cyst.

MRI using T1-weighted imaging with and without fat suppression will confirm tumour fat content with signal loss demonstrated on fat-suppressed imaging (Fig. 19), and will help differentiate from a haemorrhagic cyst or endometrioma. In- and out-of-phase chemical shift imaging can also demonstrate tiny

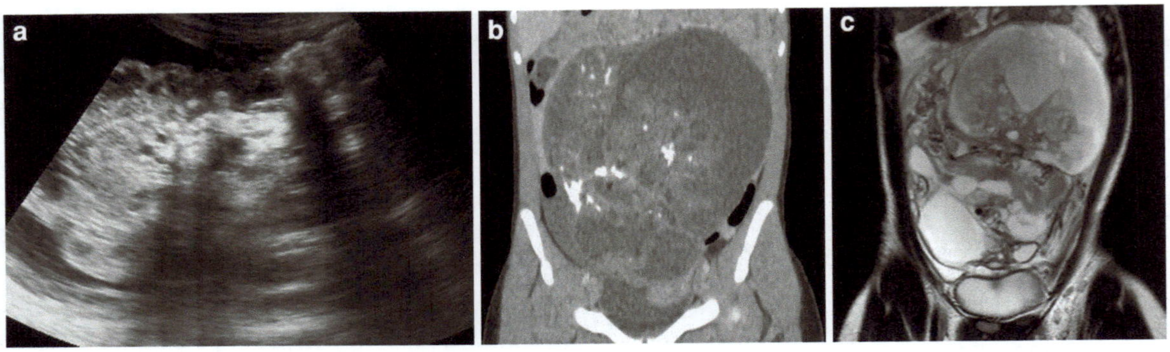

Fig. 20 Germ cell tumour. **a** Longitudinal US, **b** contrast-enhanced CT coronal reformatted image and **c** coronal T2-weighted HASTE MR image of a large abdominopelvic germ cell tumour with fatty components and dystrophic calcifications

amounts of intralesional fat with signal loss on out-of-phase imaging (Outwater et al. 2001).

Pre-contrast CT imaging is not routinely indicated. Contrast-enhanced CT is often used where the availability of MRI is limited. CT has one clear advantage in demonstrating calcifications (Fig. 20) or teeth which are typically located in non-enhancing mural nodules. Fat attenuation content is observed in most cases. CT is relatively poor at demonstrating cyst septa or walls compared with ultrasound and MRI.

8 Ovarian/Adnexal Torsion

Adnexal torsion is an acute surgical emergency. Prompt recognition and early intervention is required to prevent comprise of long-term fertility. Ovarian torsion results from partial or complete twisting of the ovarian vascular pedicle causing obstruction to venous and lymphatic outflow. If rotation of the ovarian vascular pedicle about its axis is sufficient to compromise arterial inflow, ovarian ischaemia and eventually infarction may occur (Graif and Itzchak 1988). A pathologic lead point acts as fulcrum potentiating torsion.

Adnexal torsion may involve the ovary, fallopian tube or both. There is a slight right sided preponderance. The mean age of presentation is around 10 years. Approximately 10% of cases occur neonatally or in utero. In all cases a lead point such as an ovarian cyst, teratoma or tumour should be actively sought as the underlying cause, outside the infantile period the likelihood of a lead point is low and

Table 9 Main gray-scale imaging findings of ovarian or tubo-ovarian torsion

Unilaterally enlarged ovary
8–12 mm peripheral cysts (cyst fluid-debris levels are pathognomonic)
Ascites
Heterogeneous adnexal cystic structure
Abnormal medial location of ovary
Hydrosalpinx in fallopian tube torsion

increases with age. The paediatric adnexa are more mobile than adults. Developmental abnormalities such as an absent mesosalpinx or redundant fallopian tube predispose to twisting of normal adnexa which is a more common finding in children.

The clinical presentation is fairly non-specific and consists of lower abdominal and pelvic pain, usually of acute onset and severe in nature. Pain typically localises to the affected lower quadrant and may be intermittent. Loss of appetite, nausea and vomiting are commonplace. A tender mass is a common clinical finding. These presenting symptoms are similar to those encountered in acute appendicitis with an associated inflammatory mass.

US is the imaging modality of choice to evaluate children with suspected torsion (Fig. 21). Recognition of the typical gray-scale imaging appearances (Table 9) is key to making the diagnosis. It must be noted however that these appearances are fairly non-specific. The differential includes HOC, ovarian tumour, paratubal cyst, tubo-ovarian abscess and endometrioma; pathologies which are more commonly encountered in postmenarchal adolescents.

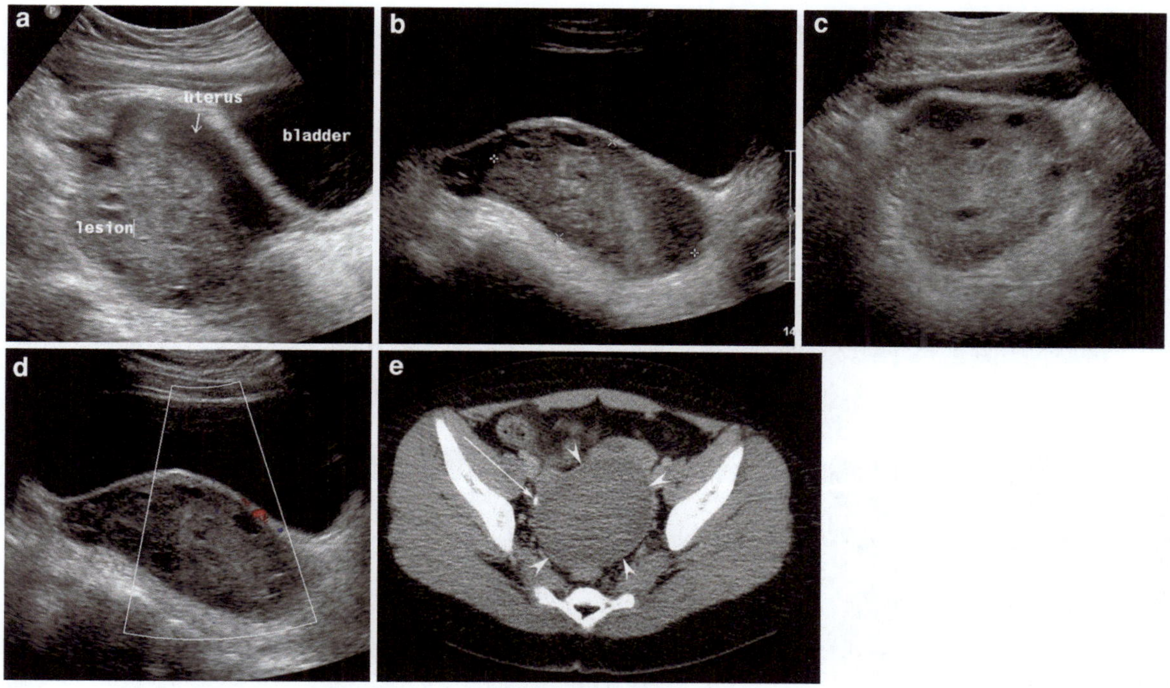

Fig. 21 Surgically proven adnexal torsion. **a–b** Longitudinal and **c** transverse US imaging in an 11-year old girl showing an enlarged echogenic torsed ovary with several peripheral non-ovulatory follicles located in the midline above the fundus of the uterus. **d** Colour Doppler imaging revealed absence of flow in this solid lesion. The presence of arterial flow does not exclude torsion. The contralateral ovary was normal. The adnexal volume ratio (symptomatic ovarian volume divided by the contralateral asymptomatic ovarian volume) was 10.2. **e** Axial contrast-enhanced CT of the same girl showing the torsed ovary (*arrowheads*) and *right* ureter (*arrow*)

Unilateral adnexal enlargement is an important diagnostic clue. Using the adnexal volume ratio (AVR) which compares the volume a pathologic adnexa to the normal contralateral ovary, a median value of 12 was seen in a retrospective surgical case series of proven torsion (Servaes et al. 2007). In the same study an AVR cut-off value of 20 yielded a positive predictive value (PPV) of 70% (AVR > 20) and negative predictive value (NPV) of 90% (AVR < 20) for an associated mass. The best negative predictor of torsion in menarcheal girls is an adnexal volume < 20 ml, with a NPV of 100% (Linam et al. 2007). Vascular congestion as result of impaired circulation is thought to account for the increase in volume.

In 74% of patients with ovarian torsion, spherical anechoic cysts measuring up to 2.5 cm in diameter (typical range 8–12 mm) have been found in the periphery of the enlarged ovary (Fig. 21) (Graif and Itzchak 1988). Transudation of fluid into the follicles as part of generalised vascular congestion is thought to account for the peripheral multifollicular enlargement. The presence of fluid-debris levels in the follicular cysts is considered pathognomonic for torsion (Kiechl-Kohlendorfer et al. 2006).

Amputation of a torsed ovary has been demonstrated and is characterised by the finding of a cystic mass with a partially calcified mural nodule (Currarino and Rutledge 1989). Rarely bowel obstruction may result from adhesions caused by a torsed necrotic ovary (Jeanty et al. 2010). In the neonate the presence of an adnexal cyst with a fluid-debris level has been used to define a complicated cyst either resulting from haemorrhage and/or torsion (Nussbaum et al. 1988).

Colour Doppler US is an important adjunct to the diagnosis of torsion but the sensitivity and specificity of transabdominal colour and power Doppler in children to date has not been encouraging. Torsion may be partial and sufficient only to impede venous

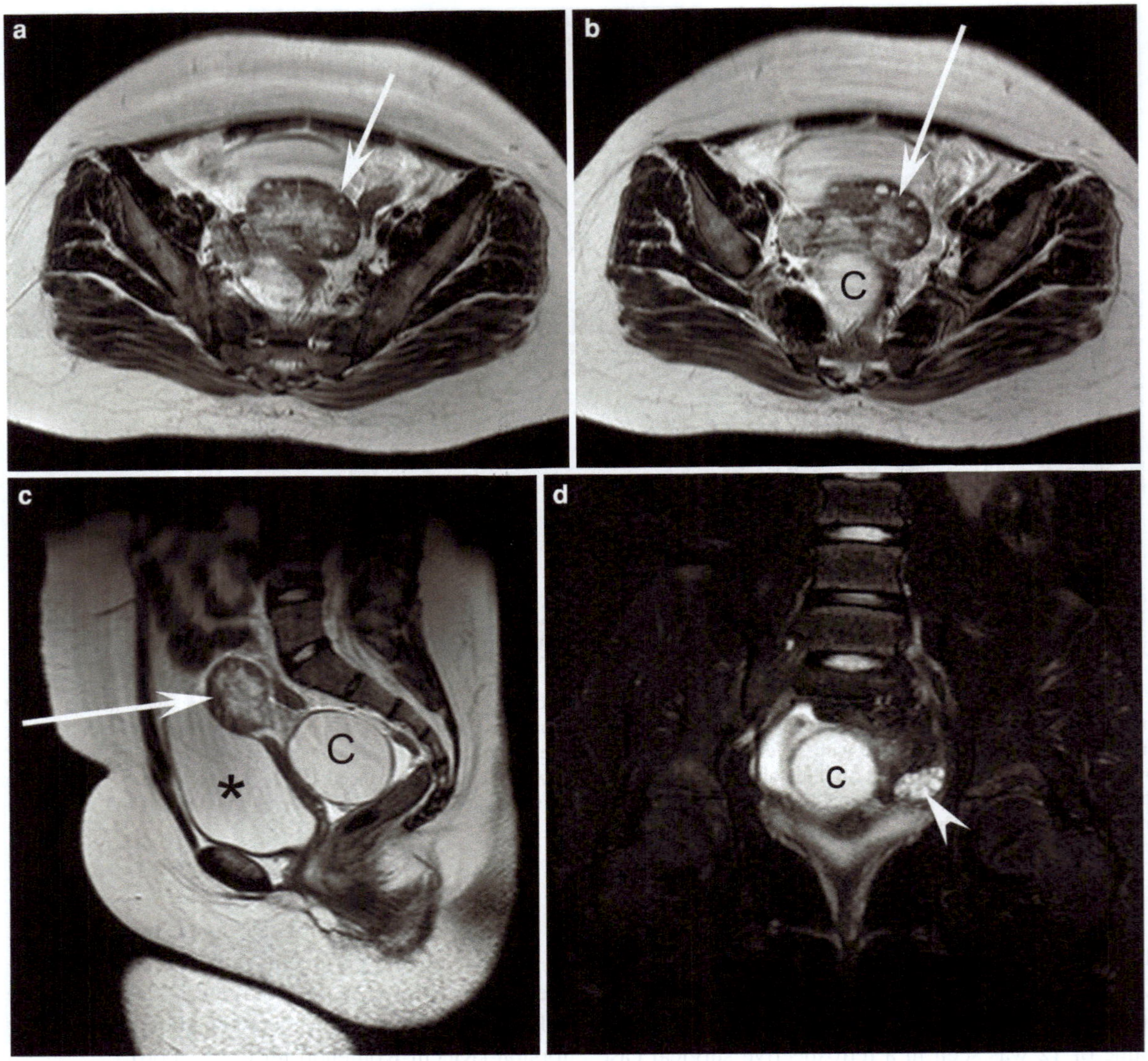

Fig. 22 Ovarian torsion. MR imaging of a 12-year old premenarchal girl presenting with a one-day history of sudden onset acute right iliac fossa pain. **a–b** Axial T2-weighted-TSE, **c** sagittal T2-weighted and **d** coronal fat-suppressed T2-weighted imaging showing unilateral enlargement of the *right* ovary (*arrow*) measuring 6.7 × 6.0 × 3.3 cm with an oedematous medulla and prominent peripheral nonovulatory follicles—*string of pearls sign*. The torsed ovary was located in the midline superior to the uterine fundus and adjacent to the urinary bladder (*). The lead point in this case was a 5 cm right ovarian cyst (C). The left ovary was normal (*arrowhead*). Trace pelvic free fluid was present. Surgical treatment involved prompt laparoscopic detorsion and oophoropexy, with ovarian cyst drainage and deroofing. The appendix was normal on pre-operative imaging and at surgery

outflow. During the recovery phase in intermittent torsion, either venous or arterial flow may be detected with de-twisting of the vascular pedicle. Ovarian flow may be normal or even increased in intermittent torsion. A normal colour Doppler study does exclude torsion due to the presence of collateral blood supply; typically there is dual supply from both the ovarian and uterine arteries (Peña et al. 2000). It should be noted that absence of blood flow in an adnexal mass with the characteristic gray-scale findings is highly suggestive of torsion (Albayram and Hamper 2001).

Colour Doppler US has been used to predict adnexal viability. Transvaginal 3D-power Doppler US has been advocated in assessing for ovarian torsion but clearly its use should only be considered in sexually active adolescents. The presence of arterial

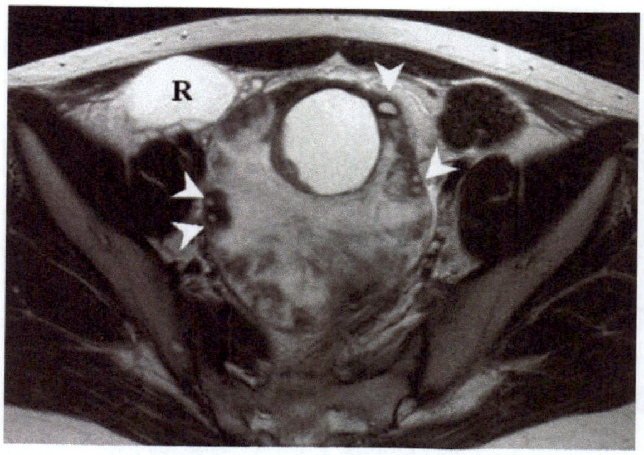

Fig. 23 Massive ovarian oedema (MOO). Axial T2-weighted MR image of a 15 year girl with acute abominopelvic pain and left ovarian torsion. The left ovary is markedly enlarged and contains follicles (*arrowheads*). The right ovary (R) is normal. Image reproduced from Yamashiro et al. 2008 with permission from Springer publishers

blood flow alone in the torsed pedicle is predictive of non-viability, but in patients with either venous or both arterial and venous blood flow is indicative of ovarian viability (Kupesic and Plavsic 2010). The presence of a 'whirlpool-sign' has been described in adult ovarian torsion (Vijayaraghavan 2004).

The CT features suggestive of adnexal torsion include an enlarged ovary (Fig. 21), typically seen as a heterogeneous cystic mass, a peripheral cystic mass in pure tubal torsion, uterine deviation towards the torsed pedicle, smooth wall thickening of the twisted adnexal cystic mass and ascites (Chang et al. 2008). Although CT may show features suggestive of adnexal torsion, the initial diagnostic yield of CT is less than that of US (Chiou et al. 2007). Whilst MRI is the cross-sectional imaging modality of choice for assessing adnexal masses it should not unnecessarily delay surgical management. MRI is useful for problem solving where the sonographic findings are indeterminate for torsion (Van Kerkhove et al. 2007) and there is prompt availability of MRI. MRI will also show an enlarged adnexal mass, with peripheral stromal microcysts (Fig. 22) and non-enhancing necrotic tissue. MRI will also reveal the presence of a lead point. On diffusion weighted imaging (DWI) the torsed ovary shows restricted diffusion with low apparent diffusion coefficient (ADC) values (Kilickesmez et al. 2009).

Laparoscopy remains the gold standard in the assessment of the female with acute pelvic pain and treatment of adnexal torsion. Surgical treatment includes laparoscopic de-torsion with ovarian tissue salvage (Breech and Hillard 2005). The torsed ovary may be successfully reperfused despite macroscopic appearances of early necrosis (Emonts et al. 2004). Adnexectomy is undertaken for non-viable tissue.

8.1 Massive Ovarian Oedema

Massive ovarian oedema (MOO) is a very rare non-neoplastic entity characterised by marked ovarian stromal oedema. Young women of child-bearing age are the group most likely to be affected. A few cases have been reported in prepubertal girls with precocious puberty (Kanumakala et al. 2002; Moon et al. 2009). Vaginal bleeding or masculinisation are rare presenting features. The clinical presentation is typically one of massive solid enlargement of the ovary and abdominal pain. Recognition of MOO is important as the condition is often mistaken for malignancy leading to unnecessary oophorectomy. Primary MOO typically occurs in the setting of chronic incomplete or intermittent ovarian torsion with secondary obstruction of venous and lymphatic drainage.

The typical US and MR findings of MOO (Fig. 23) are unilateral ovarian enlargement with oedematous stroma containing several small peripherally located follicles or 'microcysts' (Kramer et al. 1997; Umesaki et al. 2000). Haemorrhage and necrosis are recognised features of complete adnexal torsion but are not usually seen in MOO (Tamai et al. 2006). Contrast-enhancement is typically preserved in the stroma and cyst walls in MOO, whilst absent in most cases of established adnexal torsion (Tamai et al. 2006; Umesaki et al. 2000). Absence of contrast-enhancement is a marker of non-viable ovarian tissue following necrosis and infarction.

8.2 Isolated Fallopian Tube Torsion

Fallopian tube torsion typically occurs in the context of tubo-ovarian torsion. Isolated fallopian tube torsion (IFTT) is very rare with an incidence around 1–1.5 cases per million and occurs in adolescents and women of reproductive age. Only small cases series have been published in the literature (Harmon et al. 2008). Most cases are unilateral and right sided.

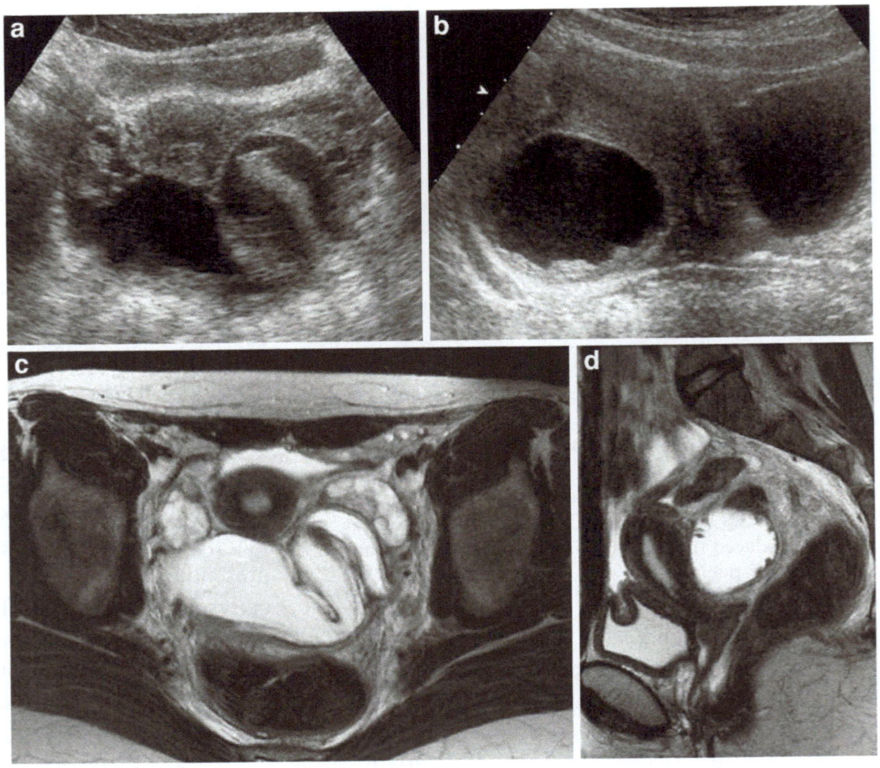

Fig. 24 Isolated fallopian tube torsion. **a** Transverse and **b** longitudinal images show a dilated, fluid-containing serpiginous left fallopian tube. The enlarged fimbriated end extends towards the midline and the uterus. Mucosal folds are visible on the inner border of tube wall. The ovaries are normal bilaterally. **c** Axial and **d** sagittal T2-weighted images of the dilated thick-walled *left* fallopian tube containing T2-hyperintense fluid. Mucosal folds are noted on the inner aspect of the tube wall. Images reproduced from Orazi et al. (2006) with permission from Springer publishers

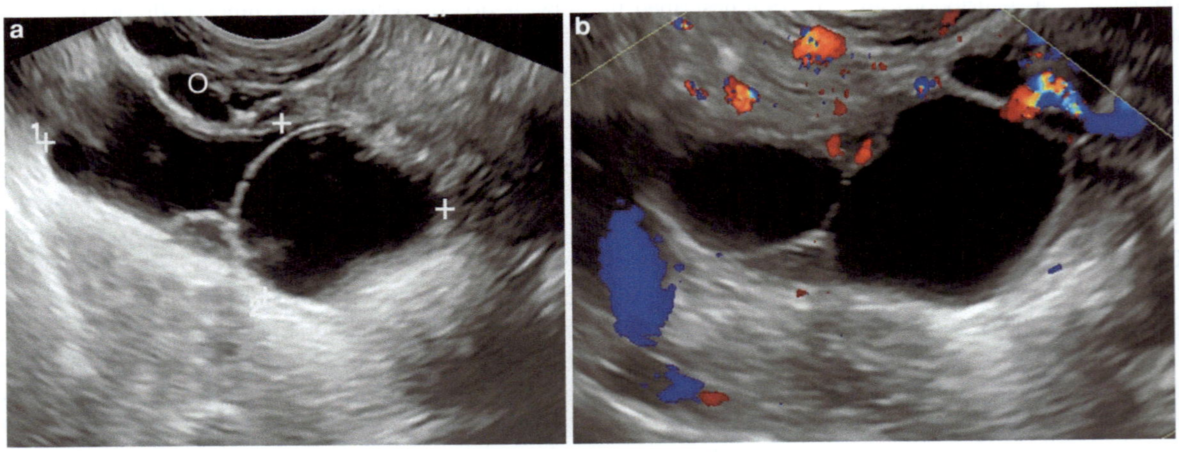

Fig. 25 Transvaginal US imaging showing a multiloculated peritoneal inclusion cyst (PIC). **a** Gray-scale image of the PIC (*between callipers*) adjacent to the ipsilateral ovary (O), **b** corresponding colour Doppler image. *Images courtesy of Dr. Helen R. Nadel MD, DABR, FRCPC Vancouver, Canada*

The aetiology of tubal torsion is not fully understood but includes excessive redundant length of the mesosalpinx, spiral course of the fallopian tube, premenstrual congestion of the fallopian tube or fallopian tube hypermotility (Merlini et al. 2008). Risk factors for acquired tubal torsion include prior tubal injury, hydrosalpinx, haematosalpinx, PID or para-adnexal cysts.

The diagnosis should be considered in girls with acute onset pelvic pain where imaging demonstrates a midline pelvic cystic mass, typically in the pouch of Douglas or superior to the uterus in the presence of a

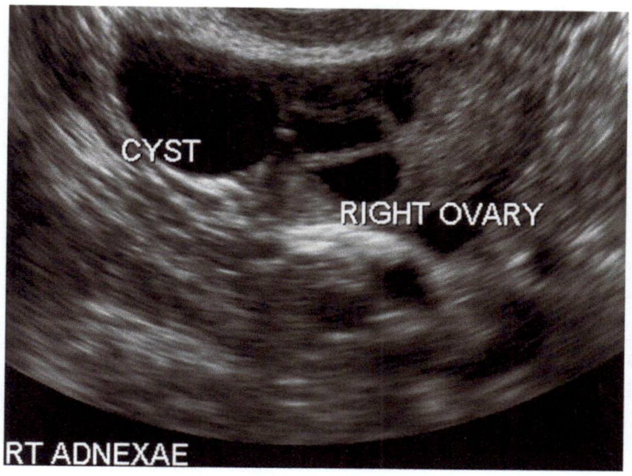

Fig. 26 Paraovarian cyst. (Hydatid cyst of Morgagni) Transverse US image of the right adnexa showing an anechoic cyst which is distinctly separate from the adjacent ovary

normal ipsilateral ovary (Fig. 24). Free fluid or haemoperitoneum may also be present. As the diagnosis is rarely made prospectively the affected tube is often not viable at surgery.

9 Peritoneal Inclusion Cyst (PIC)

The ovary produces physiologic free fluid during ovulation which is normally absorbed by the adjacent peritoneum. PICs result from pathology which gives rise to localised adhesions, these impair peritoneal fluid absorption. The causes of PIC include prior PID, pelvic surgery, trauma and rarely endometriosis. Fluid accumulates in the adhesions adjacent to the active ovary resulting in a benign complex cystic mass in which the healthy ovary becomes entrapped by loculated fluid. Symptoms tend to relate to mass effect and include pelvic fullness, abdominopelvic pain, and localised tenderness with or without a palpable mass.

The characteristic imaging features of a PIC include a normal-appearing ovary enveloped by loculated fluid (Fig. 25). This appearance has been referred to as a 'spider in a web' in which the ovary lies centrally or laterally and is the 'spider' which is surrounded by a 'web' of fluid locules (Jain 2000; Kim et al. 1997). The cyst typically shows eccentric margins with a bizarre configuration which conforms to the borders of the peritoneal wall and adjacent viscera. The cyst fluid is typically anechoic but can be echogenic if there is proteinaceous material or haemorrhage present. The cyst wall septations may be complete or incomplete and are typically less than 3 mm thick and do not exceed 6 mm (Savelli et al. 2004). A specific sign on transvaginal US for PIC is the 'flapping sail' sign which describes the appearances of a septum when displaced by the US probe. PIC may mimic a paraovarian cyst, hydrosalpinx or a cystic malignant tumour (Jain 2000). Other differentials include lymphangioma or rarely a benign peritoneal mesothelioma. The treatment of PICs is controversial, but in general conservative therapy is advocated.

10 Paraovarian/Paratubal Cysts

Paraovarian and paratubal cysts histologically are mesothelial, mesonephric or paramesonephric in origin. A mesonephric cyst (Wolffian cyst, hydatid cyst of Morgagni, Kobelt cyst, cyst of the organ of Rosenmüller), paramesonephric cyst or mesothelial cyst typically arise in the mesosalpinx in the superior free border of the round ligament between the fallopian tube and ovary. Paraovarian cysts are rare in children but can be seen in postmenarchal adolescents. The cysts are typically solitary, small, round or ovoid, thin-walled and contain anechoic content. Larger cysts can reach up to 8 cm and cause pain. Acute pain occurs following haemorrhage or torsion. A key sonographic feature is the presence of a normal ipsilateral ovary separate from the paraovarian cyst (Fig. 26) (Kim et al. 1995). This imaging clue can also be demonstrated on MR or CT. The presence of a soft tissue component with flow within the cyst is indicative of a neoplasm rather than a paraovarian cyst.

11 Hydrosalpinx

The normal fallopian tube contains a small amount of physiologic endoluminal fluid which is not demonstrable on US or cross-sectional imaging. Although this fluid is directed towards the uterine fundus by ciliary motility, the majority is discharged into the peritoneal cavity via its fimbrial portion.

Hydrosalpinx refers to a dilated fluid-filled fallopian tube which may occur in isolation but usually results from tubular injury or occlusion. It is rare in children and often occurs in the context of PID in adolescents. Hydrosalpinx itself does not cause pain. The main differentials for hydrosalpinx are PIC or

Table 10 Comparative sonographic findings of paraovarian cysts, hydrosalpinges and peritoneal inclusion cysts

Diagnosis	Paraovarian cysts	Hydrosalpinges	Peritoneal inclusion cysts
Ipsilateral ovary	Yes	Yes	Yes
Morphology	Ovoid	Tubular	Irregular
Proper wall	Yes	Yes	No
Papillae	Yes	No	Yes
'Beads-on-a-string'	No	Yes	No
Complete septa	Rare	No	Frequent
Incomplete septa	No	Frequent	Rare
'Flapping sail sign'	No	No	Yes
'Split sign'	Yes	Yes	No

After Savelli et al. (2006)

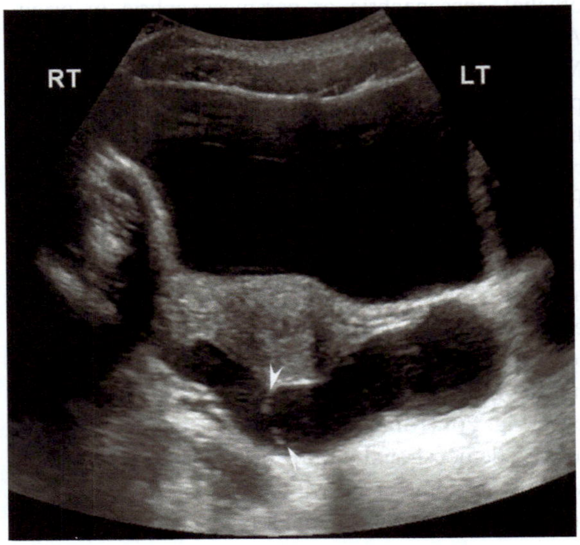

Fig. 27 Hydrosalpinx. Transverse sonogram of a dilated fluid-filled fallopian tube with incomplete septa (plicae) showing the 'waist sign' (*arrowheads*). Hydrosalpinx can resemble a complex adnexal multicystic mass

paraovarian cyst. The key sonographic features of these entities are summarised in Table 10.

Sonographically hydrosalpinx resembles fluid-filled tubular structures. Differentiation from bowel loops is possible when peristalsis is noted. Dilated ureters may appear similar. Colour Doppler imaging will confirm flow in a blood vessel. US features which may enable identification of hydrosalpinx include dilated tubules with incomplete septa (Fig. 27). Another feature is the presence of diametrically opposed indentations in the lumen of a tubular fluid-filled structure also referred to as the 'waist sign' (Timor-Tritsch et al. 1998). The 'string of beads sign' is a feature of chronic hydrosalpinx in which there are small echogenic nodules within the wall of the thin, chronically distended tube and are thought to represent effaced salpingeal folds (Timor-Tritsch et al. 1998).

On ultrasound the fallopian tube fluid content and wall thickness may assist in defining the underlying cause. Anechoic content is suggestive of serous fluid, low-level internal echoes may relate to proteinaceous fluid. A thick-walled tube with internal debris with or without an accompanying tubo-ovarian abscess is suggestive of a pus-filled tube referred to as pyosalpinx. US cannot reliably differentiate between haemorrhage and pus. An ectopic pregnancy or endometrioma is associated with a blood-filled tube referred to as haematosalpinx.

Hydrosalpinx on MRI appears as a dilated fluid-filled tubular structure, which depending on the degree of infolding can resemble confluent S- or C-shaped cysts in cross-section (Fig. 28). Hydrosalpinx is distinct from the ipsilateral ovary and can be traced from the upper outer margin of the uterine fundus. This imaging clue is useful in CT but the ovary can often be difficult to identify. MR imaging is also superior in characterising the fluid content of hydrosalpinx. In simple hydrosalpinx the fluid is isointense to CSF on all pulse sequences. Proteinaceous fluid will have higher T1 signal. Blood has variable signal depending on its age but is typically low-signal on T2-weighted imaging and high signal intensity on T1-weighted imaging and may be associated with endometriosis or

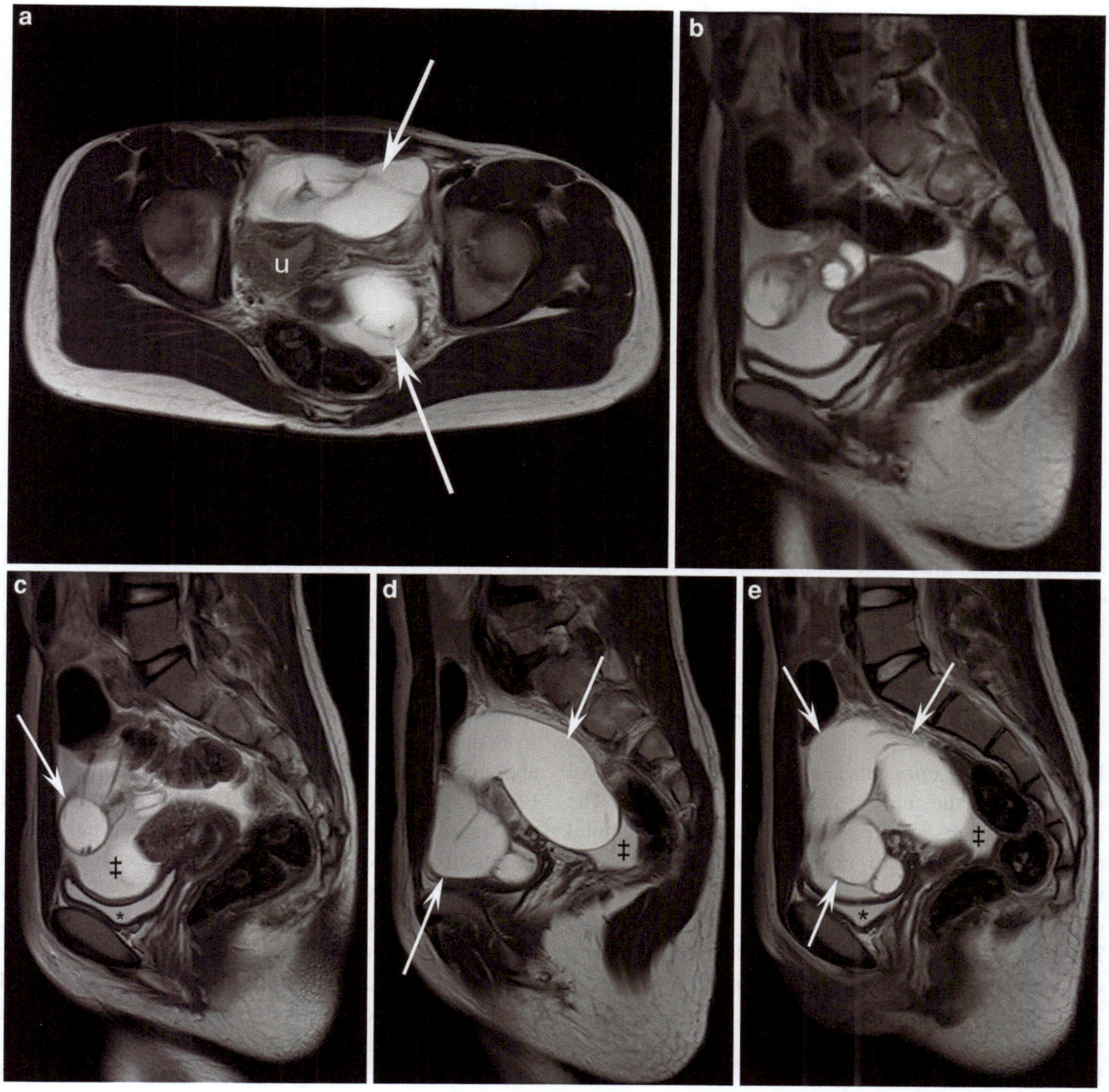

Fig. 28 Hydrosalpinges. Representative T2-weighted TSE MR imaging, **a** axial image showing bilateral isointense fluid-filled, dilated tortuous tubular structures in the adnexa (*arrows*) **b–e** Sagittal T2-weighted TSE imaging showing hydrosalpinges (*arrows*) with incompletely effaced submucosal and mucosal plicae and adjacent dependent free fluid (‡). Urinary bladder (*), uterus (u)

ectopic pregnancy. On T2-weighted imaging the presence of incomplete folds or septa are characteristic of hydrosalpinx (Rezvani and Shaaban 2011). Thickened longitudinal folds produce a characteristic "cogwheel" appearance when imaged in cross-section which are considered pathognomonic for hydrosalpinx (Benjaminov and Atri 2004). These may become effaced or absent in severe tubular dilatation. Wall thickening is indicative of an inflammatory process. A dilated thick-walled fallopian tube which exhibits heterogeneous signal intensity content may indicate the presence of pyosalpinx. Contrast may demonstrate enhancing internal septae, fallopian tube walls and a tubo-ovarian abscess complex (see tubo-ovarian

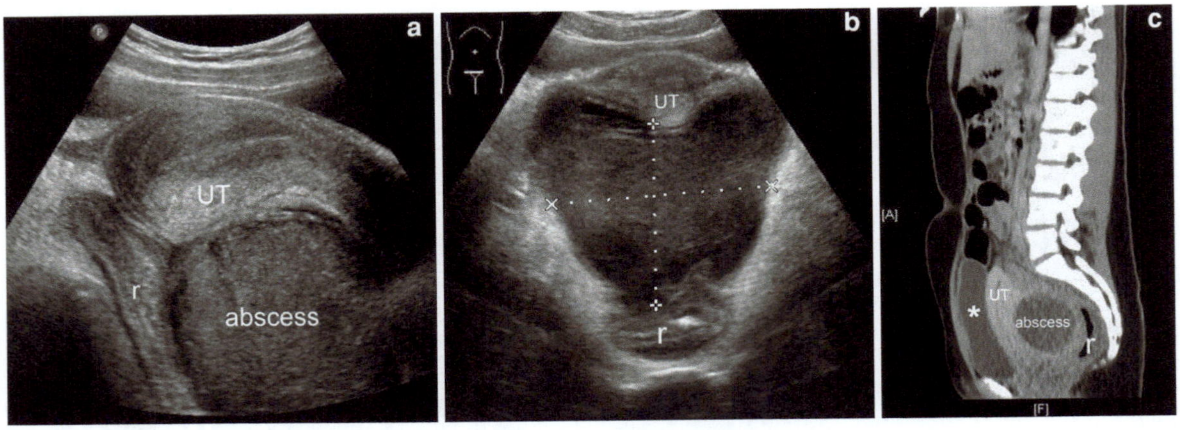

Fig. 29 Imaging showing a pelvic abscess lying between the uterus (UT) and rectum (r). **a** Longitudinal and **b** transverse US images, **c** sagittal reformatted contrast-enhanced CT image. (*) Urinary bladder. The collection resolved with US-guided transrectal drainage

abscess). Fallopian tube malignancy in children is exceedingly rare but should be considered where there is a solid enhancing component.

12 Pelvic Inflammatory Disease

Pelvic inflammatory disease (PID) is a microbial infection of the upper gynaecological tract. The aetiology is typically related to an ascending genital tract infection or can result from a blood borne infection in a sexually active female. There are small cases series and numerous case reports of rare instances of PID in virginal adolescents where endogenous aerobic and anaerobic bacteria can result in ascending genital tract infection. The most common causative organisms in the sexually active adolescent population aged between 15 and 19 years are *Neisseria gonorrhoeae* and/or *Chlamydia trachomatis* (Workowski and Berman 2010). Rare causes include actinomycosis and tuberculosis. Uncomplicated cases may remain silent and only present in later life with subfertility. The management of younger children with suspected sexually transmitted disease inevitably raises child protection concerns and requires close liaison between the treating clinicians, child protection and family services.

PID involvement may range from any combination of endometritis, salpingitis, pyosalpinx, oophoritis, tubo-ovarian abscess, peritonitis and perihepatitis (Fitz-Hugh-Curtis syndrome). Disseminated peritonitis can be complicated by peritoneal adhesions resulting in mechanical small-bowel obstruction. PID is often bilateral. Unilateral pelvic inflammation should increase the clinical suspicion for direct extension of a localised inflammatory process such as an appendiceal, Crohn's or postsurgical abscess (Fig. 29).

Patients with acute PID may present with lower abdominal pain, pelvic discharge, fever with elevated ESR or C-reactive protein level. Physical examination may reveal adnexal tenderness; cervical excitation tenderness may also be elicited. In many cases the clinical presentation may be non-specific and imaging with ultrasound is requested to identify an underlying cause.

Imaging typically appears normal in the acute phase of uterine infection. In severe or advanced presentations, the US findings of uterine involvement include endometrial thickening with or without endometrial fluid and gas. The normal contours and zonal anatomy of the uterus may become indistinct. Involvement of the fallopian tubes results in dilated inflamed thick-walled tubes (Fig. 30) distended with exudates and pus resulting in variable echotexture content and fluid-debris levels. Differentiation between blood and pus can be difficult on US and clinical correlation is required, MRI should be considered if there is doubt about the diagnosis. Free fluid either excessive or complex in nature is a common associated finding.

Ovarian involvement results in enlarged ovaries with indistinct borders. Extrauterine tubo-ovarian complexes consist of inflamed enlarged ovaries and

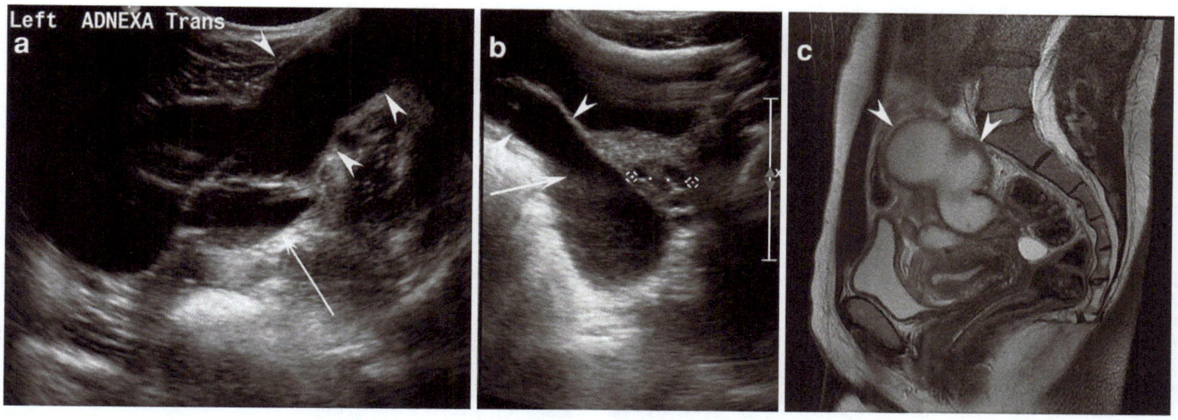

Fig. 30 Salpingitis. **a–b** Transverse US showing debris (*arrow*) within the dependent portion of a thick-walled dilated fallopian tube (*arrowheads*). **c** Sagittal T2-weighted TSE MR image showing the fluid-filled tube with wall thickening (*arrowheads*) suggestive of pyosalpinx. Intravenous gadolinium was not administered as the patient had impaired renal function. Laparoscopic verification is usually indicated

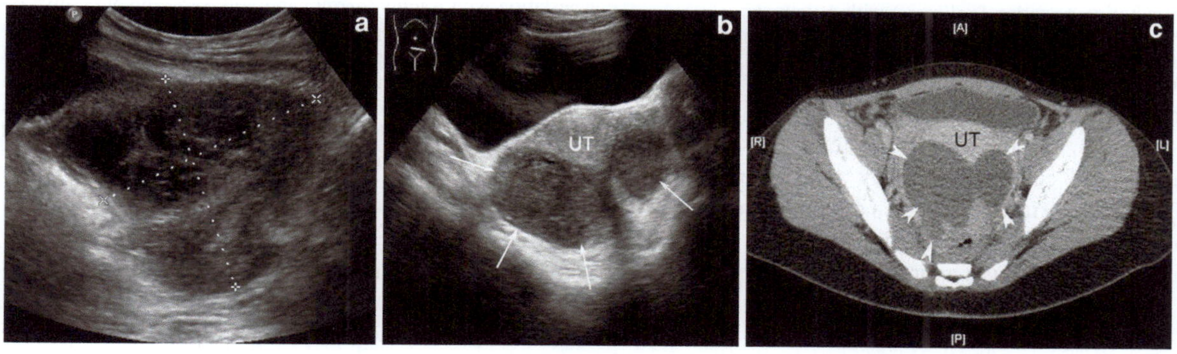

Fig. 31 Pelvic inflammatory disease with a tubo-ovarian abscess. **a** Longitudinal US of a tubo-ovarian abscess complex (*between callipers*). **b** Transverse US showing debris laden distended fallopian tubes (*arrows*) behind the uterus (UT). **c** Axial contrast-enhanced CT showing the tubo-ovarian complex (*arrowheads*)

distended fallopian tubes with preserved anatomy. These may break down into tubo-ovarian abscesses (TOA). TOA appear as complex, multilocular masses with variable internal echotexture and septations (Fig. 31). Differentiation of TOA from tumour or an endometrioma on imaging can be difficult and may require clinical or laparoscopic correlation.

13 Pregnancy

Rates of teenage pregnancy are high in the so-called developed nations (UNICEF 2001). The highest rates are observed in New Zealand, the USA and the UK. For these nations reducing teenage pregnancy rates is a key part of public health policy. Pregnant adolescents may present to healthcare providers with amenorrhoea related to a concealed pregnancy (Fig. 32), or with vaginal bleeding or acute abdominopelvic pain as result of a complication of pregnancy. It is important for the diagnosis of pregnancy or a pregnancy-related complication to be made promptly so that the affected individual can be referred onwards to receive expert obstetric and antenatal care. The role of the paediatric radiologist is to evaluate the pelvis and adnexa in the context of the serum β-hCG level. In practical terms once pregnancy is suspected, an initial abdominopelvic US may be undertaken, but it is normal practice in our department to refer the patient to an obstetric

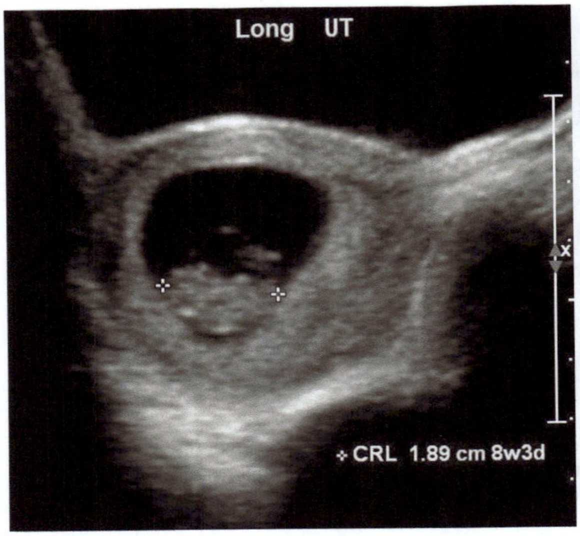

Fig. 32 Longitudinal US in a 14-year old showing a live intrauterine gestation (*callipers*) with a yolk sac

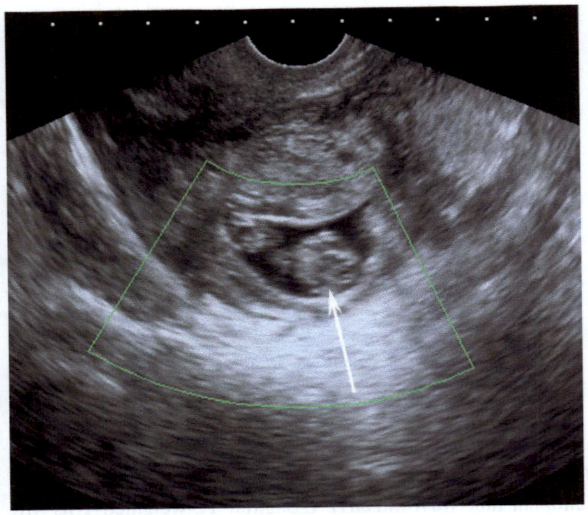

Fig. 33 Ectopic pregnancy. Transvaginal sonography (TVS) of the left adnexa in an 18-year old showing an ectopic gestation with a fetus (*arrow*) and yolk sac—this was alive on colour Doppler sonography. The diagnosis of ectopic pregnancy can be challenging. Correlation with the serum β-hCG is essential. Transabdominal sonography (TAS) is less sensitive in the diagnosis of ectopic gestation than TVS. TAS may show an empty uterus with thickened endometrium. Intrauterine and ectopic gestations can rarely co-exist

sonologist regardless of whether an intrauterine gestation has been confirmed.

In this section we will briefly look at the US imaging of ectopic pregnancy and molar pregnancy. Though rare in adolescents, anticipation and recognition of these entities is important to prevent unnecessary delay in appropriate further management.

13.1 Ectopic Pregnancy

Ectopic pregnancy, also referred to as an extrauterine gestation occurs when a fertilised ovum becomes implanted outside the endometrium. Most ectopic gestations are located in the ampullary portion of the fallopian tube, but rarely can occur elsewhere including the ovary, cervix, uterine cornua or abdominopelvic cavity.

Although ectopic pregnancy is uncommon in adolescents it remains a leading cause of morbidity and mortality in the first trimester of pregnancy. The diagnosis should always be considered in adolescents presenting with pelvic pain or vaginal bleeding and positive pregnancy test. Risk factors relate to prior fallopian tube injury with genital tract infection the most common cause. Typical organisms include *Neisseria gonorrhoeae* and *Chlamydia trachomatis* (Menon et al. 2007). Previous ectopic pregnancy and tubal surgery are more common in adults (Vichnin 2008).

Haemodynamically stable patients with emergency first trimester complications should have an intrauterine pregnancy confirmed by ultrasound (Barnhart et al. 1994). As with any sonographic technique the ability to make the diagnosis is dependent upon local clinical expertise, availability of appropriate scanning equipment and the gestational age of the pregnancy. Referral to a specialist obstetric service should always be made where possible or necessary.

Co-existing intrauterine and ectopic gestations are very rare. The demonstration of an intrauterine gestation does not conclusively exclude the diagnosis of ectopic pregnancy. Careful evaluation of the adnexae is still indicated (Levine 2007). Although an empty uterus with a positive pregnancy test is highly suggestive of ectopic pregnancy, alternative diagnoses include spontaneous abortion or early intrauterine gestation. Transabdominal ultrasound cannot reliably diagnose intrauterine pregnancies under 6 week's gestation. Transvaginal ultrasound can detect intrauterine pregnancies at approximately 4–5 weeks. Transvaginal ultrasound should be performed if an intrauterine pregnancy or ectopic pregnancy is not identifiable transabdominally.

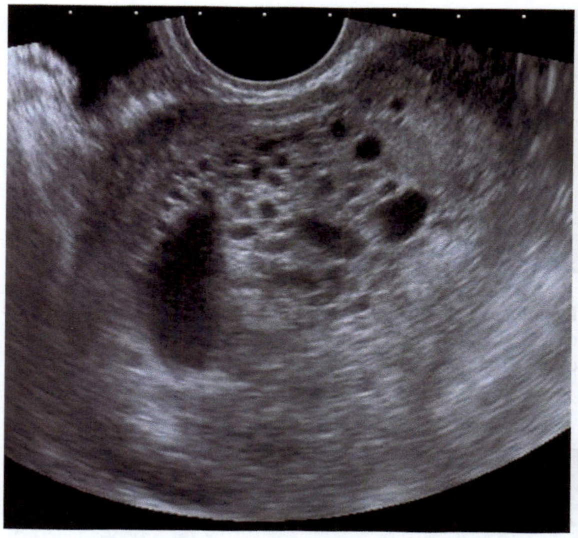

Fig. 34 Molar pregnancy. Transvaginal US showing the typical features of a molar gestation. An echogenic mass distending the uterine cavity is shown containing a '*vesicular pattern*' of multiple small cysts resembling '*grape-like clusters*'

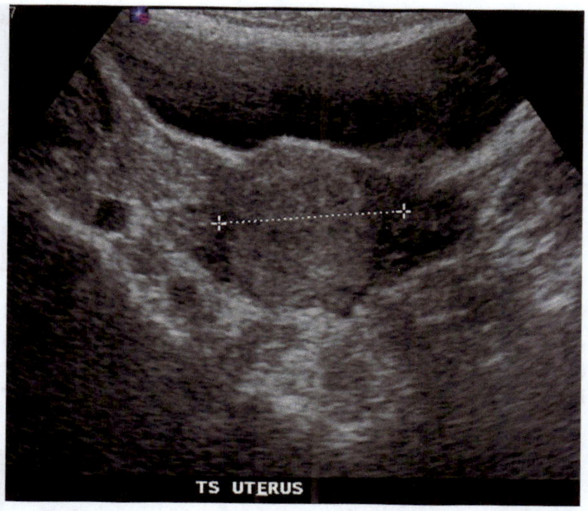

Fig. 35 Endometrioma. Transverse US showing an ovarian mass (*between callipers*) with diffuse low-level fine internal echoes in keeping with an endometrioma

Correlation with serum beta-human chorionic gonadotropin (β-hCG) levels is helpful. β-hCG levels rise in a predictable fashion in the first trimester. If this pattern is not seen, an abnormal intrauterine gestation or ectopic pregnancy should be considered. With appropriate β-hCG levels transvaginal ultrasound is usually diagnostic in most cases. Ectopic pregnancy should be suspected when no intrauterine gestation sac is seen with transabdominal sonography and the patient's β-hCG level exceeds 6,500 mIU per mL (6,500 IU per L) or with transvaginal ultrasonography with a β-hCG level in excess of 1,500 mIU per mL (1,500 IU per L) (Condous et al. 2005; Mol et al. 1999). Combining transvaginal ultrasound with serial quantitative β-hCG measurements is approximately 96% sensitive and 97% specific for diagnosing ectopic pregnancy (Gracia and Barnhart 2001).

Common ultrasound findings include an adnexal mass or cyst, a thick-walled and dilated fallopian tube also referred to as an adnexal ring sign, haematosalpinx, haemoperitoneum and extrauterine gestational sac containing a yolk sac (Fig. 33) with or without an embryo. Anechoic free fluid in the pouch of Douglas is a non-specific finding, but echogenic free fluid has a high PPV for the presence of a bleeding or ruptured ectopic pregnancy (Frates et al. 1994).

13.2 Gestational Trophoblastic Neoplasia

Gestational trophoblastic neoplasia (GTN) is a spectrum of placental lesions that arise from abnormal conceptions. These consist of excessive trophoblast tissue, cystic degeneration of the chorionic villi and contain no viable embryo. Recognition of GTN is important to ensure referral to an appropriate tertiary centre. GTN include complete hydatiform moles (CHM) and partial hydatiform moles (PHM). Around 15% of CHM and 5% of PHM undergo malignant transformation either as an invasive mole, placental site trophoblastic tumour (PSTT), epithelioid trophoblastic tumours (ETTs), and non-metastatic or metastatic choriocarcinoma (Aghajanian 2011). The risk is lowest in young patients.

The chromosomal pattern of most CHM is usually 46XXdiploid, occuring when a single haploid sperm fertilises an ovum devoid of a nucleus and maternal genes that then undergoes subsequent duplications. CHM comprise of syncytiotrophoblastic and cytotrophoblastic cells. Gross pathological specimens classically resemble a 'bunch of grapes', as a result of chorionic villus swelling (Seckl and Newlands 2002). The US appearances of CHM reflect the macroscopic findings but occasionally molar pregnancies can have very unusual sonographic appearances. In the first trimester CHM can appear as a large echogenic mass with multiple small macrocystic spaces within the

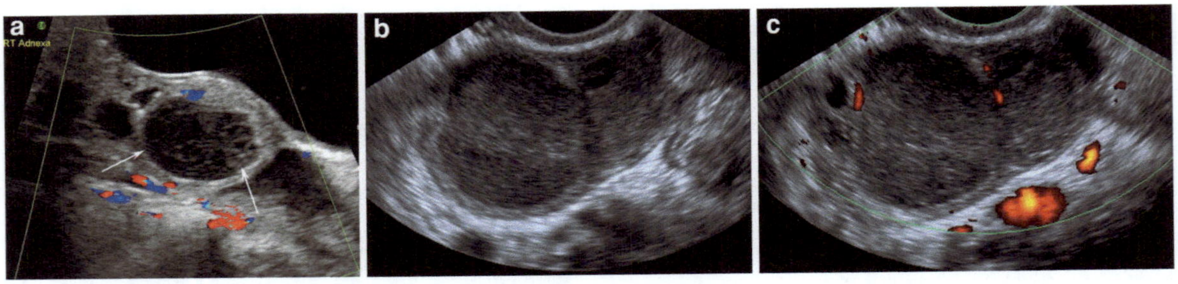

Fig. 36 Endometrioma. **a** Transabdominal colour Doppler US showing a cystic mass with soft tissue components (*arrows*) due to organising haematoma and a fluid-debris level from clot lysis. **b–c** Corresponding transvaginal US imaging. **c** Power Doppler US shows flow within the thin septa. The septa can be of variable thickness. The differential includes haemorrhagic cyst or tumour such as a dermoid

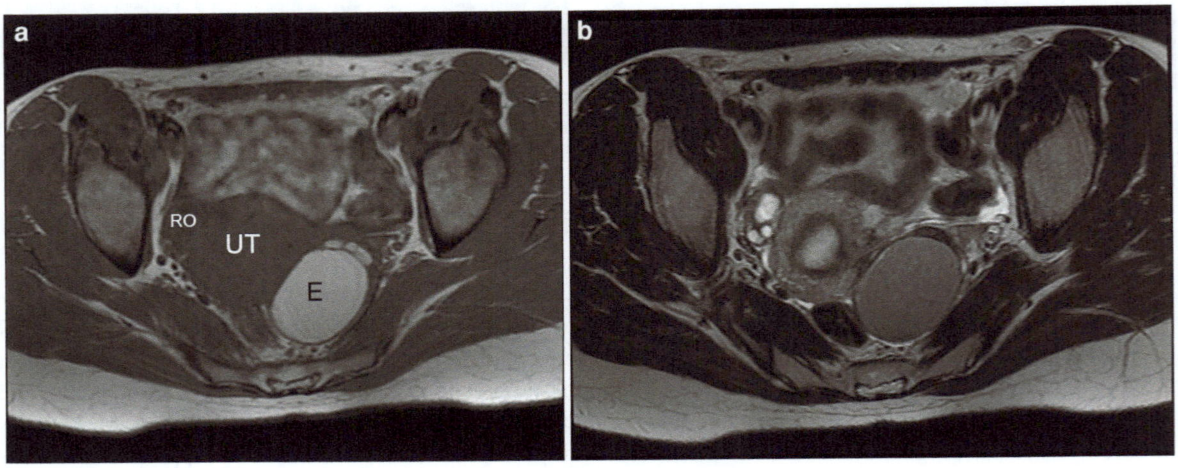

Fig. 37 Endometrioma MR imaging. **a** Axial T1-weighted TSE showing hyperintense left adnexal endometrial cyst (E). **b** axial T2-weighted TSE imaging showing corresponding lower T2 signal or 'shading' in the smaller peripheral deposits (*arrows*). The largest endometriomal cyst (E) is of intermediate T2 signal. The signal intensity can vary depending on the age of the blood products and the iron and protein content. (UT) uterus, (RO) right ovary

endometrial cavity (Fig. 34). Marked myometrial colour Doppler flow signal and low impedance waveforms in the uterine arteries are recognised imaging features (Allen et al. 2006). Involvement of the myometrium constitutes an invasive molar pregnancy. Imaging cannot reliably differentiate between an invasive mole and malignant extrauterine choriocarcinoma.

Staging and clinical risk factor scoring of GTN is based on the International Federation of Gynecology and Obstetrics (FIGO) classification (FIGO 2009; Kohorn 2001). Initial management is surgical evacuation with histopathological evaluation of the products of conception. Chemotherapy is indicated where incomplete evacuation is achieved or serum β-hCG levels persist. In most cases treatment is curative and fertility is preserved.

14 Endometriosis

Endometriosis is defined as the presence of functioning endometrial glandular tissue and stroma outside of the uterine cavity. An ectopic focus of extrauterine endometrial tissue within an ovary is referred to as an endometrioma (also known as a chocolate cyst or endometriod cyst), deposits elsewhere are referred to as endometriosis. While endometriosis in adolescents is not uncommon, endometriomas are much less so.

The precise aetiology of endometriosis is unknown. Competing theories include the role of retrograde menstruation with transvenous or translymphatic spread of ectopic endometrium (Sampson 1940). Structural abnormalities of the Müllerian ducts have

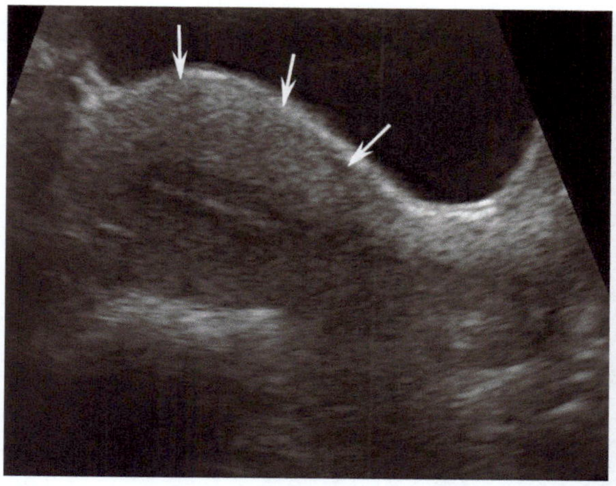

Fig. 38 Diffuse adenomyosis. Longitudinal US image in a 22-year old woman showing uterine enlargement and heterogeneity of the anterior myometrium (*arrows*). There is discrepancy of the depth of the anterior uterine wall which is thicker than the posterior wall, there is also loss of definition of the junctional zone. Affected areas typically show increased vascularity on colour Doppler US

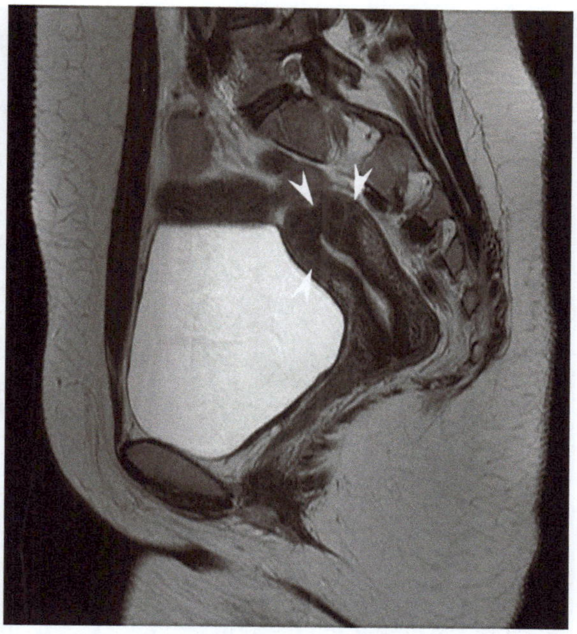

Fig. 39 Focal adenomyosis. Sagittal T2-weighted TSE MR image showing thickening of the junctional zone exceeding 12 mm (*arrowheads*)

also been implicated (Sanfilippo et al. 1986). An alternative theory has postulated the role of coelemic metaplastic differentiation of pelvic tissues resulting in endometrium-like deposits. Hereditary and local endometrial factors are currently the subject of ongoing investigation.

Endometriosis is not seen in prepubertal girls but is an important cause of chronic cyclic and noncyclic pelvic pain in the postmenarchal adolescent. It is associated with dysmenorrhoea, intermenstrual abdominal and pelvic pain, back pain, cyclic dysuria, dyschezia and deep dyspareunia (Giudice and Kao 2004). The reported incidence of endometriosis in adolescents varies but LAUFER and colleagues reported that 67% of adolescents undergoing laparoscopy for pelvic pain refractory to conservative medical therapy of non-steroidal anti-inflammatories and oral contraceptives were found to have endometriosis (Laufer et al. 1997).

Endometrioma possess the same steroid receptors as normal endometrium. They are capable of synchronously responding to the oestrogens driving the menstrual cycle in concert with the uterine endometrium. Endometrioma may therefore undergo repeated intracystic internal bleeding, which in the absence of normal drainage by the uterine cavity and vagina induces a localised inflammatory response with fibrosis and neovascularization.

Endometriosis develop in the dependent portions of the pelvis. The most common locations include the ovaries, uterine ligaments and within the pouch of Douglas. Other sites include the pelvic peritoneum, fallopian tubes, rectosigmoid, urinary bladder, cervix and vagina. Extraperitoneal Endometriosis deposits are rare but can be found in lymph nodes, skin, breast, lung or central nervous system. Endometriosis can also develop in abdominal surgical scars. Complications of endometriosis typically ensue following endometrioma rupture which can present as acute abdominal pain. The resulting fibrotic adhesions giving rise to bowel and ureteric obstruction and predispose to infertility.

The staging of endometriosis disease burden is based on surgical findings usually at laparoscopy according to the revised American Fertility Society classification (AFS 1985). Serum markers of disease activity such as Ca125 to date have not been shown to be clinically useful in adolescents. Pathologically endometrioma contain endometrial glandular or stromal tissue with blood breakdown products—typically

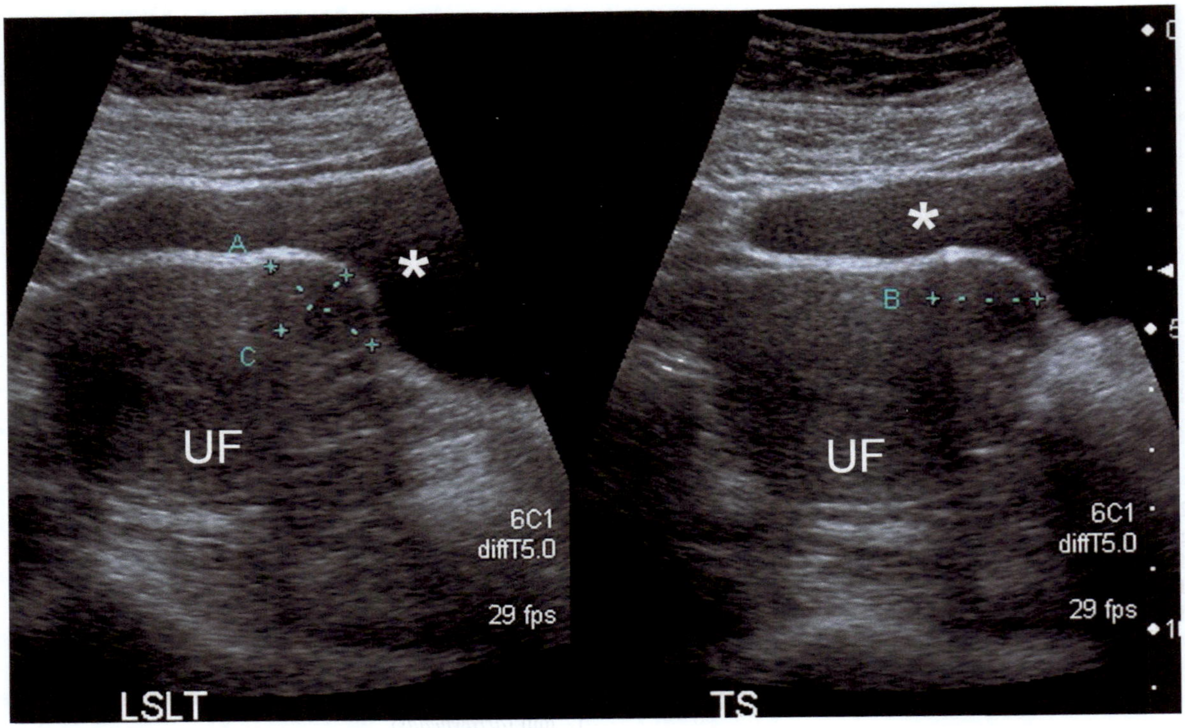

Fig. 40 Uterine fibroid (leiomyoma). Composite US images of a 19-year old nulliparous Afro–Caribbean lady showing a small well-defined intramural uterine leiomyoma (*between callipers*). Streaky shadowing is seen deep to the fibroid centred on the uterine fundus (UF). The fibroid produces greater mass effect on the outer uterine contour and distorts the adjacent urinary bladder (*). Bright texture where present may indicate high fat content and is suggestive of a lipoleiomyoma

haemosiderin deposits. These characteristics make imaging with MRI particularly suitable for non-invasive diagnosis and long-term surveillance. Both US and CT have a low specificity for the diagnosis of endometriomas (Potter and Chandrasekhar 2008). Transabdominal US remains the first-line imaging modality and offers a useful overview of the whole pelvis. Transvaginal ultrasound where available and appropriate to the individual affords improved near field resolution. On ultrasound an endometrioma is typically a round unilocular thick-walled cyst, with smooth margins and a homogenous 'ground glass' appearance with uniform low internal echoes (Fig. 35). A maximum of four locules may be demonstrated and no flow is seen within the papillations on colour Doppler imaging (Fig. 36) (Van Holsbeke et al. 2010). Appearances may be atypical with an anechoic cyst, fluid levels or appearances suggestive of a solid mass. The walls may show punctate echogenic foci related to calcification with acoustic shadowing (Asch and Levine 2007). Atypical endometrioma may mimic HOCs, TOA, dermoid cysts and ovarian neoplasms.

MRI is a useful problem solving tool in selected patients based on symptoms, response to treatment and ultrasound findings. MRI is helpful in characterising sonographically indeterminate adnexal masses and confirming the organ of origin. As blood breakdown products are T1 hyperintense 8 days following a bleed, MRI should not be scheduled earlier than day eight of the menstrual cycle (Kinkel et al. 2006) with imaging ideally undertaken around day 8–12. A typical protocol includes a sagittal T2-weighted sequence with T2-weighted images and T1-weighted images without fat suppression in two planes (axial and coronal planes along the axis of the uterus) (Spencer et al. 2010). Axial T1-weighted fat-suppressed images are also obtained; fat containing lesions will suppress whereas T1 hyperintense haemorrhagic lesions will not. A characteristic feature of endometrioma on MRI is the 'shading' sign, the cystic endometrioma shows high signal on T1-weighted spin-echo imaging with

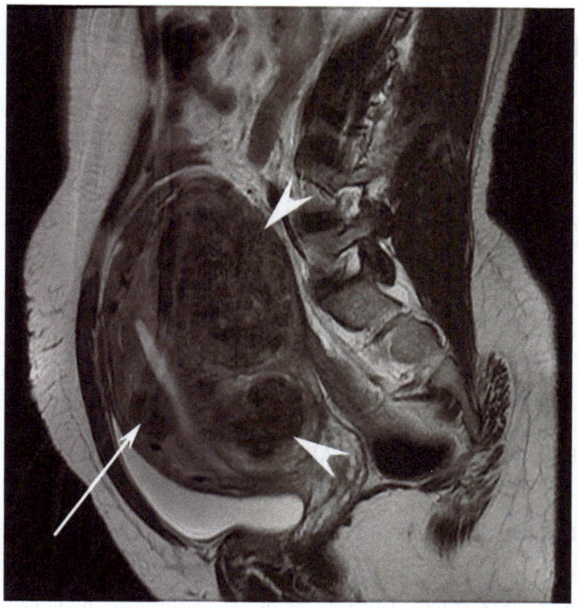

Fig. 41 Multiple fibroid uterus. Sagittal T2-weighted TSE MRI showing a small fibroid in the anterior uterine wall (*arrow*) and larger fibroids in the posterior wall (*arrowheads*). Fibroids can calcify, undergo cystic change, reach a large size, pedunculate or necrose on outstripping the blood supply

corresponding loss of signal on T2-weighted spin-echo imaging (Fig. 37). Suspicious solid elements should be assessed with intravenous gadolinium (Spencer and Ghattamaneni 2010). Anterior and posterior saturation bands are applied. Prior 6 h fasting and IV antiperistaltic agents are helpful. Magnetic resonance urography should be considered if there is ureteric dilatation. Steady state free precession imaging can be used to evaluate bowel strictures.

15 Adenomyosis

Adenomyosis is an exceptionally rare cause of dysmenorrhoea in the adolescent female population and is defined by the presence of ectopic endometrial glandular tissue within the uterine myometrium. Involvement may be localised such as when confined to a discrete adenomyotic cyst (adenomyoma) or diffuse. The speculated aetiology is presumed to be due to invagination of the uterine endometrium into the uterine myometrium, with hormonal activation of endometrial rests within the myometrium or iatrogenic endometrial implantation.

A prospective imaging diagnosis is unusual in this age group, the diagnosis is typically made at histology after hysterectomy. On ultrasound adenomyosis appear as areas of myometrial hypoechogenicity resulting from smooth muscle hyperplasia. Intramyometrial adenomyotic cysts may contain fluid-debris levels and appear highly vascular. Diffuse involvement results in loss of definition of the uterine junctional zone (JZ) (Fig. 38). While US is a useful screening tool MRI is the reference standard and has higher sensitivity and PPV. On T2-weighted images, adenomyosis typically appears as a poorly demarcated low-signal intensity lesion with uterine enlargement (Takeuchi and Matsuzaki 2011). The MR-imaging characteristics of adenomyosis include (1) small foci of heterotopic endometrial tissue (2) maximal JZ thickness $\geq$8–12 mm on sagittal T2-weighted imaging (Fig. 39) (3) Ratio JZ max/total myometrial thickness >40% (Kissler et al. 2008).

16 Uterine Leiomyoma

Uterine leiomyomas (also known as myoma, fibroid, fibroleiomyoma) are the most common benign tumours of the uterus in adult females but are exceptionally rare in adolescents. They are often asymptomatic and an incidental finding on imaging. The US findings are variable and depend on the size, number and composition of the fibroids. Intramural fibroids are typically round or ovoid in outline and appear well—circumscribed (Fig. 40). Each tumour contains variable amounts of smooth muscle, fibrous tissue and calcification and may contain hypoechoic, isoechoic or hyperechoic elements relative to the uterine myometrium. Fibroids may reach a very large size in adolescents and undergo cystic necrosis. MRI is useful in depicting intact bilateral ovaries and confirming the intramural fibroid (Fig. 41). Treatment is with myomectomy aiming to preserve fertility, recurrence is recognised (Wright and Laufer 2011).

17 Pelvic Free Fluid

Pelvic free fluid is not an uncommon finding in the child with abdominal pain. Interpretation of the presence of free fluid requires knowledge of the patient's symptoms, physical examination findings and the results of laboratory investigations and other ultrasound findings.

Free intraperitoneal fluid typically accumulates in the most dependent region of the pelvis, the rectouterine pouch of Douglas. On US small quantities anechoic of free fluid (<5 ml) should be considered physiologic, similarly on CT a volume of up to 5 mL with a mean attenuation value of <20 HU can be considered physiologic. Free fluid may accumulate as a result of rapid hydration.

A collection of more than 10 mL should raise concern about the possibility of a pathologic process (Jones 1997). Subtle pathological collections of free fluid can be demonstrated between the superior junction of bladder and the uterus on ultrasound (Nyberg et al. 1984). Haemoperitoneum is a well-recognised finding in blunt abdominopelvic trauma with solid visceral, bowel or mesenteric injury. Haemoperitoneum is also a complication of a ruptured ovarian cyst, endometriosis and ectopic pregnancy. Haemoperitoneum is a positive predictive factor for ectopic pregnancy in the setting of a positive serum β-hCG level (Jeffrey and Laing 1982). Pelvic free fluid is an important ancillary finding in acute appendicitis, abdominal visceral perforation and PID.

18 Conclusion

Pelvic pain is a relatively common presentation in children and adolescents, with a myriad of causes both gynaecological and non-gynaecological in origin. Assessment of paediatric abdominal pain can prove a diagnostic challenge. Children may be limited in their ability to give an accurate history. Parents or guardians may also have difficulty interpreting the complaints of small children. In some cases no specific cause can be found, but being reassured that there is no serious underlying problem that can be helpful. Ultrasonography is well established as the primary initial investigation of choice with MRI, if required providing excellent anatomic detail to further delineate structural anomalies and pathology. Familiarity with the imaging features of commonly associated conditions aids in the rapid diagnosis and immediate management of the patient.

References

AFS (1985) Revised American fertility society classification of endometriosis: 1985. Fertil Steril 43:351–352

Aghajanian C (2011) Treatment of low-risk gestational trophoblastic neoplasia. J Clin Oncol 29:786–788

Albayram F, Hamper U (2001) Ovarian and adnexal torsion: spectrum of sonographic findings with pathologic correlation. J Ultrasound Med 20:1083–1089

Allen SD, Lim AK, Seckl MJ (2006) Radiology of gestational trophoblastic neoplasia. Clin Radiol 61:301–313

Apley J, Naish N (1958) Recurrent abdominal pains: a field survey of 1000 school children. Arch Dis Child 33:165–170

Asch E, Levine D (2007) Variations in appearance of endometriomas. JUM 26:993–1002

Baltarowich OH, Kurtz AB, Pasto ME et al (1987) The spectrum of sonographic findings in hemorrhagic ovarian cysts. Am J Roentgenol 148:901–905

Barnhart K, Mennuti MT, Benjamin I et al (1994) Prompt diagnosis of ectopic pregnancy in an emergency department setting. Obstet Gynecol 84:1010–1015

Beller MJ (1998) The "tip of the iceberg" sign. Radiology 209:395–396

Benjaminov O, Atri M (2004) Sonography of the abnormal fallopian tube. Am J Roentgenol 183:737–742

Blask AR, Sanders RC, Rock JA et al (1991) Obstructed uterovaginal anomalies: demonstration with sonography. Part II. Teenagers. Radiology 179:84–88

Borders RJ, Breiman RS, Yeh BM et al (2004) Computed tomography of corpus luteal cysts. J Comput Assist Tomogr 28:340–342

Brandt ML, Helmrath MA (2005) Ovarian cysts in infants and children. Semin Pediatr Surg 14:78–85

Breech LL, Hillard PJ (2005) Adnexal torsion in pediatric and adolescent girls. Curr Opin Obstet Gynecol 17:483–489

Chang HC, Bhatt S, Dogra VS (2008) Pearls and pitfalls in diagnosis of ovarian torsion. Radiographics 28:1355–1368

Chiou SY, Lev Toaff AS, Masuda E et al (2007) Adnexal torsion: new clinical and imaging observations by sonography, computed tomography and magnetic resonance imaging. J Ultrasound Med 26:1289–1301

Cicchiello LA, Hamper UM, Scoutt LM (2011) Ultrasound evaluation of gynecologic causes of pelvic pain. Obstet Gynecol Clin N Am 38:85–114

Condous G, Okaro E, Khalid A et al (2005) The accuracy of transvaginal ultrasonography for the diagnosis of ectopic pregnancy prior to surgery. Hum Reprod 20:1404–1409

Currarino G, Rutledge JC (1989) Ovarian torsion and amputation resulting in partially calcified, pedunculated cystic mass. Pediatr Radiol 19:395–399

Emonts M, Doornewaard H, Admiraal JC (2004) Adnexal torsion in very young girls: diagnostic pitfalls. Eur J Obstet Gynecol Reprod Biol 116:207–210

FIGO (2009) Current FIGO staging for cancer of the vagina, fallopian tube, ovary, and gestational trophoblastic neoplasia. Int J Gynaecol Obstet 105:3–4

Forcier M (2009) Emergency department evaluation of acute pelvic pain in the adolescent female. Clin Ped Emerg Med 10:20–30

Frates MC, Brown DL, Doubilet PM et al (1994) Tubal rupture in patients with ectopic pregnancy: diagnosis with transvaginal ultrasound. Radiology 191:769–772
French L (2008) Dysmenorrhoea in adolescents: diagnosis and treatment. Paediatr Drugs 10:1–7
Giudice LC, Kao LC (2004) Endometriosis. Lancet 364:1789–1799
Glastonbury CM (2002) The shading sign. Radiology 224:199–201
Gracia CR, Barnhart KT (2001) Diagnosing ectopic pregnancy: decision analysis comparing six strategies. Obstet Gynecol 97:464–470
Graif M, Itzchak Y (1988) Sonographic evaluation of ovarian torsion in childhood and adolescence. Am J Roentgenol 150:647–649
Harel Z (2008) Dysmenorrhoea in adults. Ann NY Acad Sci 1135:185–195
Harmon J, Binkovitz L, Binkovitz L (2008) Isolated fallopian tube torsion: sonographic and CT features. Pediatr Radiol 38:175–179
Harms D, Zahn S, Göbel U et al (2006) Pathology and molecular biology of teratomas in childhood and adolescence. Klin Padiatr 218:296–302
Helmrath MA, Shin CE, Warner BW (1998) Ovarian cysts in the pediatric population. Semin Pediatr Surg 7:19–28
Hernon M, McKenna J, Busby G, Sanders C, Garden A (2010) The histology and management of ovarian cysts found in children and adolescents presenting to a children's hospital from 1991 to 2007: a call for more paediatric gynaecologists. BJOG 117:181–184
Hillen TI, Grbavac SL, Johnston PJ et al (1999) Primary dysmenorrhoea in young Australian women: prevalence impact, and knowledge of treatment. J Adolesc Health 25:40–45
Hutton L, Rankin R (1979) The fat–fluid level: another feature of dermoid tumors of the ovary. J Clin Ultrasound 7:215–216
Islam S, Yamout SZ, Gosche JR (2008) Management and outcomes of ovarian masses in children and adolescents. Am Surg 74:1062–1065
Jain KA (2000) Imaging of peritoneal inclusion cysts. Am J Roentgenol 174:1559–1563
Jain KA (2002) Sonographic spectrum of hemorrhagic ovarian cysts. J Ultrasound Med 21:879–886
Jeanty C, Frayer EA, Page R et al (2010) Neonatal ovarian torsion complicated by intestinal obstruction and perforation, and review of the literature. J Pediatr Surg 45:e5–e9
Jeffrey RB, Laing FC (1982) Echogenic clot: a useful sign of pelvic hemoperitoneum. Radiology 145:139–141
Jones HW (1997) Pelvic pain: overview. In: Fleischer AC, Javitt MC, Jeffrey RB, Jones HW (eds) Clinical gynecologic imaging. Lippincott-Raven, Philadelphia, pp 245–248
Kanumakala S, Warne GL, Stokes KB et al (2002) Massive ovarian edema causing early puberty. J Pediatr Endocrin Metabol 15:861–864
Kawamoto S, Sato K, Matsumoto H et al (2001) Multiple mobile spherules in mature cystic teratoma of the ovary. Am J Roentgenol 176:1455–1457
Kiechl-Kohlendorfer U, Maurer K, Unsinn KM et al (2006) Fluid-debris level in follicular cysts: a pathognomonic sign of ovarian torsion. Pediatr Radiol 36:421–425
Kilickesmez O, Tasdelen N, Yetimoglu B et al (2009) Emerg Radiol 16:399–401
Kim JS, Woo SK et al (1995) Sonographic diagnosis of paraovarian cysts: value of detecting a separate ipsilateral ovary. Am J Roentgenol 164:1441–1444
Kim JS, Lee HJ, Woo SK et al (1997) Peritoneal inclusion cysts and their relationship to the ovaries: evaluation with sonography. Radiology 204:481–484
Kinkel K, Frei KA, Balleyguier C et al (2006) Diagnosis of endometriosis with imaging: a review. Eur Radiol 16:285–298
Kissler S, Zangos S, Kohl J et al (2008) Duration of dysmenorrhea and extent of adenomyosis visualized by magnetic resonance imaging. Eur J Obstet Gynecol Reprod Biol 137:204–209
Kohorn EI (2001) The new FIGO 2000 staging and risk factor scoring system for gestational trophoblastic disease: description and critical assessment. Int J Gynecol Cancer 11:73–77
Kontoravdis A, Hassan E, Hassiakos D et al (1999) Laparoscopic evaluation and management of chronic pelvic pain in adolescence. Clin Exp Obstet Gynecol 26:76–77
Kramer LA, Lalani T, Kawashima A (1997) Massive edema of the ovary: high resolution MR findings using a phased-array pelvic coil. J Magn Reson Imaging 7:758–760
Kupesic S, Plavsic BM (2010) Adnexal torsion: color Doppler and three-dimensional ultrasound. Abdom Imaging 35:602–606
Laufer MR, Goitein L, Bush M et al (1997) Prevalence of endometriosis in adolescent girls with chronic pelvic pain not responding to conventional therapy. J Pediatr Adolesc Gynecol 10:199–202
Levine D (2007) Ectopic pregnancy. Radiology 245:385–397
Linam LE, Darolia R, Naffaa LN et al (2007) US findings of adnexal torsion in children and adolescents: size really does matter. Pediatr Radiol 37:1013–1019
Malde HM, Kedar RP, Chadha D et al (1992) Dermoid mesh: a sonographic sign of ovarian teratoma. Am J Roentgenol 159:1349–1350
Menon S, Sammel MD, Vichnin M et al (2007) Risk factors for ectopic pregnancy: a comparison between adults and adolescent women. J Pediatr Adolesc Gynecol 20:181–185
Merlini L, Anooshiravani M, Vunda A (2008) Noninflammatory fallopian tube pathology in children. Pediatr Radiol 38:1330–1337
Mol BW, Van der Veen F, Bossuyt PM (1999) Implementation of probabilistic decision rules improves the predictive values of algorithms in the diagnostic management of ectopic pregnancy. Hum Reprod 14:2855–2862
Moon RJ, Mears A, Kitteringham LJ et al (2009) Massive ovarian oedema: an unusual abdominal mass in infancy. Pediatr Blood Cancer 53:217–219
Nussbaum AR, Sanders RC, Hartman DS et al (1988) Neonatal ovarian cysts: sonographic-pathologic correlation. Radiology 168:817–821
Nyberg DA, Laing FC, Jeffrey RB (1984) Sonographic detection of subtle pelvic collections. Am J Roentgenol 143:261–263
Olpin JD, Heilbrun M (2009) Imaging of Mullerian duct anomalies. Clin Obstet Gynecol 52:40–56

Orazi C, Inserra A, Lucchetti MC et al (2006) Isolated tubal torsion: a rare cause of pelvic pain at menarche. Sonographic and MR findings. Pediatr Radiol 36:1316–1318

Orazi C, Lucchetti MC, Schingo PM et al (2007) Herlyn-Werner-Wunderlich syndrome: uterus didelphys, blind hemivagina and ipsilateral renal agenesis. Sonographic and MR findings in 11 cases. Pediatr Radiol 37:657–665

Outwater EK, Siegelman ES, Hunt JL (2001) Ovarian teratomas: tumour types and imaging characteristics. Radiographics 21:475–490

Panteli C, Curry J, Kiely E et al (2009) Ovarian germ cell tumours: a 17-year study in a single unit. Eur J Pediatr Surg 19:96–100

Patel MD, Feldstein VA, Filly RA (2005) The likelihood ratio of sonographic findings for the diagnosis of hemorrhagic ovarian cysts. J Ultrasound Med 24:607–614

Peña JE, Ufberg D, Cooney N et al (2000) Usefulness of Doppler Sonography in the diagnosis of ovarian torsion. Fertil Steril 73:1047–1050

Potter AW, Chandrasekhar CA (2008) US and CT evaluation of acute pelvic pain of gynecologic origin in nonpregnant premenopausal patients. RadioGraphics 28:1645–1659

Prada Arias M, Muguerza VR, Montero SM et al (2005) Uterus didelphys with obstructed hemivagina and multicystic dysplastic kidney. Eur J Pediatr Surg 15:441–445

Quinn SF, Erickson S, Black WC (1985) Cystic ovarian teratomas: the sonographic appearance of the dermoid plug. Radiology 155:477–478

Rezvani M, Shaaban AM (2011) Fallopian tube disease in the nonpregnant patient. Radiographics 31:527–548

Sampson J (1940) The development of the implantation theory for the origin of peritoneal endometriosis. Am J Obstet Gynecol 40:549–557

Sanfilippo JS, Wakim NG, Schikler KN et al (1986) Endometriosis in association with uterine anomaly. Am J Obstet Gynecol 154:39–43

Savelli L, Deiaco P, Ghi T et al (2004) Transvaginal sonographic appearance of peritoneal pseudocysts. Ultrasound Obstet Gynecol 23:284–288

Savelli L, Ghi T, De Iaco P et al (2006) Paraovarian/paratubal cysts: comparison of transvaginal sonographic and pathological findings to establish diagnostic criteria. Ultrasound Obstet Gynecol 28:330–334

Seckl MJ, Newlands ES (2002) Gestational trophoblastic tumours. In: Shaw RW, Soutter WP, Stanton SI (eds) Gynaecology, 3rd edn. Churchill Livingstone, Edinburgh, pp 653–664

Servaes S, Zurakowski D, Laufer MR et al (2007) Sonographic findings of ovarian torsion in children. Pediatr Radiol 37:446–451

Spencer J, Ghattamaneni S (2010) MR Imaging of the sonographically indeterminate adnexal mass. Radiology 256:677–694

Spencer JA, Forstner R, Cunha TM, ESUR female imaging subcommittee, et al. (2010) ESUR guidelines for MR imaging of the sonographically indeterminate adnexal mass: an algorithmic approach. Eur Radiol 20:25–35

Svanberg L, Ulmsten U (1981) The incidence of primary dysmenorrhoea in teenagers. Arch Gynecol 230:133–137

Takeuchi M, Matsuzaki K (2011) Adenomyosis: usual and unusual imaging manifestations, pitfalls, and problem-solving MR imaging techniques. RadioGraphics 31:99–115

Talerman A (2003) Germ cell tumors of the ovary. In: Altchek A, Deligdisch L, Kase NG (eds) Diagnosis and management of ovarian disorders, 2nd edn. Academic Press, Amsterdam, pp 95–110

Tamai K, Koyama T, Saga T et al (2006) MR features of physiologic and benign conditions of the ovary. Eur Radiol 16:2700–2711

Templeman CL, Fallat ME (2005) Benign ovarian masses. Semin Pediatr Surg 14:93–99

Timor-Tritsch IE, Lerner J, Monteagudo A et al (1998) Transvaginal sonographic markers of tubal inflammatory disease. Ultrasound Obstet Gynecol 12:56–66

Umesaki N, Tanaka T, Miyama M et al (2000) Successful preoperative diagnosis of massive ovarian edema aided by comparative imaging study using magnetic resonance and ultrasound. Obstet Gynecol 89:97–99

UNICEF (2001) A league table of teenage births in rich nations. Innocenti Report Card No. 3. Florence: UNICEF Innocenti Research Centre. www.unicef-icdc.org/publications/index.html [accessed 08/2011]

Van Holsbeke C, Van Calster B, Guerriero S et al (2010) Endometriomas: their ultrasound characteristics. Ultrasound Obstet Gynecol 35:730–740

Van Kerkhove F, Cannie M, Op de Beeck K et al (2007) Ovarian torsion in a premenarcheal girl: MRI findings. Abdom Imaging 32:424–427

Vichnin M (2008) Ectopic pregnancy in adolescents. Curr Opin Obstet Gynecol 20:475–478

Vijayaraghavan SB (2004) Sonographic whirlpool sign in ovarian torsion. J Ultrasound Med 23:1643–1649

Yamashiro T, Inamine M, Kamiya H et al (2008) Massive ovarian edema with torsion: unusual hemorrhage and the recovery of contrast enhancement. Emerg Radiol 15:115–118

Workowski KA, Berman S (2010) Center for disease control: sexually transmitted diseases guidelines, 2010. MMWR 59(RR-12):1–116

Wright KN, Laufer MR (2011) Leiomyomas in adolescents. Fertil Steril 95:2434.e15-7

Gynaecological Neoplasia

Kieran McHugh, Kirsteen McDonald, and Edwin Jesudason

Contents

1 **Introduction** 210

2 **Ovarian Germ Cell Tumours** 210
2.1 Epidemiology 210
2.2 Pathology 211
2.3 Clinical Presentations 211
2.4 Imaging Investigations 213
2.5 Surgical Management 214
2.6 Prognosis 214

3 **Non-germ Cell Ovarian Tumours** 214
3.1 Primary Tumours 214
3.2 Secondary Tumours 218

4 **Non-neoplastic Ovarian Lesions** 218

5 **Rhabdomyosarcoma** 218
5.1 Epidemiology 218
5.2 Pathology 218
5.3 Clinical Presentation 220
5.4 Imaging Investigations 220
5.5 Treatment and Prognosis 221

6 **Other Lesions** 221

References 222

Abstract

Gynaecological neoplasms in childhood are not common and malignancies are rare. Whilst the age standardised rate for all cancers in UK girls (0–14 years) is 127 per million, the rate of malignant germ cell tumours (GCTs) is only 2 per million. The commonest paediatric gynaecological tumours are GCTs of the ovary and rhabdomyosarcoma of the uterus, vagina and cervix. Ovarian tumours in childhood are more commonly benign than malignant. Between 1991 and 2000, the United Kingdom National Registry of Childhood Tumours recorded 126 ovarian tumours and 37 arising in the rest of the female reproductive tract amongst girls aged 0–14. Of the ovarian tumours, there were 112(89%) GCTs, 6(5%) carcinomas, 6(5%) lymphomas, 1(1%) neuroblastoma and 1(1%) mesothelioma. Amongst the non-ovarian reproductive tract tumours, there were 19(51%) rhabdomyosarcomas, 12(32%) GCTs, 5(14%) carcinomas and 1(3%) other sarcoma. Tumours usually associated with adults, such as squamous cell carcinomas of the cervix, are also rarely seen in adolescent patients. Imaging is useful before surgery in determining tumour origin, characteristics, extent, local invasion and distant spread. Ultrasound is the first line imaging modality for any newly diagnosed or suspected pelvic mass lesion, followed ideally when necessary by MRI. MRI avoids the radiation associated with CT scanning, gives excellent tissue contrast, and should be the next line of investigation when a mass is discovered.

K. McHugh (✉)
Great Ormond Street Hospital for Children, London, WC1N 3JH, UK
e-mail: mchugk@gosh.nhs.uk

K. McDonald
Barts and The London NHS Trust, West Smithfield, London, EC1A 7BE, UK

E. Jesudason
Children's Hospital Los Angeles, University of Southern California, Los Angeles, USA

E. Jesudason
Alder Hey Children's Hospital and University of Liverpool, Eaton Road, Liverpool, L12 2AP, UK

G. Mann et al. (eds.), *Imaging of Gynecological Disorders in Infants and Children*, Medical Radiology. Diagnostic Imaging, DOI: 10.1007/174_2010_126,

Abbreviations

GCT	Germ cell tumour
CCG	Children's cancer study group
ADC	Apparent diffusion coefficient
PET/CT	Positron emission tomography—computed tomography
STIR	Short-tau inversion recovery
EST	Endodermal sinus tumour
AFP	Alpha fetoprotein
POG	Pediatric oncology group
RMS	Rhabdomyosarcoma
MOO	Massive ovarian oedema
TNM	Tumor-node-metastasis
IRS	Intergroup rhabdomyosarcoma study
IVC	Inferior vena cava
T1W	T1-weighted
T2W	T2-weighted
CT	Computed tomography
MRI	Magnetic resonance imaging
UK	United Kingdom

1 Introduction

Gynaecological neoplasms in childhood are not common and malignancies are rare (Stiller 2008). Whilst the age standardised rate for all cancers in UK girls (0–14 years) is 127 per million, the rate of malignant germ cell tumours (GCTs) is only 2 per million. The commonest paediatric gynaecological tumours are GCTs of the ovary and rhabdomyosarcoma of the uterus, vagina and cervix. Ovarian tumours in childhood are more commonly benign than malignant (Panteli et al. 2009). Between 1991 and 2000, the United Kingdom National Registry of Childhood Tumours recorded 126 ovarian tumours and 37 arising in the rest of the female reproductive tract amongst girls aged 0–14. Of the ovarian tumours, there were 112(89%) GCTs, 6(5%) carcinomas, 6(5%) lymphomas, 1(1%) neuroblastoma and 1(1%) mesothelioma. Amongst the non-ovarian reproductive tract tumours, there were 19(51%) rhabdomyosarcomas, 12(32%) GCTs, 5(14%) carcinomas and 1(3%) other sarcoma (Stiller 2008). Tumours usually associated with adults, such as squamous cell carcinomas of the cervix, are also rarely seen in adolescent patients (Yang et al. 2009). Imaging is useful before surgery in determining tumour origin, characteristics, extent, local invasion and distant spread. Ultrasound is the first line imaging modality for any newly diagnosed or suspected pelvic mass lesion, followed ideally when necessary by MRI. MRI avoids the radiation associated with CT scanning, gives excellent tissue contrast, and should be the next line of investigation when a mass is discovered (Riccabona 2008). CT has the advantage that it is quicker and may obviate the need for sedation or general anaesthesia in smaller children but the radiation burden may preclude its use, in general, unless MRI is unavailable. PET/CT is still not commonly used in paediatric oncology imaging, but early experience has shown avid FDG uptake in paediatric abdominal neoplasms including ovarian tumours (Murphy et al. 2008). Currently, PET/CT is primarily used to identify residual or recurrent tumour in difficult cases. Nevertheless, imaging alone cannot reliably differentiate benign and malignant lesions, nor can it necessarily always distinguish the pelvic organ of origin. Surgery remains an integral part of disease staging and local control for most of these neoplasms. Fertility-sparing procedures are achievable in part because of the adjuvant therapies now available for residual disease.

2 Ovarian Germ Cell Tumours

2.1 Epidemiology

Delineating the epidemiology of ovarian GCTs in childhood is complicated by variation in the definition of childhood by age. In some series, women up to 19 years are included (Brookfield et al. 2009), in others only children of 14 years and below are counted (Stiller 2008). Approximately 80% of ovarian masses in childhood are benign (including epithelial cysts and teratomas) (Rescorla 2008); the rates of malignancy reported in the literature range from 16 to 24% (Billmire et al. 2004). GCTs represent almost 80% of childhood ovarian neoplasms (Brookfield et al. 2009); an estimated 25% are malignant (Rescorla 2008); they are rare below 5 years of age (Brookfield, et al. 2009) with a peak incidence around 12 years (Billmire et al. 2004).

2.2 Pathology

GCTs are considered to originate from primordial germ cells which migrate to the urogenital ridges in the retroperitoneum, where they are incorporated into the gonads before descent (West et al. 2009). Therefore, GCTs can arise in the gonads or anywhere along normal or aberrant migration pathways. Extra-gonadal tumours are usually located in the midline, i.e. anterior mediastinum, retroperitoneum, or sacrococcygeal regions (Talerman 1985). GCTs containing derivatives of two or three germ layers are typically teratomas. The most common teratomas are mature and benign. Mature teratomas contain different tissue types, including hair, skin and teeth. Immature teratomas are potentially malignant and typically contain primitive neuroepithelium (Harms et al. 2006). GCTs that contain derivatives of only a single-germ layer include dysgerminomas and endodermal sinus tumours (EST). EST are also referred to as yolk sac tumours and characteristically secrete alpha fetoprotein (AFP). In a US study by the Pediatric Oncology Group (POG) and Children's Cancer Study Group (CCG) between 1990 and 1996, 131 malignant ovarian GCTs were identified: there were 39 teratomas with EST, 25 pure EST, 23 pure dysgerminoma, 21 teratomas with other malignant elements, 10 with multiple malignant elements (but without teratoma), two choriocarcinoma and two gonadoblastoma (where sex chromosome anomalies may occur) (Billmire et al. 2004). In a European two-centre study of ovarian GCTs, bilateral disease was found in 3 of 66 patients across a range of benign and malignant histology (De Backer et al. 2006). Spread of malignant GCTs mainly occurs locally to bladder, rectum, uterus or pelvic peritoneum. Spread can also be via the lymphatic system, and haematogenously to the liver or lungs. Peritoneal seeding is more common with immature teratomas (Fig. 1). Pre-operative imaging may detect lymph node enlargement, and spread to the peritoneum, omentum, liver or lungs.

2.3 Clinical Presentations

Patients with ovarian GCTs present most commonly with symptoms related to the effects of the primary tumour with sub-acute abdominal pain, or an abdominal or pelvic mass (Panteli et al. 2009) (Fig. 2). Children with peritoneal metastases and ascites may also present with abdominal distension. Presentations with poor appetite, urinary symptoms, menstrual changes and weight loss have also been reported (Schultz et al. 2005). Presentations with an acute abdomen may follow tumour torsion and/or rupture. Torsion rates vary widely between series and may depend on the distinction between clinically evident torsion and that noted only at operation (Panteli et al. 2009; Schultz et al. 2005). The degree of ovarian ischaemia probably depends on the extent of vascular compromise. The latter may progress from veno-lymphatic obstruction with oedema to arterial thrombosis and ovarian necrosis or haemorrhagic infarction. Untreated, this can be associated with peritonitis and even death. Early diagnosis is therefore advantageous. Ultrasound in this setting can be non-specific, showing thickening of the mass wall. Doppler ultrasound may show a twisted vascular pedicle (the 'whirlpool sign') and can detect changes in arterial and venous flow (Vijayaraghavan 2004). However, as the obstruction can be variable, ultrasound imaging may be normal. The most specific findings on CT or MRI are a twisted vascular pedicle and a thickened fallopian tube. Other non-specific findings include increased ovarian volume, mass wall thickening and ascites.

Tumour rupture may be associated with torsion, infection or trauma. Rupture causes an acute or chronic peritoneal inflammatory response. Imaging may demonstrate the discontinuity of the tumour wall, distortion or flattening of the tumour, and ascites with omental infiltration, if it is chronic.

Less commonly, ovarian GCTs may present due to effects of secondary disease and, still more rarely, precocious puberty (Panteli et al. 2009) or paraneoplastic syndromes. An example of the latter with clinical implications for imaging is the rare problem of hypercalcaemia in the presence of an ovarian dysgerminoma (Matthew et al. 2006; Nelken et al. 1978). Whilst the mechanisms for such hypercalcaemia vary (e.g. production of parathyroid hormone-related peptide or 25-hydroxyvitamin D-1α-hydroxylase (Evans et al. 2004)), the renal failure that attends hypercalcaemia may preclude use of intravenous contrast agents for cross-sectional imaging. At the same time, prompt tumour excision or debulking is a key part of controlling the hypercalcaemia (Matthew et al. 2006; Okoye et al. 2001). However, as the pre-operative imaging and

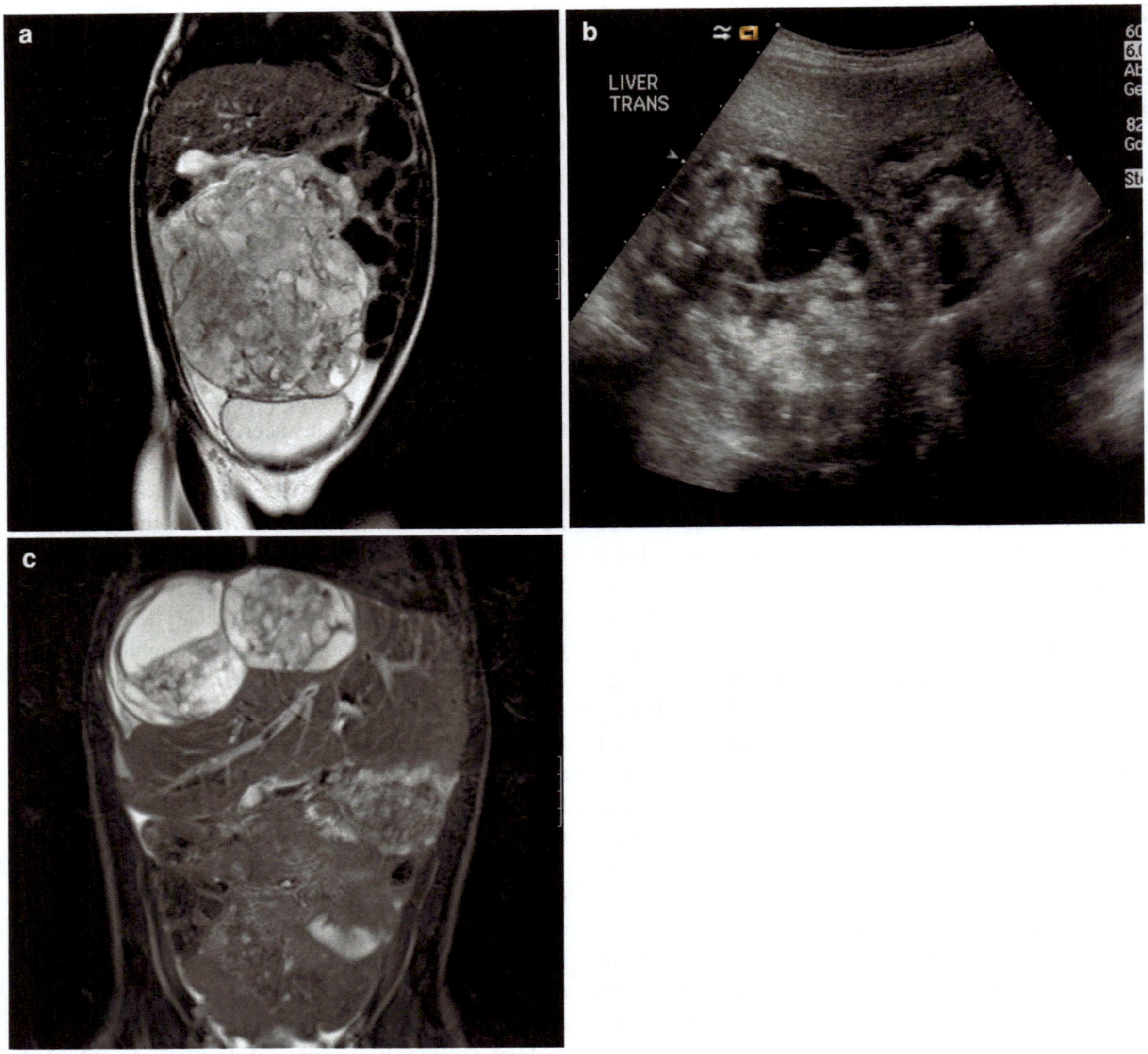

Fig. 1 Imaging of an 8-year-old girl originally presenting with an abdominal mass. Ultrasound and **a** MRI showed a multicystic mass with a few small solid areas. A moderate amount of ascites was present. At surgery, the entire peritoneal surface was studded with smaller similar foci. The large mass was removed and on histological assessment was a mature germ cell tumour (GCT). Biopsy of a few of the small, but innumerable, peritoneal lesions also showed mature GCT. These smaller GCT lesions were not visible on pre-operative imaging, even in retrospect. Abdominal distension had developed by routine follow-up 3 months later. **b** Ultrasound and **c** MRI now showed new large right-sided perihepatic masses. These were removed and again found to be mature GCT. Surgical resection of the recurrent lesions in this case was mandated to reduce potential complications of abdominopelvic organ compression and mechanical obstruction and further to evaluate for malignant degeneration

intra-operative photography demonstrates (Figs. 3, 4), non-contrast scanning may substantially fail to display the relevant vascular anatomy associated with the tumour(s). Again, this rare example illustrates a further potential benefit of using MRI rather than CT (when the former is reasonably available).

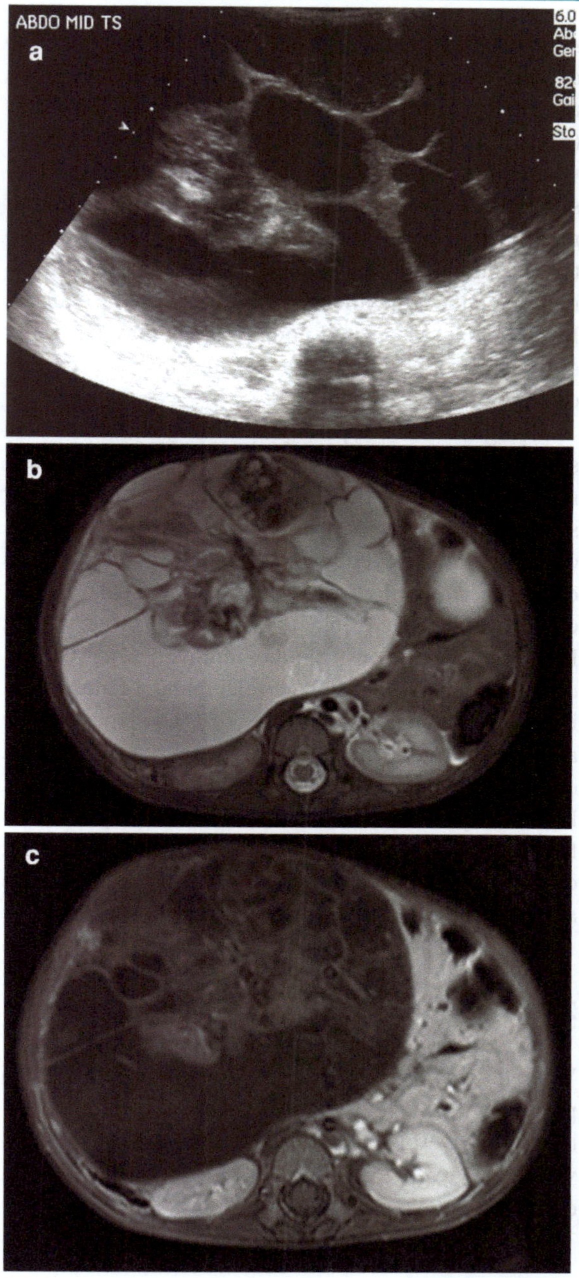

Fig. 2 Imaging of a 2-year-old girl with a right-sided ovarian teratoma which contained focal immature elements. **a** Transverse ultrasound scan of the mid-abdomen showed a large multi-loculated cystic abdominal mass with some solid components; **b** Axial STIR sequence of the same patient showing a predominantly high signal loculated mass, with intermediate signal components, in keeping with a cystic mass containing solid elements; **c** Axial T1-weighted image post-contrast at same level as **b**. The mass is mainly low signal with mild enhancement of the solid components and septa

Table 1 Staging of paediatric ovarian germ cell tumours

Stage	Characteristics
Stage I	Limited to one or both ovaries. Peritoneal washings normal. Tumour markers return to normal after appropriate half-life decline
Stage II	Microscopic residual disease or positive lymph nodes. Peritoneal washings normal. Tumour markers either normal or showing evidence of malignancy
Stage III	Lymph node involvement. Gross residual disease or biopsy only. Contiguous visceral involvement. Peritoneal washings positive. Tumour markers either normal or showing evidence of malignancy
Stage IV	Distant metastases

2.4 Imaging Investigations

Initial investigation of a child with the presenting features described above should be transabdominal ultrasound of the abdomen and pelvis in the presence of a full bladder (Fig. 2a) (De Silva et al. 2004). Transvaginal ultrasound is rarely practically possible or indicated in girls in the paediatric age range. Sonographically, benign tumours appear as large predominantly cystic masses, with an echogenic tubercle, which may contain hair, teeth, or fat. Malignant tumours appear more solid, and may demonstrate central necrosis with thickened irregular walls and septa, and increased vascularity. Benign GCTs are well demonstrated on MRI (Outwater et al. 2001; Saba et al. 2009). The fat component shows typically high signal on T1W imaging, and low signal on fat suppression sequences. Calcification may not be visible or may be seen as signal drop out on all MR sequences. The fluid component appears as high signal on T2W images and low or intermediate on T1W images. Fat–fluid levels may be present. Malignant GCTs have more solid components which appear as low or intermediate signal on T1W images, and intermediate or high signal on T2W images (Figs. 2b and c). There is variable contrast enhancement of the solid components. Fibrovascular septa appear as low or intermediate signals on T1W images and enhance markedly post-gadolinium administration. Benign tumours demonstrate different attenuation characteristics on CT depending on the tissue present. Fat has very low attenuation (< 0 Hounsfield Units), calcification has high attenuation and fluid has low attenuation. Malignant tumours have larger soft tissue components which enhance, and irregular walls and septa. There may be central areas of low attenuation due to haemorrhage or necrosis.

It is not generally possible to identify different tumour types from imaging, but one small study has shown the presence of dilated blood vessels in EST on post-contrast CT scans, which correlates with abundant vessels seen on microscopy (Choi et al. 2008). Similarly, on CT scans, characteristic stippled calcifications have been described in dysgerminoma; these contrast with the coarse 'bony' calcifications often seen in teratomata (Ratani et al. 2004) (Fig 1.12). In general, the more solid a tumour appears on imaging, the more likely it is to be either malignant or an immature teratoma.

2.5 Surgical Management

Accurate staging is based on the histological findings of the resected tumour and tumour markers, as outlined in Table 1 (Billmire et al. 2004; Rescorla 2008). Alongside surgical staging, complete resection and adjuvant chemotherapy are recommended for malignant tumours (Billmire et al. 2004; Rescorla 2008). Raised tumour markers and/or a predominantly solid lesion are indicative of malignancy. In these circumstances, laparotomy is performed to accomplish tumour excision where involvement is limited to the ovary, unilateral salpingo-oophorectomy suffices and can be readily achieved via a cosmetically acceptable Pfannenstiel approach (Billmire et al. 2004; Rescorla 2008). Given the high cure rates, surgery has more recently taken greater account of fertility-sparing strategies. Historical operations undertaken in adults which included hysterectomy and excision of the contralateral ovary, have no place in routine paediatric practice (Brookfield et al. 2009; Cass et al. 2001). In cases where retroperitoneal nodal masses are present and persist despite chemotherapy, they may be excised along with the primary through a more extensive higher incision (Figs. 3 and 4). Pre-operative imaging allows the surgeon to site the incision optimally and is invaluable in counselling both patient and parents before surgery. Nevertheless, it may be difficult to distinguish unilateral from bilateral ovarian involvement using imaging alone (Fig. 3). In cases where imaging indicates tumour invasion of adjacent structures, multi-disciplinary consideration is given to debulking surgery and further adjuvant therapy in an attempt to preserve adjacent organs such as the uterus (Figs. 3 and 4) (Jawaid et al. in press). Even in cases where imaging indicates that tissue planes are preserved, this does not guarantee straightforward tumour mobilisation. Perioperative examination under anaesthesia (abdominal and rectal) can give further information on the attachments of the tumour to be excised. In particular, associated nodal masses may be firmly secured by overlying vessels and require careful extirpation (Figs. 3 and 4).

Benign tumours typically feature cystic rather than solid masses (Fig. 5). These lesions require surgical resection only. In these circumstances, tube-sparing surgery can be used (De Backer et al. 2006). With overwhelmingly cystic lesions, laparoscopic excision can be performed (Karpelowsky et al. 2009). Small cysts are removed intact in an endosurgery bag. Larger cystic lesions can be removed after careful drainage that avoids spillage (e.g. using a fenestration in an adherent bag) (Rescorla 2008). The laparoscopic approach confers the potential benefits of improved cosmesis and rapid recovery when compared to full laparotomy; however, the multidisciplinary team is first required to make a very conservative judgement on the likelihood of malignancy on the basis of the available pre-operative imaging (Fig. 6).

2.6 Prognosis

With the majority of patients (approximately 75%) present with Stage 1 disease, and with a few exceptions, the overall prognosis is good with a 95% survival rate, even for Stage 3 or 4 tumours (Billmire et al. 2004).

3 Non-germ Cell Ovarian Tumours

3.1 Primary Tumours

Stromal cell origin tumours (including Sertoli–Leydig cell and granulosa-thecal cell tumours) represent about 10% of ovarian malignancies in adolescents (Schneider et al. 2003). They are derived from the sex cord of the fetal gonad, and may contain fibroblasts, theca, Leydig, Sertoli or granulosa cells. In the Kiel Pediatric

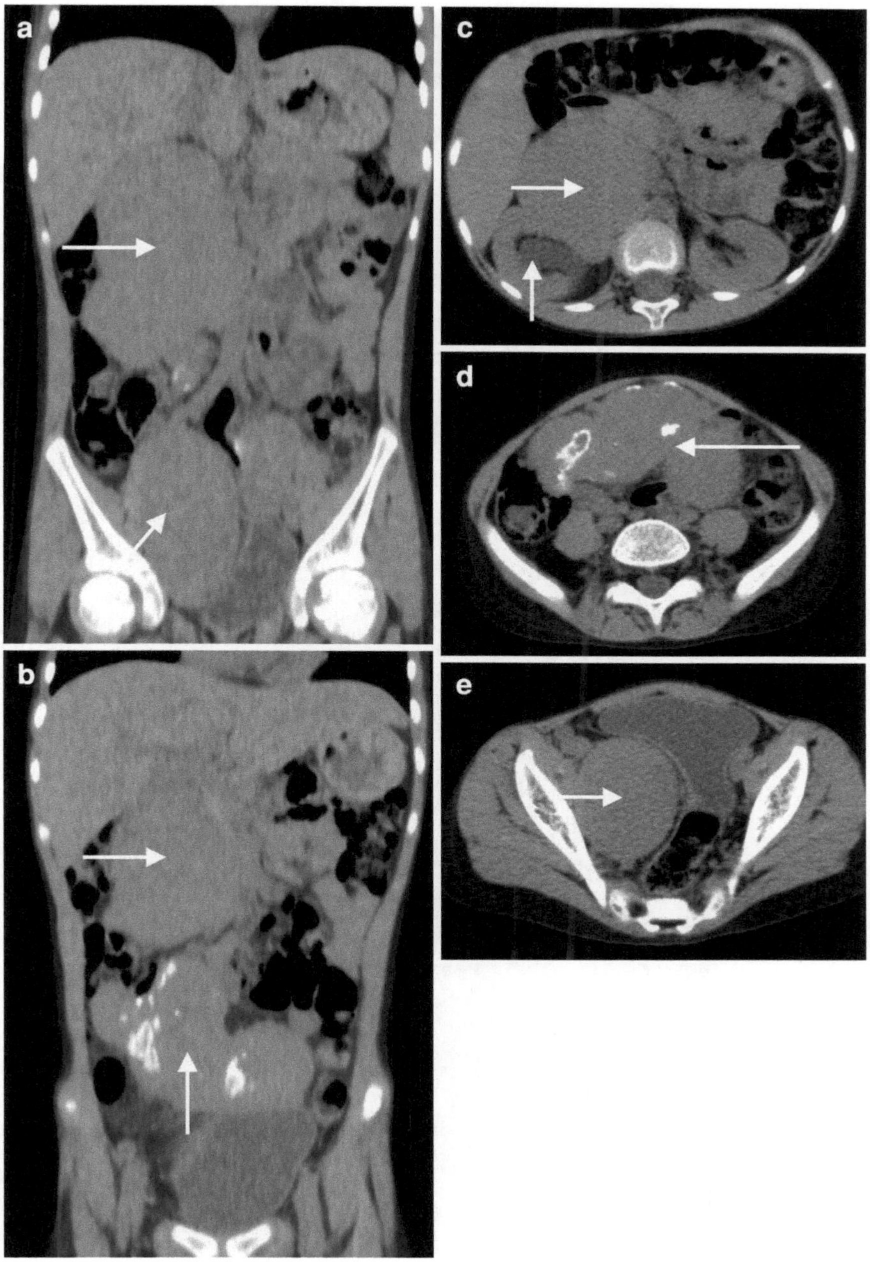

Fig. 3 Pre-operative emergency CT scan of prepubertal patient with ovarian dysgerminoma, hypercalcaemia and renal failure (precluding contrast administration). **a** Coronal view showing the retroperitoneal mass (*horizontal arrow*) and pelvic mass (*oblique arrow*) and their relation to the aortic bifurcation; **b** Coronal view showing the retroperitoneal mass (*horizontal arrow*) and ovarian lesion (*vertical arrow*); Transverse views showing (*arrowed*) the retroperitoneal mass and associated hydronephrosis (**c**), the ovarian mass (**d**) and pelvic mass (**e**). Note the non-contrast scan gives little information on the related vascular anatomy. MRI should ideally be obtained

Tumor Registry, 72 patients with these rare tumours were identified over a 20-year period. Amongst these, they described 48 juvenile granulosa cell tumours, 14 Sertoli–Leydig tumours, five sclerosing stromal tumours, two sex cord tumors with annular tubules, two thecomas and one steroid cell tumor (Schneider et al. 2003). Median age at presentation varied from 7 years for juvenile granulosa cell tumours to almost 14 years for Sertoli–Leydig tumours and thecomas. Most tumours are hormonally active: endocrine symptoms were present in 61% of granulosa cell tumours (typically oestrogen-led pseudoprecocious puberty) and 45% of Sertoli–Leydig tumours (normally androgen-driven virilisation) (Schneider et al. 2003).

Endocrine symptoms and signs were more common in the rarer variants. Bilateral disease was unusual (2 of 48 granulosa cell tumours and 1 of 14 Sertoli–Leydig tumours) and most children presented

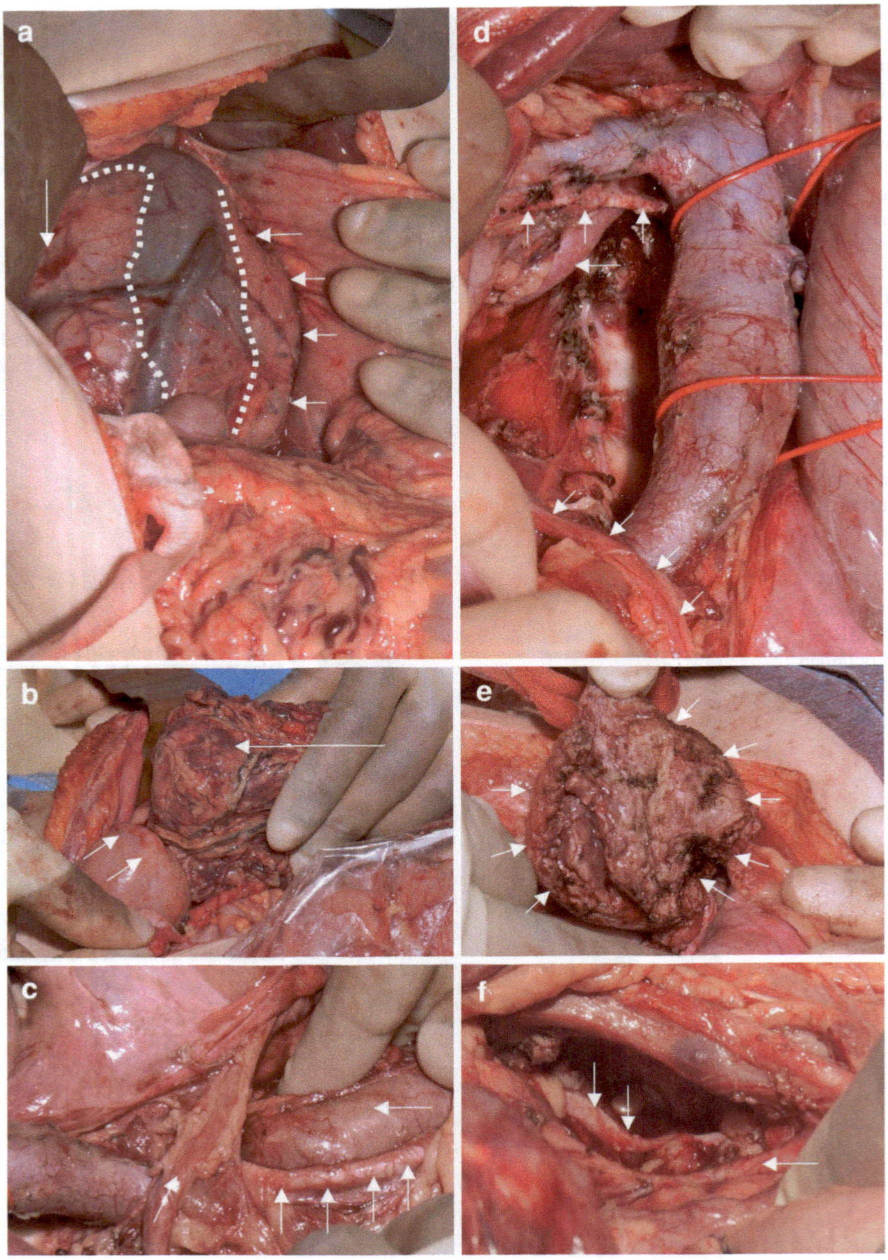

Fig. 4 Intraoperative photographs of the same patient as shown in Fig. 3, with ovarian dysgerminoma, hypercalcaemia and renal failure. These pictures illustrate the limitations of emergency non-contrast CT in identifying vascular anatomy and tissue planes. She was referred to the surgical oncology service after CT. However, MRI may have been a preferable modality in this instance. **a** The right retroperitoneal mass (*arrows*) with the renal veins and inferior vena cava (IVC: *dotted lines*) chronically effaced over the surface; **b** Omental covered right ovarian mass (*horizontal arrow*) extending to and filling the uterus (external margin demonstrated by *oblique arrows*); **c** Superior pole of pelvic mass (*horizontal arrow*) lying between right internal iliac (not seen) and external iliac (*vertical arrows*) arteries with adjacent right ureter (*oblique arrow*) crossing the ipsilateral common iliac vessels. **d** IVC, right renal vein and renal artery (*vertical arrows*), right kidney (*horizontal arrow*) and ipsilateral ureter (*oblique arrows*) after excision of the retroperitoneal mass. Pre-operative scans had not shown that the mass had displaced the arterial structures posteriorly whilst the venous ones were moved anteriorly; **e** tumour-involved uterus opened out along its right hand margin with the edges arrowed. This involvement was not predicted on the scans. The uterus was repaired and retained in a fertility-sparing approach; **f** Right obturator nerve (*vertical arrows*) and external iliac artery (*horizontal arrow*) seen after pelvic mass excision

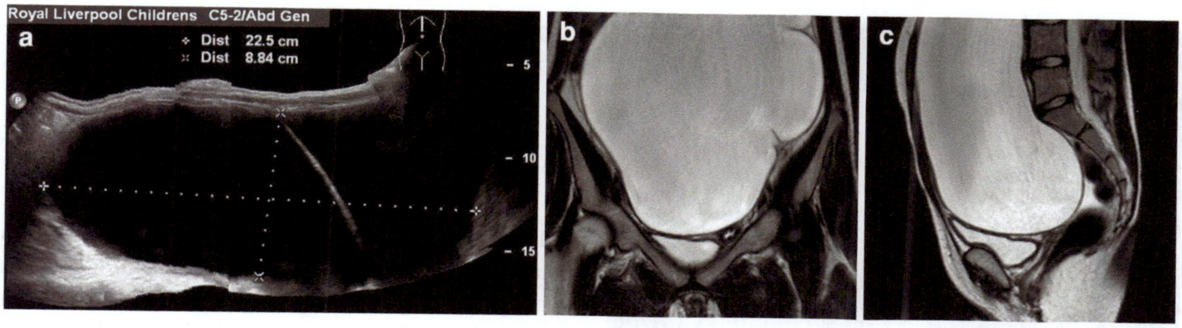

Fig. 5 Imaging of a 14-year-old girl with a short history of increasing abdominal distension and discomfort. **a** Panoramic ultrasound showing a large multicystic mass arising from the pelvis occupying most of the abdominopelvic cavity. She was immediately transferred to the MRI scanner but was unable to tolerate a complete examination. **b** Coronal and **c** sagittal T2-weighted MRI showing a massive, well- circumscribed, thin-walled pelvic cyst. This was excised without rupture of the cyst and confirmed to be a mature cystic teratoma

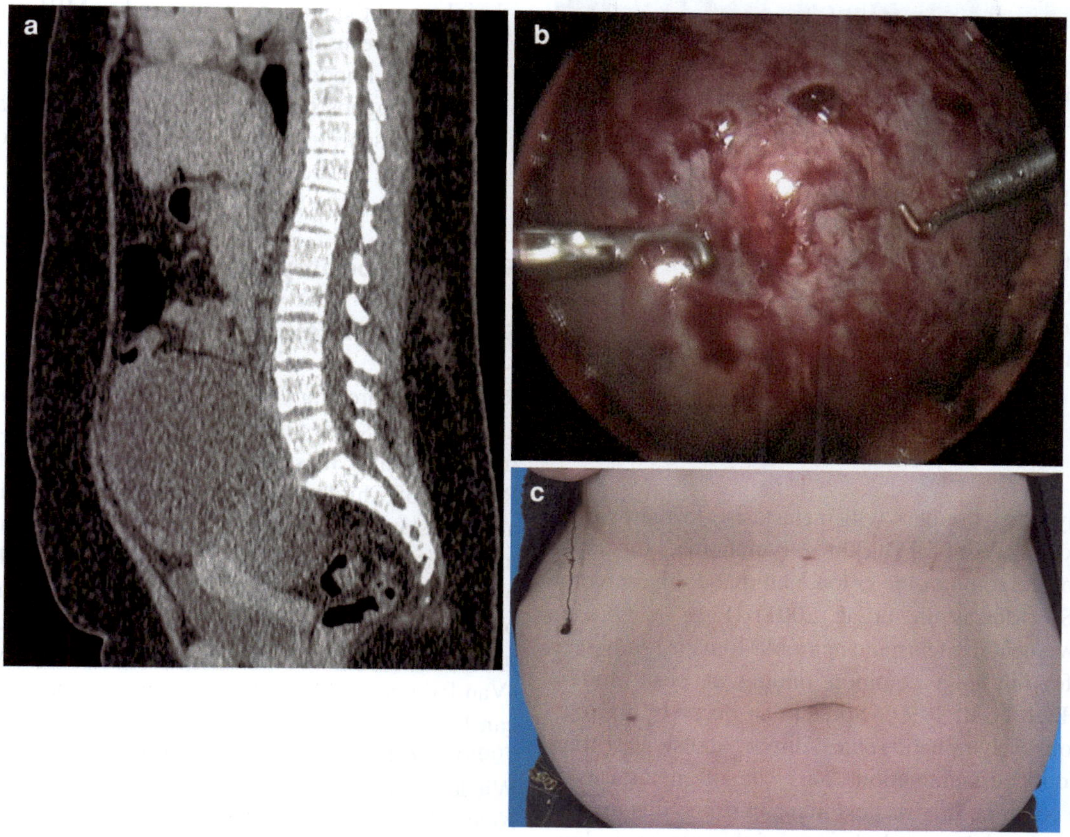

Fig. 6 Imaging and peri-operative pictures for a postpubertal patient with a torted right ovarian cyst: This patient had an emergency CT having presented with acute abdominal pain and normal tumour markers. She was then referred to the surgical oncology service. **a** Sagittal CT view of the pelvic mass (prior ultrasound confirmed a huge fluid filled cyst); **b** Laparoscopic view of the large torted ovarian cyst. Removal was accomplished endosurgically after careful cyst drainage via the umbilicus; **c** Post-operative view of the abdomen showing the recent port sites and umbilicus. Laparoscopic excision allowed early mobilisation and rapid hospital discharge in a patient where full laparotomy may have necessitated a large incision and longer in-patient stay. Histology showed no malignant features

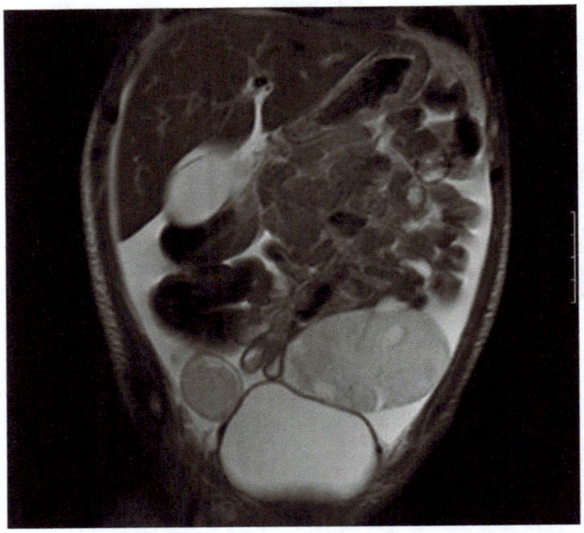

Fig. 7 Coronal T2W image shows bilateral pelvic masses, proven on biopsy to be metastases from a rhabdomyosaroma of the skull base

with Stage 1 disease (Schneider et al., 2003). However, late recurrence (~10 years later) has been reported (Schneider et al. 2003). Epithelial ovarian tumours are the most common type in adults, but account for less than 5% of malignant ovarian tumours in childhood (Ind and Shepherd 2003).

3.2 Secondary Tumours

Rarely other tumours will metastasise to the ovaries, including Wilms', Burkitt's lymphoma, mucinous adenocarcinoma of the colon, and rhabdomyosarcoma (RMS) (McCarville et al. 2001) (Fig. 7). Ovarian involvement in metastatic neuroblastoma is rarely seen in life, but is a common finding at post mortem (McHugh et al. 1999). Spread can occur by haematogenous or lymphatic routes, direct extension, or transcoelomic dissemination. This site of metastases is more common in girls post menarche, and this may be due to the rich vascularisation of the ovaries in hormonally active girls. However, secondary ovarian tumours can also occur in the pre-pubertal age group. It has been reported that secondary tumours are more likely to be bilateral than primary ovarian tumours (56 vs. 20%) (McCarville et al. 2001). Therefore the presence of bilateral ovarian tumours should raise suspicion of an occult primary tumour elsewhere. It should be noted that these rarer ovarian masses cannot be reliably distinguished from malignant GCTs by imaging.

4 Non-neoplastic Ovarian Lesions

Massive ovarian oedema (MOO) is a rare benign enlargement of the ovary, which typically occurs in post-pubertal girls and young women, but has been reported in infants (Moon et al. 2009). The underlying aetiology is not well understood. Patients may present with an abdominal mass and precocious puberty, although the endocrine disturbance can be variable. Ovarian torsion is a recognised complication. Multiple enlarged follicles may be seen in the periphery of the mass on ultrasound or MRI, and are thought to be useful diagnostically (Umesaki et al. 2000). It is important to consider MOO in the differential diagnosis of children with ovarian masses, as ovarian-sparing surgery and contralateral oophoropexy are the treatment of choice.

5 Rhabdomyosarcoma

5.1 Epidemiology

Rhabdomyosarcoma (RMS) is the 3rd commonest extra-cranial solid tumour in childhood, and arises from primitive mesenchyme. In the UK National Registry of Childhood Tumours (1991–2000), it had an age standardised annual rate of about four per million in girls with a peak incidence in the 1–4 year old age group (Stiller 2008). It is the most common paediatric tumour of the non-ovarian reproductive tract. Some 30% involve the genitourinary system (Van Rijn et al. 2008). They are mostly sporadic, but can be associated with Li Fraumeni (Sedlacek et al. 1998), Gorlin (Cajaiba et al. 2006) and Beckwith–Wiedemann syndrome (Cohen 2005) as well as Neurofibromatosis type 1 (Brems et al. 2009).

5.2 Pathology

There are five main pathological types: embryonal, botyroid, alveolar, undifferentiated and pleomorphic (the latter mostly occurring in adults) (Parham and

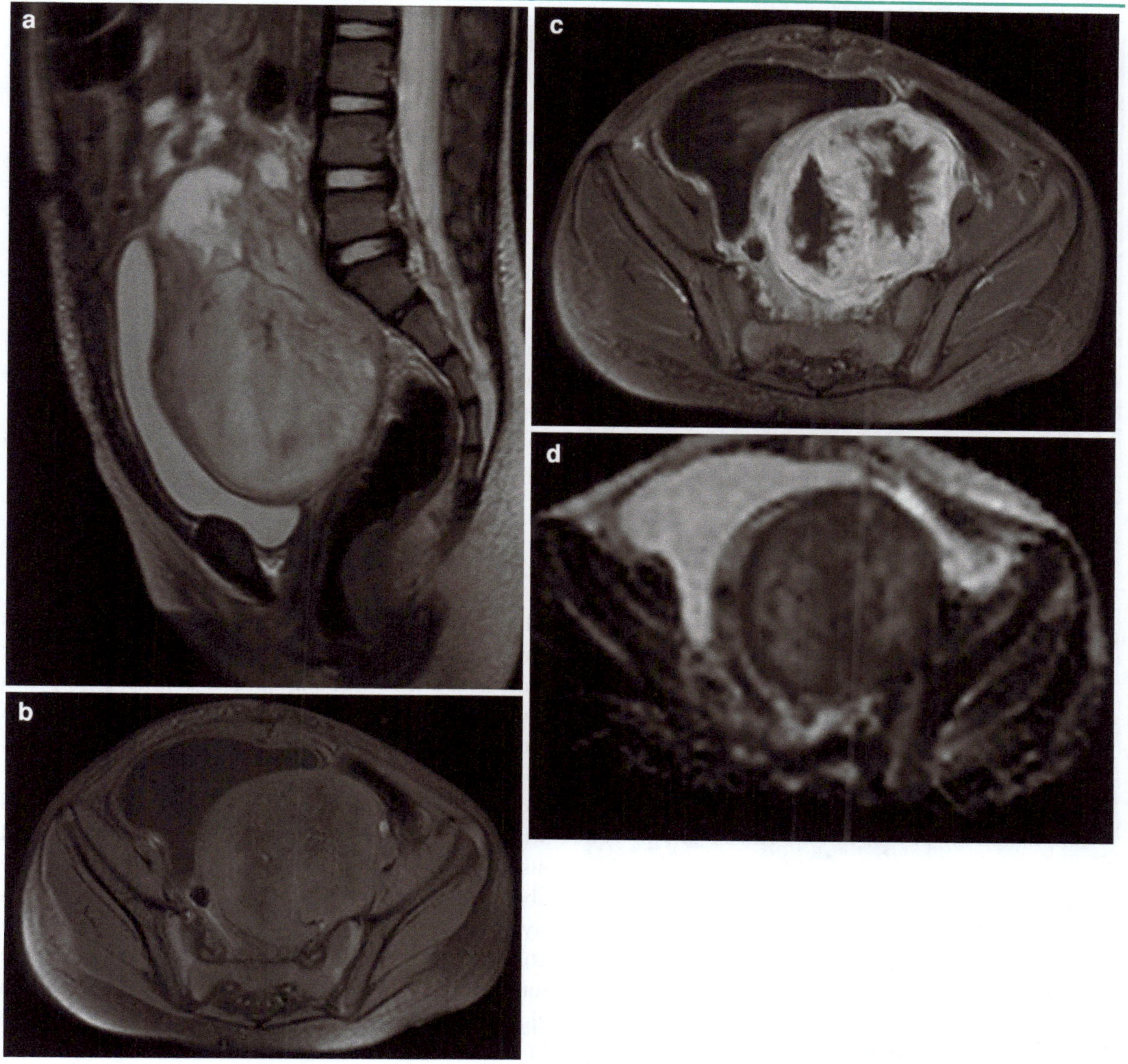

Fig. 8 Imaging of a 3-year-old girl with an embryonal rhabdomyosarcoma arising from the uterus or vagina. **a** Sagittal T2 weighted image shows the tumour is intermediate signal arising posterior to the bladder and anterior to the rectum, with clear planes between them; **b** Axial T1-weighted fat saturated image of the same patient. The mass is low/intermediate signal, and displaces the bladder laterally; **c** Axial T1-weighted image post-contrast at same level as B, showing marked contrast enhancement of the mass, with low signal centrally; **d** Axial apparent diffusion coefficient (ADC) map at same level as (**b**) and (**c**), showing heterogeneous but predominantly low signal, in keeping with a cellular (and thus likely malignant) tumour

Ellison 2006). Genetic changes associated with different histiotypes may influence tumour behaviour (Parham et al. 2007). The botyroid subtype rarely metastasises, is chemoresponsive and has the best prognosis. Embryonal RMS has intermediate prognosis, whilst alveolar and undifferentiated RMS have the worst prognosis. Female genital tract RMS is botyroid in 55% of patients and embryonal in 35% (Ind and Shepherd 2003). Vaginal or uterine RMS is more common in patients under 10 years of age, and cervical or vulval RMS occurs most commonly in adolescents (Ind and Shepherd 2003). Vaginal

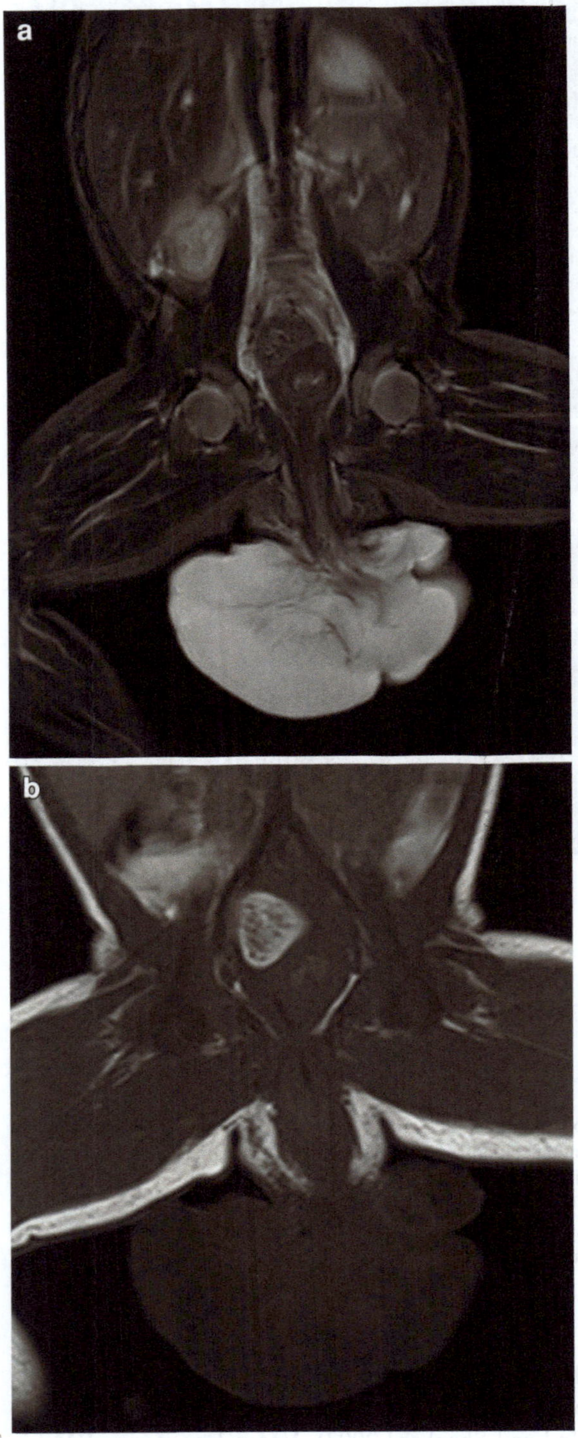

Fig. 9 Imaging of a 1 day old girl with an exophytic vaginal embryonal rhabdomyosarcoma. **a** Coronal STIR image which demonstrate homogenous high signal, with a few low signal septa. **b** Coronal T1-weighted image of same patient, at the same level. The tumour is low T1 signal

tumours are invariably the botyroid type of RMS. Lung and bone are the most common sites for distant metastatic spread which is present in 10–20% patients. A further 10% of patients with pelvic primaries have loco-regional lymph nodal disease spread (Ind and Shepherd 2003; Raney et al. 2001a, b).

5.3 Clinical Presentation

Patients usually present with non-specific symptoms due to the primary disease including palpable abdominopelvic masses, vaginal bleeding or discharge, difficulty micturating or a soft tissue mass extruding from the vagina (Ind and Shepherd 2003).

5.4 Imaging Investigations

Ultrasound is the first line of investigation for patients with genitourinary symptoms, or a suspected pelvic tumour. Patients should have a full bladder when possible to allow adequate ultrasound visualisation of the pelvic organs. RMS appears as a well-defined hypoechoic heterogeneous mass, and may have increased vascularity on Doppler imaging. Any child with a pelvic mass documented on ultrasound should also have further cross-sectional imaging. MRI of the abdomen and pelvis is the preferred imaging modality, avoiding radiation, and providing excellent tissue contrast (Van Rijn et al. 2008). RMS typically has intermediate signal on T1W, and intermediate/high signal on T2W sequences, and demonstrates variable but often marked contrast enhancement (Figs. 8, 9 and 7.21). Vascular invasion can be excluded by identifying a fat plane between the tumour and vessel (Van Rijn et al. 2008).

MRI is also useful for assessing bone marrow deposits, seen as areas of abnormal signal or enhancement, and thus may lead to suspicion of metastatic marrow disease (Van Rijn et al. 2008). CT, however, is routinely necessary for diagnosing or excluding lung metastases. Most international RMS-staging protocols also include routine bone scintigraphy (Van Rijn et al. 2008). Bony metastases appear as areas of increased uptake, and should be correlated with X-rays or MRI of any documented lesion. The role of PET/CT in the staging of RMS at diagnosis is currently uncertain but it may be useful (Völker et al. 2007).

Table 2 Intergroup Rhabdomyosarcoma Study (IRS) Group staging

Group	Characteristics
Group I	Localised disease, completely resected
	A. Confined to organ of origin
	B. Tumour infiltrating outside of organ (regional nodes not involved)
Group II	Localised or regional disease with total resection of gross tumour
	A. Primary tumour grossly resected, with microscopic residual disease
	B. Primary tumour and positive nodes completely resected
	C. Primary tumour and positive nodes resected, evidence of microscopic residual disease
Group III	Incomplete resection of tumour or biopsy with macroscopic residual tumour
	A. Localised or locally extensive tumour, gross residual disease after biopsy
	B. Localised or locally extensive tumour, gross residual disease after major resection
Group IV	Distant metastases at diagnosis

Table 3 TNM Staging system (modified for genitourinary rhabdomyosarcoma)

Stage	Characteristics	Nodes*	Metastases*
Stage I	Localised, non-bladder/GU sites	N0, N1 or NX	M0
Stage II	Localised, involving unfavourable sites, i.e. bladder/prostate, < 5 cm	N0, NX	M0
Stage III	Localised, involving unfavourable sites, or > 5 cm	N1	M0
Stage IV	All sites	N0, N1	M1

**Note*: N0 no clinical involvement of regional nodes, N1 clinical involvement of regional nodes, NX node status unknown; M0 no distant metastases, M1 distant metastases

5.5 Treatment and Prognosis

Staging of RMS is based on a combination of the TNM-staging system and surgical resection (Tables 2 and 3). This staging system is used with features of tumour histology and genetics to stratify patients into risk groups, give an indication of prognosis and determine the appropriate treatment regime. Local control may involve surgery and/or brachytherapy (e.g. for vaginal rhabdomyosarcoma) with chemotherapy for local and systemic control. The overall cure rate for patients is 70%. The 3 year failure-free survival in low risk groups is 88%, intermediate risk groups, 55–76%, and high risk with distant metastases <30% (Raney et al. 2001a, b). Favourable prognostic factors include: embryonal or botyroid subtypes; tumour < 5 cm; children aged < 10 years at diagnosis; favourable anatomical sites such as the vagina; grossly complete surgical resection; and no metastases at diagnosis. Tumour relapse presents with loco regional disease in 50% and with distant metastases in the remaining 50% (Pappo et al. 1999).

6 Other Lesions

In the past, children whose mothers were given diethylstilbestrol during pregnancy had a 1 in 1000 risk of developing cervico-vaginal clear cell carcinoma in adolescence (Ind and Shepherd 2003). However, it is now over 30 years since this drug was used in pregnancy, and it is unlikely that such tumours will be seen in paediatric practice today.

Squamous cell carcinoma of the cervix is a cancer normally seen in adulthood. Recent data indicate an increasing incidence in adolescents which may be due in part to changing patterns of sexual behaviour amongst teenagers (Yang et al. 2009). The impact of mass vaccination of girls against strains of human papilloma virus on the prevalence of squamous cell carcinoma of the cervix remains to be seen. Patients typically present with inter-menstrual bleeding and are diagnosed by a cervical smear test. If the cancer is invasive then further imaging is required to assess metastases and determine the stage. Either MRI or CT scanning is used.

Benign lesions may occasionally feature in the list of differential diagnoses for suspected gynaecological neoplasia. There have been reports of children with appendicitis wrongly diagnosed with a pelvic malignancy (in particular ovarian tumours) (Baker et al. 2004). Both ultrasound and CT/MRI can fail to reliably distinguish inflammatory appendix masses from pelvic tumours. Thus, care should always be taken when communicating with parents in the context of a new mass lesion, particularly if there has been a recent febrile episode. Similarly, in younger girls and even in fetal patients, developmental lesions such as cystic duplications and lymphatic malformations should be considered in the preoperative differential diagnosis of presumed ovarian lesions (Konen et al. 2002; Meyberg-Solomayer et al. 2006).

References

Baker JL, Gull S, Jesudason EC et al (2004) Appendicitis masquerading as malignancy. Arch Dis Child 89:481–482

Billmire D, Vinocur C, Rescorla F et al (2004) Outcome and staging evaluation in malignant germ cell tumors of the ovary in children and adolescents: an intergroup study. J Pediatr Surg 39:424–429

Brems H, Beert E, de Ravel T et al (2009) Mechanisms in the pathogenesis of malignant tumours in neurofibromatosis type 1. Lancet Oncol 10:508–515

Brookfield KF, Cheung MC, Koniaris LG et al (2009) A population-based analysis of 1037 malignant ovarian tumors in the pediatric population. J Surg Res 156:45–49

Cajaiba MM, Bale AE, Alvarez-Franco M et al (2006) Rhabdomyosarcoma, Wilms tumor, and deletion of the patched gene in Gorlin syndrome. Nat Clin Pract Oncol 3:575–580

Cass DL, Hawkins E, Brandt ML et al (2001) Surgery for ovarian masses in infants, children, and adolescents: 102 consecutive patients treated in a 15-year period. J Pediatr Surg 36:693–699

Choi HJ, Moon MH, Kim SH (2008) Yolk sac tumor of the ovary: CT findings. Abdom Imaging 33:736–739

Cohen MM (2005) Beckwith-Wiedemann syndrome: Historical, clinicopathological, and etiopathogenetic perspectives. Pediatr Devel Pathol 8:287–304

De Backer A, Madern GC, Oosterhuis JW et al (2006) Ovarian germ cell tumors in children: a clinical study of 66 patients. Pediatr Blood Cancer 46:459–464

de Silva KS, Kanumakala S, Grover SR et al (2004) Ovarian lesions in children and adolescents—an 11-year review. J Pediatr Endocrinol Metab 17:951–957

Evans KN, Taylor H, Zehnder D et al (2004) Increased expression of 25-hydroxyvitamin D-1alpha-hydroxylase in dysgerminomas: a novel form of humoral hypercalcemia of malignancy. Am J Pathol 165:807–813

Harms D, Zahn S, Göbel U et al (2006) Pathology and molecular biology of teratomas in childhood and adolescence. Klin Padiatr 218:296–302

Ind T, Shepherd J (2003) Pelvic tumours in adolescence. Best Pract Res Clin Obstet Gynaecol 17:149–168

Jawaid W, Solari V, Howell L, Jesudason EC. Excision of extensive metastatic dysgerminoma to control refractory hypercalcaemia in a child at high risk for tumour-lysis syndrome. J Pediatr Surg (in press)

Karpelowsky JS, Hei ER, Matthews K (2009) Laparoscopic resection of benign ovarian tumours in children with gonadal preservation. Pediatr Surg Int 25:251–254

Konen O, Rathaus V, Dlugy E et al (2002) Childhood abdominal cystic lymphangioma. Pediatr Radiol 32:88–94

Matthew R, Christopher O, Philippa S (2006) Severe malignancy-associated hypercalcemia in dysgerminoma. Pediatr Blood Cancer 47:621–623

McCarville M, Hill D, Miller B et al (2001) Secondary ovarian neoplasms in children: imaging features with histopathologic correlation. Pediatr Radiol 31:358–364

McHugh K, Pritchard J, Dicks-Mireaux C (1999) Bilateral ovarian involvement at presentation in metastatic (stage 4) neuroblastoma. Pediatr Radiol 29:741

Meyberg-Solomayer GC, Buchenau W, Solomayer EF et al (2006) Cystic colon duplication as differential diagnosis to ovarian cyst. Fetal Diagn Ther 21:224–227

Moon RJ, Mears A, Kitteringham LJ et al (2009) Massive ovarian oedema: an unusual abdominal mass in infancy. Pediatr Blood Cancer 53:217–219

Murphy J, Tawfeeq M, Chang B, Nadel H (2008) Early experience with PET/CT scan in the evaluation of pediatric abdominal neoplasms. J Pediatr Surg 43:2186–2192

Nelken RP, Nieburg PI, Bergstrom WH et al (1978) Dysgerminoma presenting as a calcified abdominal mass with hypercalcemia. Pediatrics 61:791–793

Okoye BO, Harmston C, Buick RG (2001) Dysgerminoma associated with hypercalcemia: a case report. J Pediatr Surg 36:E10

Outwater EK, Siegelman ES, Hunt JL (2001) Ovarian teratomas: tumor types and imaging characteristics. Radiographics 21:475–490

Panteli C, Curry J, Kiely E et al (2009) Ovarian germ cell tumours: a 17-year study in a single unit. Eur J Pediatr Surg 19:96–100

Pappo AS, Anderson JR, Crist WM et al (1999) Survival after relapse in children and adolescents with rhabdomyosarcoma: a report from the Intergroup Rhabdomyosarcoma Study Group. J Clin Oncol 17:3487–3493

Parham DM, Ellison DA (2006) Rhabdomyosarcomas in adults and children: an update. Arch Pathol Lab Med 130:1454–1465

Parham DM, Qualman SJ, Teot L et al (2007) Correlation between histology and PAX/FKHR fusion status in alveolar rhabdomyosarcoma: a report from the Children's Oncology Group. Am J Surg Pathol 31:895–901

Raney RB, Anderson JR, Barr FG et al (2001a) Rhabdomyosarcoma and undifferentiated sarcoma in the first two decades of life: a selective review of intergroup rhabdomyosarcoma study group experience and rationale for Intergroup Rhabdomyosarcoma Study V. J Pediatr Hematol Oncol 23:215–220

Raney RB, Maurer HM, Anderson JR et al (2001b) The inter-group rhabdomyosarcoma study group (IRSG): major lessons from the IRS-I through IRS-IV studies as background for the current IRS-V treatment protocols. Sarcoma 5:9–15

Ratani RS, Cohen HL, Fiore E (2004) Pediatric gynecologic ultrasound. Ultrasound Q 20:127–139

Rescorla F (2008) Malignant germ cell tumors. In: Carachi R, Grosfeld J, Azmy A (eds) The surgery of childhood tumors. Springer-Verlag, Berlin, pp 261–271

Riccabona M (2008) Potential of MR-imaging in the paediatric abdomen. Eur J Radiol 68:235–244

Saba L, Guerriero S, Sulcis R, Virgilio B, Melis G, Mallarini G (2009) Mature and immature ovarian teratomas: CT, US and MR imaging characteristics. Eur J Radiol 72:454–463

Schneider DT, Janig U, Calaminus G et al (2003) Ovarian sex cord-stromal tumors—a clinicopathological study of 72 cases from the Kiel Pediatric Tumor Registry. Virchows Arch 443:549–560

Schultz KA, Sencer SF, Messinger Y et al (2005) Pediatric ovarian tumors: a review of 67 cases. Pediatr Blood Cancer 44:167–173

Sedlacek Z, Kodet R, Kriz V et al (1998) Two Li-Fraumeni syndrome families with novel germline p53 mutations: loss of the wild-type p53 allele in only 50% of tumours. Br J Cancer 77:1034–1039

Stiller C (2008) Epidemiology of childhood tumors. In: Carachi R, Grosfeld J, Azmy A (eds) The surgery of childhood tumors. Springer-Verlag, Berlin, pp 3–15

Talerman A (1985) Germ cell tumours. Ann Pathol 5:145–157

Umesaki N, Tanaka T, Miyama M et al (2000) Sonographic characteristics of massive ovarian edema. Ultrasound Obstet Gynecol 16:479–481

Van Rijn RR, Wilde JCH, Bras J, Oldenburger F, McHugh K et al (2008) Imaging findings in noncraniofacial childhood rhabdomyosarcoma. Pediatr Radiol 38:617–634

Vijayaraghavan SB (2004) Sonographic whirlpool sign in ovarian torsion. J Ultrasound Med 23:1643–1649

Völker T, Denecke T, Steffen I et al (2007) Positron emission tomography for staging of pediatric sarcoma patients: results of a prospective multicenter trial. J Clin Oncol 25:5435–5441

West J, Viswanathan S, Yabuuchi A et al (2009) A role for Lin28 in primordial germ-cell development and germ-cell malignancy. Nature 460(7257):909–913

Yang L, Fujimoto J, Qiu D et al (2009) Trends in cancer mortality in Japanese adolescents and young adults aged 15–29 years, 1970–2006. Ann Oncol 20:758–766

Breast Disorders

Gurdeep S. Mann, Asha Shivaram, and Andrew Healey

Contents

1	**Introduction**	226
2	**Embryology**	226
3	**Normal Postnatal Breast Development**	226
4	**Normal Anatomy**	227
5	**Imaging Techniques**	228
5.1	Ultrasound	228
5.2	Cross-Sectional Modalities	228
5.3	Mammography	228
6	**Normal Imaging Appearances**	229
7	**Clinical Evaluation of the Breast**	230
8	**Congenital Disorders**	230
8.1	Supernumerary Breast Tissue	230
9	**Developmental Disorders**	231
9.1	Premature Thelarche	231
10	**Breast Asymmetry**	231
10.1	Absent and Underdeveloped Breast Tissue	231
10.2	Breast Asymmetry in Chest Wall Deformities & Scoliosis	232
11	**Symmetrical Disorders of Breast Size**	233
11.1	Macromastia	233
11.2	Virginal Hypertrophy	233
11.3	Bilateral Small Breasts	233
12	**Inflammatory Masses**	233
12.1	Breast Abscess	233
13	**Cystic Lesions**	235
13.1	Breast Cyst	235
13.2	Retroareolar Cyst	235
13.3	Galactocele	236
13.4	Mammary Duct Ectasia	236
13.5	Fibrocystic Disease	236
13.6	Haematoma	237
14	**Vascular Anomalies**	237
14.1	Lymphangioma	237
14.2	Haemangioma	238
15	**Solid Breast Masses**	238
15.1	Management of Solid Breast Masses	238
15.2	Benign Neoplastic Lesions	239
15.3	Malignant Masses	241
16	**Nipple Discharge**	243
17	**References**	243

Abstract

Breast pathology in children and adolescents is rare. Nevertheless, it is useful for medical practitioners involved in the care of this age group to have practical knowledge of physiological breast development, its normal variation, and the different types of breast lesion encountered in clinical practice. This chapter focuses on the imaging of breast development and specific disorders of the breast encountered in the paediatric and adolescent population.

Abbreviations

FSH	Follicular stimulating hormone
LH	Luteinizing hormone
IMA	Internal mammary artery
LTA	Lateral thoracic artery

G. S. Mann (✉), and A. Healey
Department of Paediatric Radiology, Alder Hey Children's Hospital NHS Foundation Trust, Liverpool, UK
e-mail: gurdeep.mann@alderhey.nhs.uk

A. Shivaram
Department of Radiology, Royal Liverpool and Broadgreen University Hospitals NHS Trust, Liverpool, UK

G. Mann et al. (eds.), *Imaging of Gynecological Disorders in Infants and Children*, Medical Radiology. Diagnostic Imaging, DOI: 10.1007/174_2010_125,

MHz	Megahertz
US	Ultrasound
CT	Computed tomography
PET	Positron emission tomography
MRI	Magnetic resonance imaging
IPT	Isolated premature thelarche
CSF	Cerebrospinal fluid
STIR	Short tau inversion recovery
MRA	Magnetic resonance angiography
MRV	Magnetic resonance venography
CI	Confidence Interval
RMS	Rhabdomyosarcoma

1 Introduction

Breast pathology in children and adolescents is rare. Nevertheless, it is useful for medical practitioners involved in the care of this age group to have practical knowledge of physiological breast development, its normal variation, and the different types of breast lesion encountered in clinical practice.

This chapter focuses on the imaging of breast development and specific disorders of the breast encountered in the paediatric and adolescent population.

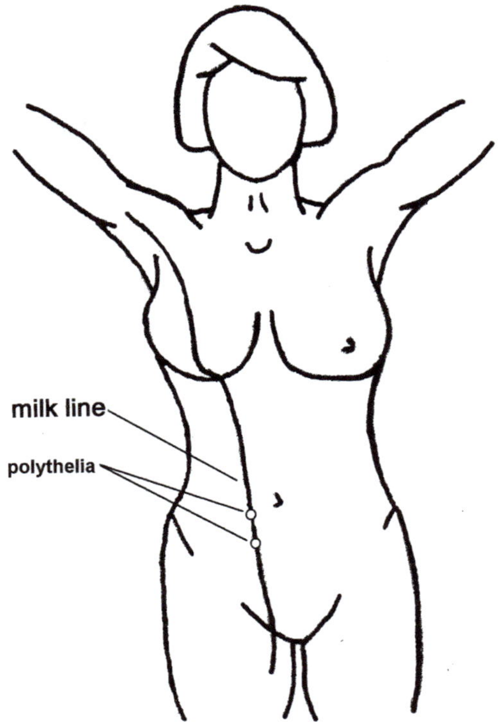

Fig. 1 The 'milk lines' are paired lines found in both sexes and correspond to the embryologic mammary ridges, formed by thickening of the ventral fetal epidermis. They extend from the upper limbs to the lower limbs. Accessory breast tissue may develop along the milk lines

2 Embryology

Mammary gland development begins in the fetus and is only complete in the postpartum adult female. During the fifth fetal week, paired ectodermal mammary ridges develop on the ventral surface of the embryo. These are also referred to as the milk lines (Fig. 1) that extend convexly from the axillae to the medial groins. By the tenth fetal week, the mammary ridges involute, leaving small bilateral pectoral ridges referred to as the primary mammary buds. Primary mammary buds are the precursors of the lactiferous ducts and mammary glands and lie at the level of the fourth intercostal spaces. These proliferate by successive elongation and branching. By the twelfth week, secondary mammary buds develop and are the precursors of the adult breast lobules.

In the fifth fetal month, each mammary bud develops around 15–20 solid cord-like primary lactiferous ducts. The areola derived from ectoderm also develops at this time. The pectoral mesenchyme differentiates into supporting fibrous and adipose tissue. By the 8 month, the lactiferous ducts canalise draining into the retroareolar ampullae. Simultaneously, a small depressed pit in the overlying skin develops eventually giving rise to the nipple which appears shortly after birth.

3 Normal Postnatal Breast Development

The breasts in pre-pubertal children are composed of epithelial-lined ducts. In the term neonatal breast, these ducts may enlarge subject to transient hormonal influences, principally maternal oestrogens and neonatal prolactin secretion (Mckiernan and Hull 1981). Palpable bilateral subaroelar nodules are not an uncommon finding and can persist for the first 6–12 months of life (Garcia et al. 2000). Thereafter,

Table 1 Tanner Breast staging (adapted from Marshall and Tanner 1969 with Permission from BMJ publishing group Ltd)

Breast stage	Age (years)		Clinical findings
1	<10	Prepubertal preadolescent	Elevation of the breast papillae only
2	10–11.5	Visible breast bud	Elevation of the breast bud and papillae to form a small mound
3	11.5–13		Further enlargement of the breast and areola. The areola darkens and the Montgomery's tubercles appear.
4	13–15		Elevation of areola and papilla to form a secondary mound
5	>15	Mature stage	Areolar recession results in projection of the nipple only

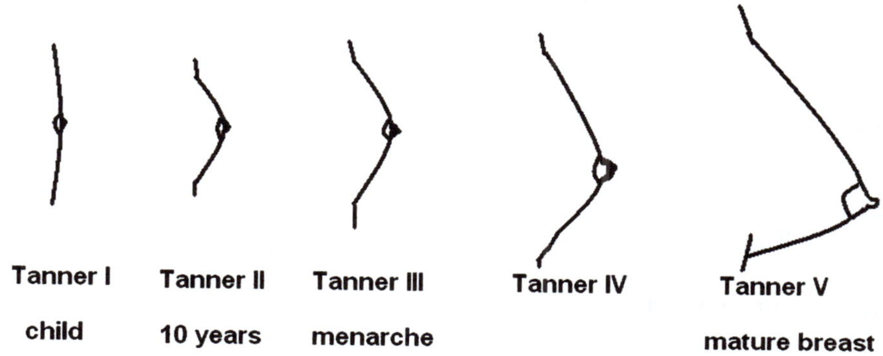

Fig. 2 The Tanner stages of breast development during puberty (adapted from Marshall and Tanner 1969 with Permission from BMJ publishing group Ltd)

the breasts remain relatively quiescent until the onset of thelarche-pubertal breast development that is normally seen between the ages of 8–13 years. Thelarche is also referred to Tanner stage 2 (see Table 1) breast development, heralding the development of a 'breast bud' when breast stroma and glandular tissue become apparent and grow in proportion to the child but no lobular development is present.

Rapid growth of the breasts occurs following the onset of thelarche. Circulating oestrogens initiate stromal and ductal tissue growth and promote adipose tissue deposition. Ductal growth is mediated by oestrogens, prolactin and growth hormone but is independent of progesterone. Progesterones enable lobular growth and alveolar budding. The pubertal development of the female breast, referred to as the Tanner staging, is summarised in table (Fig. 2).

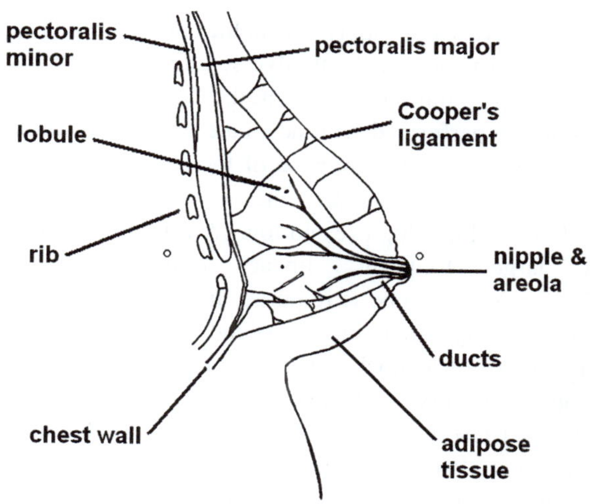

Fig. 3 Line diagram: Normal breast anatomy. Mid sagittal section of the developed female breast

4 Normal Anatomy

The breast is a modified sweat gland and principally comprises of skin, subcutaneous and mammary tissue. The mammary tissue is composed of 15–20 lobules arranged radially about the nipple. The lobules comprise of parenchyma, fibroglandular stroma and lactiferous ducts. The skin envelops and supports the breast. Fibrous suspensory ligaments of Astley Cooper anchor the breast to the pectoral fascia (Fig. 3). The areola contains epidermal glands including the sebaceous Montgomery gland.

The principle muscles supporting muscles are the pectoralis major, pectoralis minor, serratus anterior, latissimus dorsi and aponeuroses of the rectus abdominus and external oblique muscles.

The arterial blood supply of the breast is principally derived from the internal mammary artery (IMA) and lateral thoracic arteries (LTA). Minor contributions are made by the intercostal, thoracoacromial, thoracodorsal and subscapular arteries. The central and medial breast is supplied by perforating branches of the IMA and the upper outer quadrant by the LTA. Venous drainage of the breast follows that of the chest wall and includes the tributaries of the internal thoracic, axillary and intercostal veins. The lymphatic drainage of the breast follows the venous drainage.

5 Imaging Techniques

5.1 Ultrasound

Ultrasonography (US) is the imaging modality of choice in evaluating breast disorders in children. US is non-invasive, widely available and acceptable, cost-effective and without adverse effect. No specific patient preparation is required. The examination should be performed with adequate prior explanation as to the nature and purpose of the test and with an appropriate chaperone present.

US enables high-resolution, real-time imaging. A large footprint, linear array broadband (7–17.5 MHz) probe is required. In smaller children, and for very small or superficial lesions, we also favour use of a 'hockey stick', compact linear array probe (typically 15 MHz). The latter affords high temporal resolution and submillimetre lateral spatial resolution. Panoramic imaging is useful in demonstrating the relationship of larger lesions to adjacent structures. Scanning may be performed in either the supine or erect positions with arm of the side being examined elevated behind or above the patients head. The supine position is preferred. A wedge may be placed under the scapula of the side being examined. Each breast is scanned systematically and radially in clockwise and anticlockwise directions relative to the nipple. The axillae, adjacent chest wall and supraclavicular fossae should also be evaluated for satellite lesions or adenopathy using standard transverse and longitudinal imaging planes. Both sides are assessed and if necessary comparative dual screen images obtained to compare the contralateral breast. Mobile lesions may require to be held in a fixed position to enable full evaluation.

Steerable pulsed Doppler, colour Doppler and colour power Doppler are useful to characterise lesional flow and to differentiate between solid and cyst. US guidance is used in directing targeted biopsies of solid masses and fine needle aspiration of cysts. Image-guided procedures are preferable to surgery in most cases but both may result in a poor cosmetic outcome due to resulting breast deformity (Greydanus et al. 1989).

5.2 Cross-Sectional Modalities

Cross-sectional imaging is useful in tumour staging and in particular when evaluating suspected chest wall involvement from tumours and vascular malformations. MRI is preferable; unlike adult practice, a dedicated breast coil is rarely required. PET-CT or CT may have a role in specific cases.

5.3 Mammography

Mammography is relatively contraindicated in paediatric practice. Avoidance of exposure to diagnostic radiation is important as developing glandular breast tissue is radiosensitive increasing the risk of malignancy in later life (Feig 1984). Poor image quality from dense fibroglandular mammary tissue makes mammography unsuitable for use in children and adolescents (Furnival et al. 1983). Mammography is not routinely recommended in women under 35 years of age as evidenced by retrospective observational studies which have shown mammography does not influence clinical management in this age group (Brand et al. 1993; Hindle et al.1999). Mammography is reserved for selected cases to detect microcalcifications and to evaluate discrete suspicious masses (Chung et al. 2009).

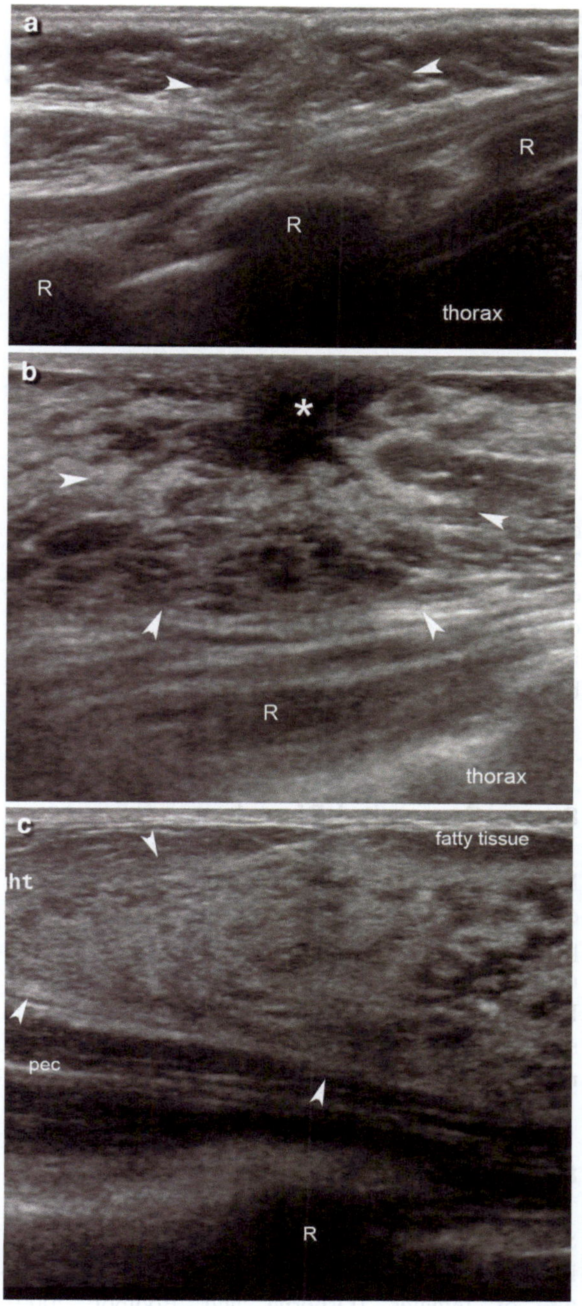

Fig. 4 Breast development. **a** Tanner stage 1. Transverse US in a two-year-old girl reveals a small slightly ill-defined subaroelar breast bud (between *arrowheads*). *R*, rib. **b** Tanner stage 3 in an 11-year-old girl showing a central hypoechoic focus (*) and echogenic breast tissue (between arrowheads). **c** Tanner stage 5 in a 15-year-old girl showing mature heterogeneous fibroglandular tissue (between *arrowheads*) and loss of the central hypoechoic area. *Pect*, pectoral muscle

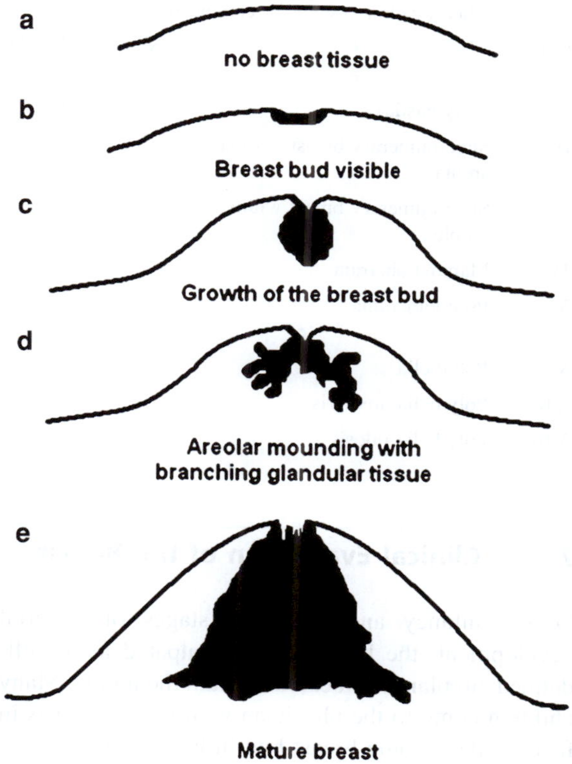

Fig. 5 Schematic representation of breast development as depicted by ultrasound (adapted from Bruni et al. 1990). (*Stage A*) absent breast bud, (*Stage B*) appearance of the glandular bud, (*Stage C*) growth of the breast bud, (*Stage D*) branching of the glandular bud (*Stage E*) mature glandular tissue demonstrating triangular morphology

6 Normal Imaging Appearances

The breast bud undergoes sequential development (Table 1) that can be correlated with US imaging appearances (Figs. 4 and 5). Prior to thelarche (Tanner breast stage 1), US of the immature breast reveals a small ill defined, heterogeneous retroareolar breast bud, comprising of echogenic fat and connective tissue. By Tanner stage 3, breast US typically reveals a more prominent breast bud with a central hypoechoic focus compared to the surrounding fat and connective tissue (Garcia et al. 2000). By Tanner stage 5, the mature adolescent breast comprises of dense, echogenic fibroglandular tissue surrounded by a thin layer of hypoechoic subcutaneous fat. The central hypoechoic focus is no longer present.

Table 2 Classification system for ectopic supernumerary breast tissue after Kajava (1915)

Class		Nipple	Areola	Mammary tissue	
I	(polymastia)	+	+	+	Complete mammary gland
II	Supernumerary breast without areola	+		+	Nipple and glandular tissue but no areola
III	Supernumerary breast without nipple		+	+	Areola and glandular tissue but absent nipple
IV	Mamma aberrata			+	Glandular tissue only
V	Pseudomamma	+	+		Nipple and areola. Glandular tissue replaced by fat
VI	Polythelia	+			Nipple only
VII	Polythelia areolaris		+		Areola only
VIII	Polythelia pilosis				Hairy patch only

7 Clinical Evaluation of the Breast

During infancy and the early stages of pubertal development, the breast can be palpated as a well-defined circular disc located beneath the nipple. Many children come to the physician with a lump that is in fact the developing breast bud in its entirety.

As the breast develops through puberty, the base of the disc broadens until the mature breast extends from 1 cm from the midline to the anterior line of the axilla, a distance of approximately 14 cm. Underdevelopment of the breast base results in tuberous breasts. The nipple and areolar are enlarged and may contain all the glandular tissue of the breast. This developmental abnormality may occur more frequently in girls undergoing pubertal induction using exogenous oestrogen. The clinical definition of the disc depends on the amount of fat both subcutaneously and infiltrated within the breast tissue. Accumulation of fat occurs during the later stages of development.

Three techniques of breast examination are used commonly in clinical practice, all of which should result in systematic palpation of all breast tissue in a consistent manner. The breast can be palpated in a radial manner moving the distal ends of the 2nd/3rd and 4th fingers (distal to the second interphalangeal joints) from the outer circumference of the breast towards the nipple, following a pattern similar to the spokes of a wheel. Circular palpation is preferred by others, palpating the breast tissue in small concentric circles or a spiral pattern inwards. Linear palpation in either a vertical or a horizontal plane is also effective. The key is that the whole of the breast tissue is covered including behind the nipple and the axillary tail of the breast. Normal glandular breast tissue has an irregular, granular texture. Examination is completed by palpation of the supraclavicular, infraclavicular and axillary lymph nodes.

8 Congenital Disorders

Most congenital anomalies of the breast are usually clinically apparent. More often, these are due to the presence of supernumerary breast tissue rather than underdevelopment or absence of breast tissue. Imaging is rarely indicated but may be required in selected cases for pre-operative planning and patient reassurance.

8.1 Supernumerary Breast Tissue

Supernumerary breast tissue results from failure of involution of the milk line (Fig. 1) and occurs in 2–6% of females (Osborne and Boolbol 2009). Approximately two-thirds of affected patients have solitary accessory breast tissue. Most occur in the thoracic or abdominal portions of the milk line that extends from the axilla to the groin. The most widely used clinical classification system for supernumerary breast tissue in current practice was first published by Kajava 1915 and is summarised in Table 2 (Kajava 1915).

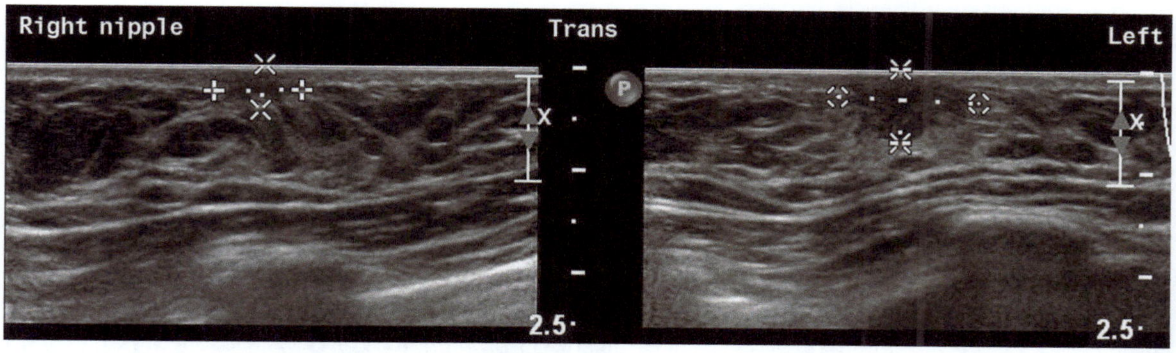

Fig. 6 Asymmetrical breast bud development. Dual screen comparison images showing asymmetrical breast bud development (between callipers) in a child with suspected left breast mass

8.1.1 Polythelia

Polythelia refers to the presence of a supernumerary nipple and is the most common form of accessory breast tissue. Most cases occur in the inframammary region and are usually sporadic, presenting as an isolated finding which is of only cosmetic concern (Fig. 1).

8.1.2 Polymastia

Polymastia results from accessory mammary glandular tissue and is the second most common form of supernumerary breast tissue (Class I and IV in Table 2). Type IV is the most common form. Typical locations include the axilla or inframammary region. Polymastia may not be noticed unless fullness is appreciated in response to the hormonal cycles of menstruation, pregnancy or lactation.

9 Developmental Disorders

9.1 Premature Thelarche

Breast development that occurs before the age of 8 years whether unilateral or bilateral is considered premature. Premature thelarche may be isolated and idiopathic, or result from premature activation of the hypothalamic–pituitary–gonadal axis (central or true precocious puberty), or more rarely from exposure to exogenous oestrogen or as a presenting feature of an oestrogen-secreting tumour. True isolated premature thelarche (IPT) compromises of breast development without progression through puberty. Bone age develops normally, no growth spurt is seen and the onset of menarche is normal.

Breast development in IPT is often atypical in appearance with relatively immature nipple development, which is frequently asymmetric and does not progress beyond Tanner stage 3 (Stanhope and Traggiai 2004) Girls with IPT have been shown to show no significant difference in pelvic US measurements when compared with age-matched controls (Haber et al. 1995); hence, pelvic US is useful in discriminating between IPT and precocious puberty.

10 Breast Asymmetry

Asymmetric breast development is common, especially in the early stages of pubertal development, and is generally of no clinical significance. Typical presentations include unilateral early development of a breast bud (Fig. 6). However, in a small minority of patients, asymmetrical breast development is the presenting feature of a breast abscesses, mass or cyst. US examination will exclude a mass and provide reassurance in most cases. Asymmetry may be seen in the rapid phases of breast growth (Tanner stages 2–4). If one breast attains Tanner stage 5, a delay of more than 3 years in attaining stage 5 in the contralateral breast indicates end-organ insensitivity and true hypoplasia.

10.1 Absent and Underdeveloped Breast Tissue

The breast fails to develop in girls with a congenital absence of glandular tissue or as a feature of delayed puberty. There are many causes of delayed puberty

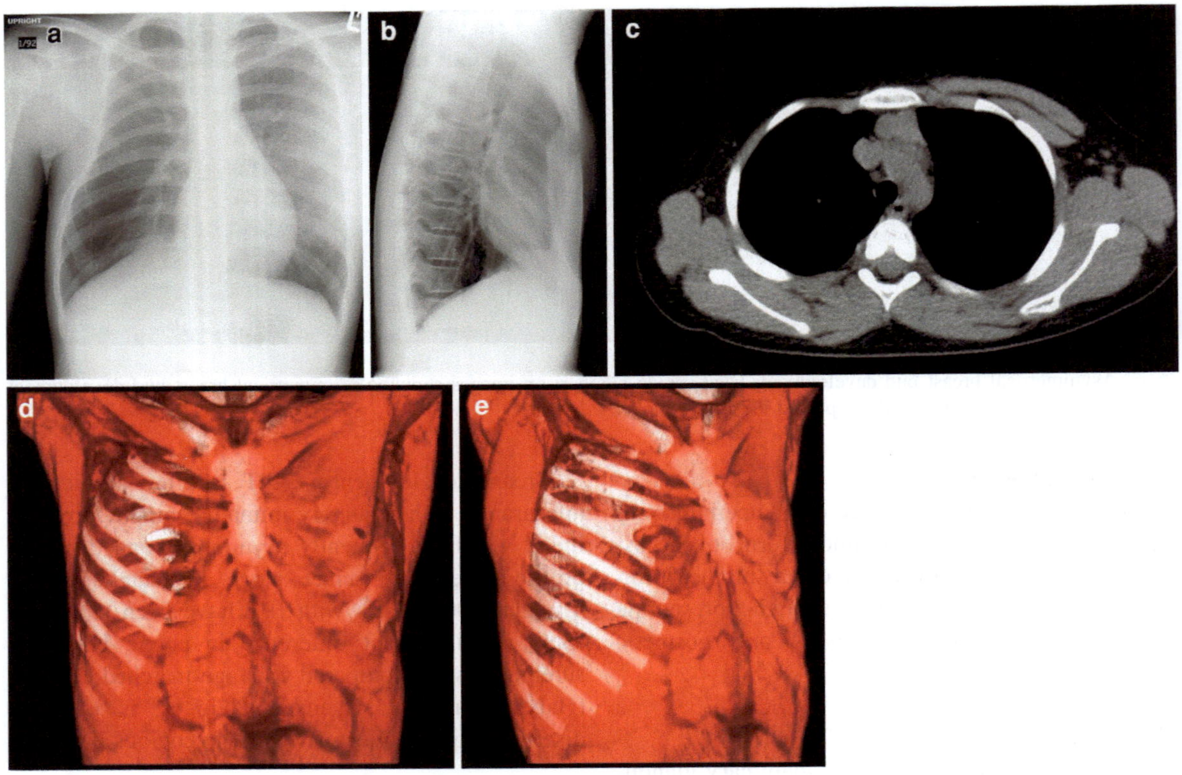

Fig. 7 **a–e** Poland's syndrome. **a** Frontal and **b** lateral chest radiographs showing deficient right pectoral soft tissues, congenital malformation of the right chest wall (hypoplastic right 3rd–6th ribs and extenuation of rib 7 with an accompanying sternal cleft. **c** Axial CT and **d–e** volume rendered imaging in another child with congenital absence of the right pectoral musculature. A bifid rib is also present

and these are discussed in detail in Delayed and Precocious Puberty.

Congenital amastia (absent mammary gland) refers to absence of glandular tissue, nipple and areola. Athelia refers to absence of the nipple and areola. Amastia is extremely rare and is generally unilateral. It occurs most commonly in association with Poland syndrome, a condition characterised by a variable expression of a wide spectrum of abnormalities. These include aplasia or hypoplasia of the nipple, areola or breast, absence of the ipsilateral sternocostal portion of the pectoralis major and minor muscles, syndactyly and accompanying rib and chest wall abnormalities (Fig. 7). Poland syndrome occurs in approximately 1 in 30,000 live births.

Bilateral breast hypoplasia can also be seen in congenital adrenal hyperplasia, Turner syndrome and delayed menarche (Delayed and Precocious Puberty). Oral oestrogen therapy may promote glandular development. Unilateral hypoplasia is not an uncommon finding on chest X-ray (Fig. 8).

10.2 Breast Asymmetry in Chest Wall Deformities & Scoliosis

Pectus deformities and scoliosis may give rise to apparent or true breast asymmetry (Denoel et al. 2009).

Pectus excavatum is the most common anterior chest wall deformity and is of unknown aetiology typically presenting in the first year of life. The deformity results from posterior depression of the sternum and costal cartilages and can be associated with scoliosis. Pectus carinatum results from anterior protrusion of the sternum and the costal cartilages and is of unknown aetiology. Around 50% of children with this deformity may develop abnormal anterior chest contour during the pubertal growth spurt (Shamberger 1996).

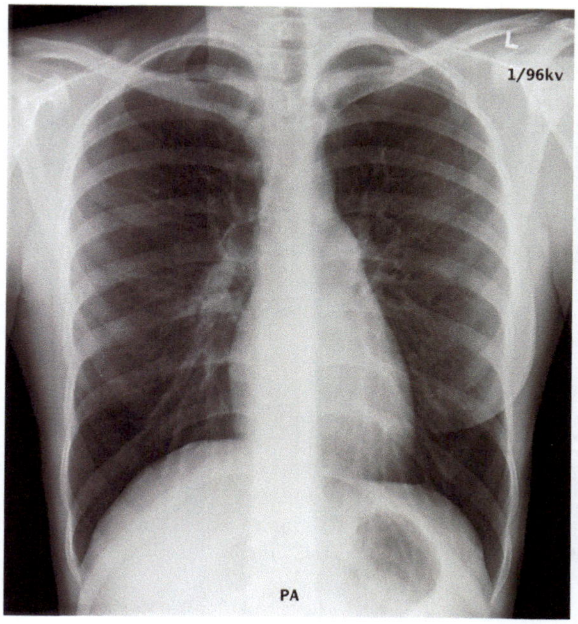

Fig. 8 Breast hypoplasia and aplasia. Frontal chest radiograph in an adolescent female with developmental hypoplasia of the right breast. The left breast was normal. True aplasia of the breast is exceedingly rare

Surgical reconstruction of the chest wall deformity maybe performed early to improve lung function and aesthetic appearances. Breast symmetry may not be achieved by chest wall reconstruction alone.

In all cases of breast asymmetry, reconstructive surgery is best performed when the contralateral breast has attained its mature configuration in order to obtain symmetry.

11 Symmetrical Disorders of Breast Size

11.1 Macromastia

The term macromastia is applied to excessively large breasts. The differential diagnosis includes juvenile or virginal hypertrophy, pregnancy, tumours and exposure to excessive levels of exogenous or endogenous oestrogen or progesterone. An association between macromastia and cannabis and D-penicillamine has also been reported (O'Hare and Frieden 2000).

11.2 Virginal Hypertrophy

Virginal hypertrophy, also referred to as juvenile hypertrophy, manifests as massive and rapid enlargement of one or both breasts disproportionate to overall body growth.

Serum oestradiol levels and the number of oestrogen receptors in the affected breast are reported to be normal (O'Hare and Frieden 2000), and excessive mammary growth results from stromal hypertrophy reflecting end-organ hypersensitivity. Virginal hypertrophy has been associate with Hashimoto's thyroiditis, rheumatoid arthritis and myasthenia gravis (Duflos et al. 2004) leading to speculation that this is an autoimmune phenomenon. Treatment with progesterone or anti-oestrogenic agents may helpful if breast growth is incomplete. When breast growth has stabilised, surgical options include reduction mammoplasty or reconstruction following mastectomy (O'Hare and Frieden 2000).

11.3 Bilateral Small Breasts

Bilateral breast hypoplasia, also termed hypomastia, is associated with connective tissue disorders, mitral valve prolapse, ovarian dysfunction, gonadal dysgenesis (Turner's Syndrome), congenital adrenal hyperplasia, hypothyroidism and androgen-secreting tumours (Greydanus et al. 1989). Treatment of the underlying condition generally results in improved breast development. Pubertal induction with oral or transdermal oestrogen can result in acceptable breast development in girls with Turner syndrome; however, surgical reconstruction of the areolar complex and augmentation mammoplasty may be necessary in some cases.

12 Inflammatory Masses

12.1 Breast Abscess

Inflammatory lesions of the breast are recognised in the neonate (Rudoy and Nelson 1975), children, and puerperal and non-pubertal adolescents (Hayes et al. 1991). A review of 751 biopsies taken from adolescents and young women presenting with a breast mass revealed around 15% were for non-lactational abscesses (Ferguson and Powell 1989). The aetiology remains

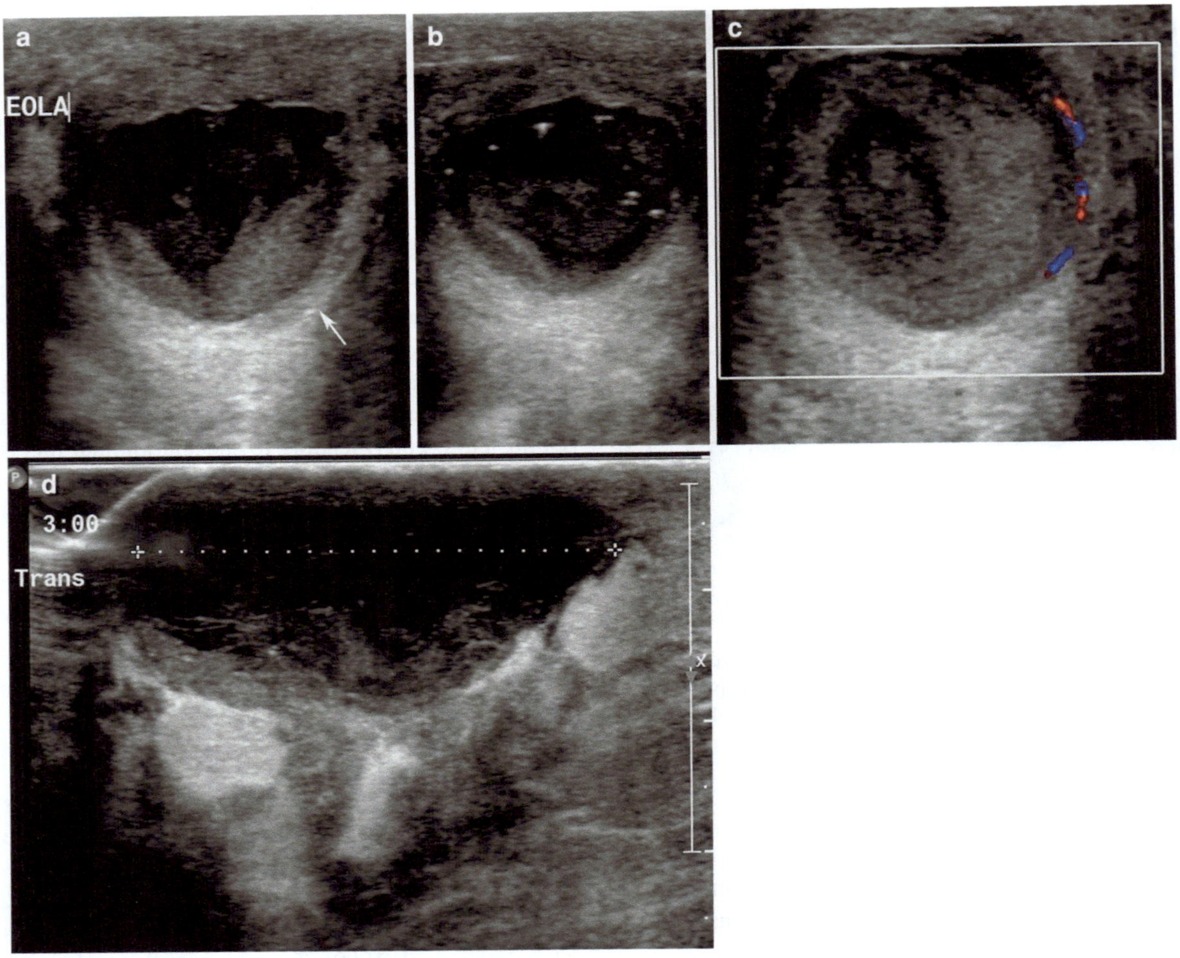

Fig. 9 Breast abscesses. **a-c** Imaging from a 16 year old girl, a Supine longitudinal view showing a complex mass with a thick wall and complex internal echoes. **b** Transverse erect view in the same patient showing a mobile fluid-debris and **c** supine longitudinal colour Doppler showing peripheral flow **d** 14 year old with a large breast abscess (between callipers)

unclear but mammary duct obstruction, infection of a retroareolar cyst, nipple abrasion and local cellulitis have all been implicated (West et al. 1995). The predominant causative organisms are staphylococci.

Clinical presentation includes focal breast tenderness, fluctuant mass, skin induration and occasionally systemic illness. US is helpful in identifying a potentially drainable abscess collection. US demonstrates the typical features of soft tissue abscesses found elsewhere in the body and include a hypoechoic cyst, internal echoes of varying complexity, posterior acoustic enhancement, fluid-debris level (Fig. 9a, b), thick wall and overlying soft tissue thickening. Colour Doppler demonstrates peripheral flow (Fig. 9c) with absent lesional flow and may show hyperaemic soft tissues (Siegel 2002).

Conservative treatment includes antibiotic therapy. Minimally invasive US-guided drainage is both therapeutic and diagnostic affording samples for microbial culture and sensitivities (Fig. 10). A 17 gauge or even 14 gauge needle is sometimes required as the infected material is often viscous. Surgical incision and drainage is preferably avoided in the developing breast bud but if required a small periareolar incision should be made and probing should be minimal to avoid later deformity (De Silva and Brandt 2006a). All parents of neonates with breast abscesses needing drainage should be warned

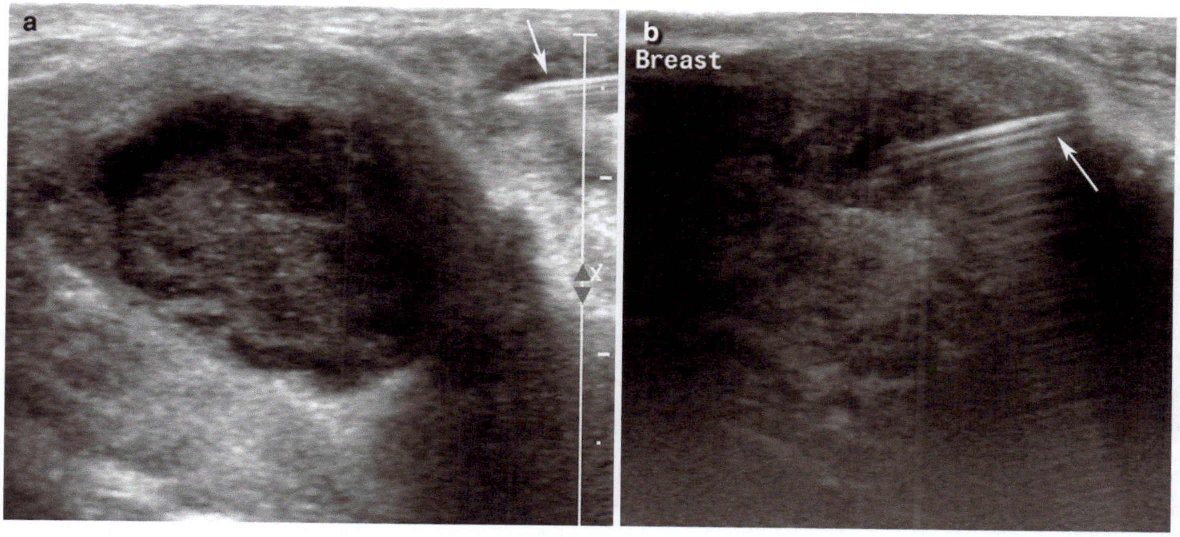

Fig. 10 Breast abscess drainage. Composite sonograms of a breast abscess (**a**) pre- (**b**) and post-US-guided drainage using an 18-G needle (*arrow*). This was performed under local anaesthetic. Prompt recovery was made following a course of oral antibiotics

that there is a possibility of asymmetrical breast development in the future.

13 Cystic Lesions

13.1 Breast Cyst

Breast cysts occur fairly commonly during adolescence. Spontaneous resolution over weeks to months is the norm; however, a small minority persist and needle aspiration may be necessary.

Breast cysts are typically solitary but can be multiple, around 1–5 cm in maximal diameter and located at or near the nipple-areola complex. Clinical presentations are fairly non-specific but include a palpable mass and local pain. Sonographically, simple cysts are anechoic, demonstrating sharply marginated borders with post-cystic acoustic enhancement (Fig. 11). Acoustic enhancement is the least consistent finding and may be absent if the cyst is small or close to the chest wall (Jackson 1990) or diminished due to attenuation from tissues anterior or posterior to the cyst. Colour Doppler flow is absent within the cyst. More complex cysts may contain septae or debris, and the differential for these appearances includes abscess and haematoma.

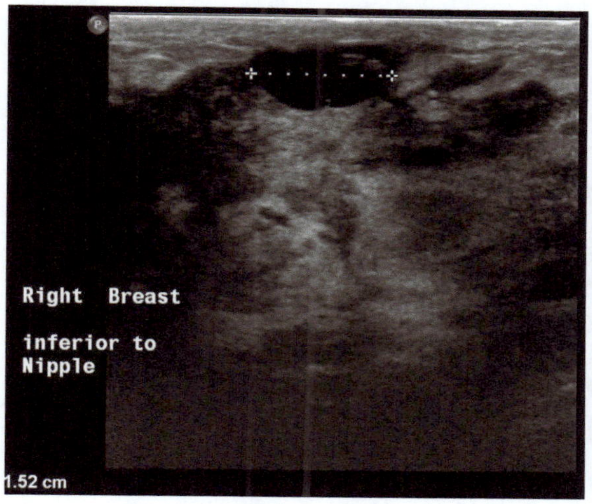

Fig. 11 Simple breast cyst. Transverse sonogram of the left breast in a 12-year-old girl presenting with a palpable, non-painful, breast lump. US reveals a thin-walled, anechoic structure with posterior acoustic enhancement and sharply marginated anterior and posterior borders. Colour Doppler interrogation revealed no internal flow

13.2 Retroareolar Cyst

Retroareolar (Montgomery) cysts (Fig. 12) arise at the edge of the areola. Approximately two-third of girls present with inflammatory mastalgia and the remainder with palpable painless nodules (Huneeus

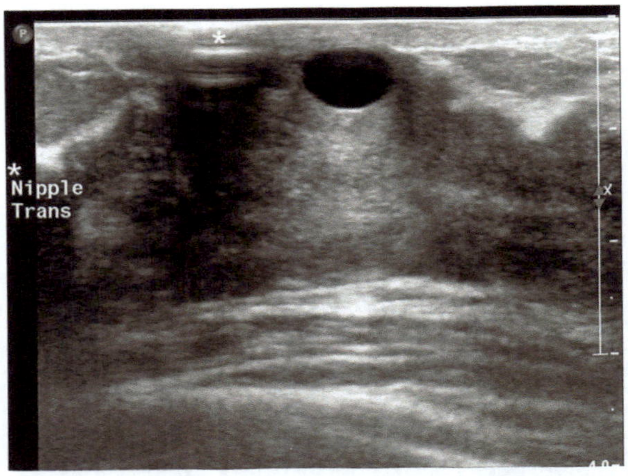

Fig. 12 Montgomery duct cyst. US showing a small well-circumscribed peri-areolar cyst with posterior acoustic enhancement

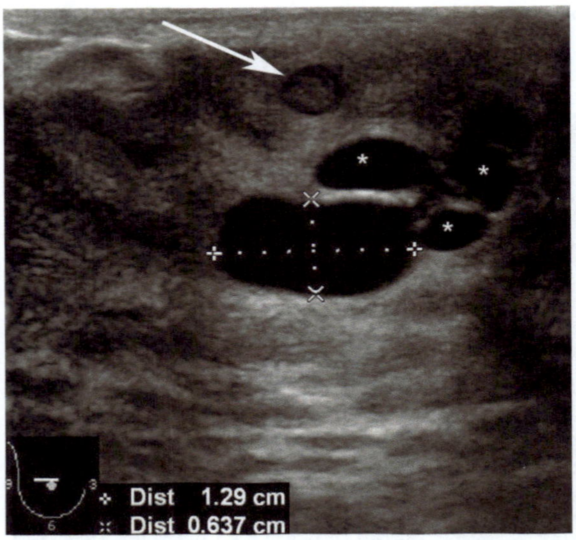

Fig. 13 Fibrocystic disease. Transverse sonogram of the right breast in a 15-year-old girl. Several tubular anechoic cystic spaces (between callipers and asterisks) of varying size are demonstrated, which show posterior acoustic enhancement, the largest cyst is between the callipers. Incidental note is of intramammary lymph node (arrow) that shows normal size and architecture

et al. 2003) that may be bilateral and do not usually exceed 2 cm in maximal diameter (Chung et al. 2009). Retroareolar cysts are usually self-limiting masses with conservative therapy including antibiotics and non-steroidal anti-inflammatory drugs (De Silva and Brandt 2006a).

13.3 Galactocele

Galactoceles usually occur in the lactating breast but can also be seen in infants or rarely in endocrinopathies affecting older children. Galactoceles may be unilateral, bilateral or multiple and present as painless enlarging masses. Cyst aspiration yields milky fluid with variable fat and water content (Welch et al. 2004). The imaging appearances reflect the cyst content; on US, water is anechoic and fat hyperechoic. A fluid–fluid level or complex cyst may be present.

13.4 Mammary Duct Ectasia

Mammary duct ectasia is rare in infants and children and results from periductal inflammation and fibrosis. The clinical presentation ranges from no symptoms, bloody nipple discharge, pain or a palpable mass, and occur most commonly in the subareolar region. If the fluid within the cyst is blood stained, it may present as a blue mass beneath the nipple. The aetiology is unknown but stasis and secondary infection of the ductules is implicated (Greydanus et al. 2006). US appearances include tubular anechoic structures, which may be hyperechoic if laden with debris.

Cystic lesions generally resolve spontaneously; however, they are susceptible to infection, and these may result in mastitis and breast abscesses. Recurrent or persistent symptoms may necessitate surgical excision.

13.5 Fibrocystic Disease

Fibrocystic disease (diffuse cystic mastopathy/mammary dysplasia) is a benign multicystic proliferative disorder of the adolescent breast, more typically seen in the third decade of life. It should be considered to be a normal variant and is observed in 50% of women of reproductive age (Templeman and Hertweck 2000). Cyclical breast pain in relation to menstrual cycle is a common complaint. Small cysts or discrete lumps may be found on clinical examination and serial breast examinations performed at different stages of the menstrual cycle differ significantly. US findings are non-specific and may include echogenic glandular tissue with multiple cysts of differing sizes and duct dilatation (Fig. 13). Malignancy in this condition has not been reported in adolescents but a persisting lump should be monitored and treated as any other persisting mass.

13.6 Haematoma

Haematomas result from blunt trauma or iatrogenic injury. The sonographic appearances are variable depending upon the timing of presentation. Acute haematomas are hyperechoic cysts that show acoustic enhancement. With clot lysis and resorption, the internal echotexture can show increasing complexity with fluid-debris levels, which become more anechoic with time (Fig. 14a). Colour Doppler reveals no internal flow (Fig. 14b). The main differential is abscess.

14 Vascular Anomalies

Haemangioma are high-flow neoplasms with an associated parenchymal mass. Lymphatic, mixed venous-lymphatic malformations and venous channels are low or absent flow lesions without an associated soft tissue mass. Both types of lesion can affect the paediatric chest wall and rarely the breast.

14.1 Lymphangioma

Cystic lymphangioma (cystic hygroma) is a benign congenital malformation of the lymphatic system. Most cystic hygromas are located in the posterior triangle of the neck or axilla and present at birth or by early childhood. The lesions are usually asymptomatic but are infiltrative and can cause local mass effect as lesions tend to span fascial planes. This accounts for the propensity for recurrence following surgical therapy.

US in macrocystic lymphatic malformations reveal multiple cysts of varying size (Fig. 15). The cysts are often thin walled and anechoic but can contain fluid-debris levels, usually following prior haemorrhage or occasionally secondary infection. Lymphatic malformations show no Doppler flow. Venous malformations may contain phleboliths. Doppler interrogation can demonstrate low flow in venous channels. MRI is the examination of choice to delineate lesion extent.

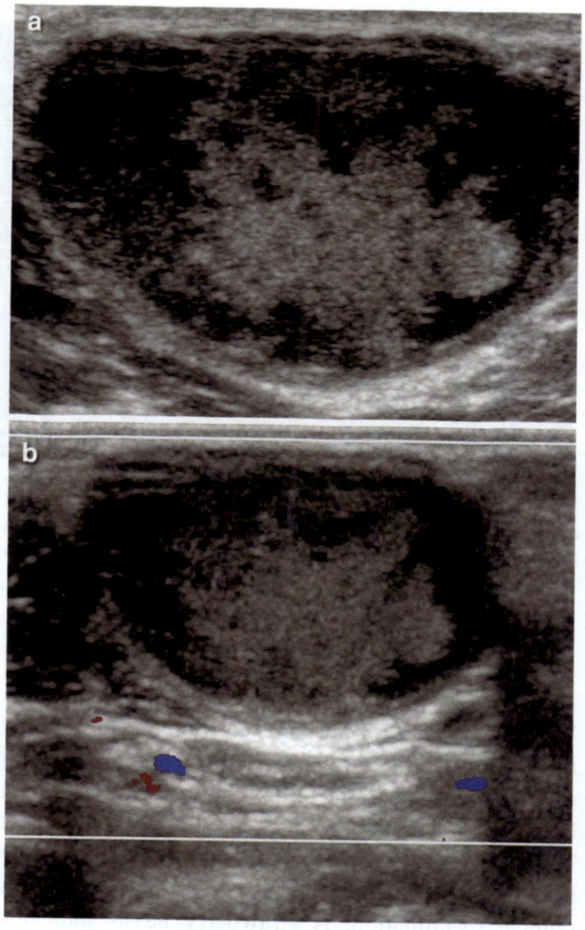

Fig. 14 Breast haematoma. Oblique sonograms of the axillary tail in a 3-year-old boy following a recent playground injury show a fairly well defined mass within the soft tissues. **a** Complex internal echoes are present in this predominately cystic mass, **b** confirmed on Doppler colour flow imaging to show posterior acoustic enhancement and no internal flow. This resolved on clinical follow-up

The fluid in the dilated lymphatic sacs tends to be isointense to CSF on all spin echo pulse sequences and bright on fat suppressed T2 STIR sequences.

Interventional radiology-based treatment in many centres has supplanted surgical treatment for vascular malformations. Symptomatic relief and reduction in lesion size can be effectively achieved with serial image-guided therapy. Picibanil (OK432) (Ogita et al. 1987) and ethibloc (Dubois et al. 1997) are effective sclerosants for lymphangiomas. Sodium tetradecyl sulphate (O'donovan et al. 1997) and ethanol are used for venous malformations (Lee et al. 2001).

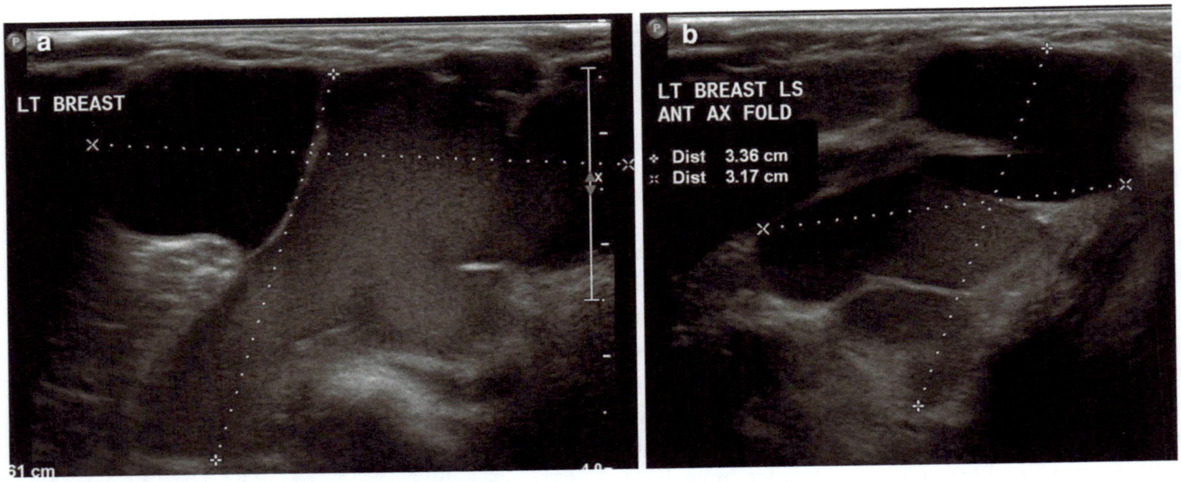

Fig. 15 Lymphangioma. Longitudinal scans (**a**) over the left anterior chest wall and (**b**) axilla in a newborn male with a fluctuant chest wall mass show a multilocular macrocystic mass with anechoic cysts and high-density fluid content. No flow is seen on Doppler imaging

14.2 Haemangioma

Haemangiomas are the most common tumour of infancy. Infantile or capillary haemangioma rarely involves the breast but is the commonest cause of a breast mass in infancy and childhood. The typical history is of growing mass presenting in the first few months of life. The diagnosis is normally made on clinical examination. A strawberry nevus indicates skin involvement. The vascular mass proliferates until the age of around 1 year and then slowly involutes. Doppler US is diagnostic in most cases (Dubois et al. 1998). Typical sonographic features include a discrete, superficial soft tissue mass with internal high-flow vascular channels (Figs. 16 and 17). MRI is confirmatory and useful in defining soft tissue extent. T1 and fat suppressed T2 (STIR) sequences in two orthogonal planes are usually adequate to define local extent, MRA and MRV and post-contrast scans are not normally required. Most lesions are isointense to muscle on T1 and homogenously or heterogeneously hyperintense on T2-weighted imaging. Flow signal voids can be seen on spin echo sequences. Fine needle biopsy is rarely indicated.

Most lesions will completely regress spontaneously. There is a risk that mammary hypoplasia may result if the breast bud is involved, either following regression or attempted surgical intervention. Rapidly growing haemangioma may necessitate resection but this may not be feasible and a course of oral corticosteroids may be trialled (Miaux et al. 1992).

15 Solid Breast Masses

15.1 Management of Solid Breast Masses

Clinical assessment of the child with a breast mass should begin with a history and physical examination. In adult practice, optimal assessment currently comprises of a 'triple screen', consisting of a physical examination, diagnostic imaging and pathological correlation. In the vast majority of children, clinical examination supplemented by US will suffice for complete diagnostic evaluation. US is most helpful in demonstrating and characterising abnormalities and directing further investigation (Bock et al. 2005).

Imaging criteria have been developed to attempt to discriminate between benign and malignant breast lesions based on high-resolution sonography, referred to as the Stavros criteria (Stavros et al. 1995). According to these criteria, a lesion should be considered malignant until proven otherwise if any one of the following features is present: marked hypoechogenicity (fat is isoechoic), microcalcifications, spiculated or angular margins, microlobulations, branching

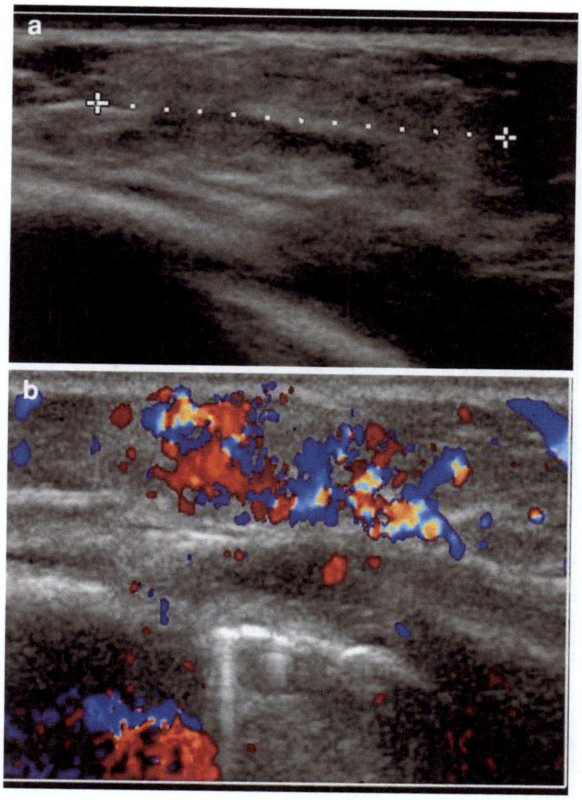

Fig. 16 Haemangioma. Transverse sonograms of the left breast in a newborn girl. **a** The left breast is enlarged and occupied by a solid mass (between callipers) within the superficial soft tissues which shows well defined margins and smooth outline. **b** Colour Doppler interrogation reveals high-flow internal vascular channels

pattern or ductal extension. A lesion is classified as benign if any one of the following criteria is present: ellipsoid shape with a thin uniform echogenic capsule, three or less gentle macrolobulations with a thin uniform echogenic capsule or uniform intense hyperechogenicity. In a retrospective study of 20 adolescent girls aged 13–19 years with sonograms depicting 21 solid masses, 15 out of 21 were correctly classified as benign according to the Stavros criteria when correlated with histopathological or clinical follow-up. All 21 masses were classified benign at final review.

The age-specific risk of breast malignancy in female children and adolescents is extremely low below 19 years of age. (Ries et al. 2005). A study of 242 adolescent girls aged 14 to 20 years with breast masses found that only 6 patients (2.5%) had malignant lesions (Elsheikh et al. 2000). Furthermore, only a third of palpable breast masses were pathological in a retrospective analysis of a cohort of children and adolescents (Kronemer et al. 2001).

The most common benign neoplastic lesions in the paediatric and adolescent breast are fibroadenoma and benign phyllodes tumours (Vade et al. 2008). The malignant potential in these lesions is exceedingly low. Other benign solid lesions include haemangioma, lymphangioma, fibroma, fat necrosis, lipoma, intraductal papilloma and intramammary lymph nodes (Boothroyd and Carty 1994). Given the low risk of malignancy in this age group, conservative management has been advocated by some for solid breast mass lesions in children. Observation for at least two menstrual cycles or serial follow-up until adulthood has been recommended (Bower et al. 1976; West et al. 1995). US-guided fine needle aspiration has also been advocated to avoid unnecessary excision biopsy for the vast majority of lesions that are benign unless they are rapidly growing (Pacinda and Ramzy 1998).

15.2 Benign Neoplastic Lesions

15.2.1 Fibroadenoma

Fibroadenomas are the most common solid breast mass excised in paediatric and adolescent surgical series (West et al. 1995; Pacinda and Ramzy 1998; Siegal et al. 1992). These benign fibroepithelial tumours develop from a single duct and show a hormonal response similar to that of normal breast tissue. Fibroadenomas typically present in the late teens as slow growing, smooth, well-circumscribed, painless, freely mobile masses resulting in breast asymmetry. The vast majority are unilateral and grow over a period of 6–12 months and then stabilise. Around 10–40% may resolve completely (Pacinda and Ramzy 1998). On US, classic fibroadenomas are well-circumscribed, hypoechoic masses with uniform homogeneity and show acoustic enhancement. They are often oval in shape but may be round or show gentle lobulation (Fig. 18). A thin echogenic capsule may be seen. Myxoid fibroadenomas typically appear as smooth high signal intensity masses on T2-weighted images, which enhance following contrast administration. The malignant potential in these lesions is exceedingly low. As described earlier, conservative management of defined fibroadenomas is safe clinical practice (Cant et al. 1995).

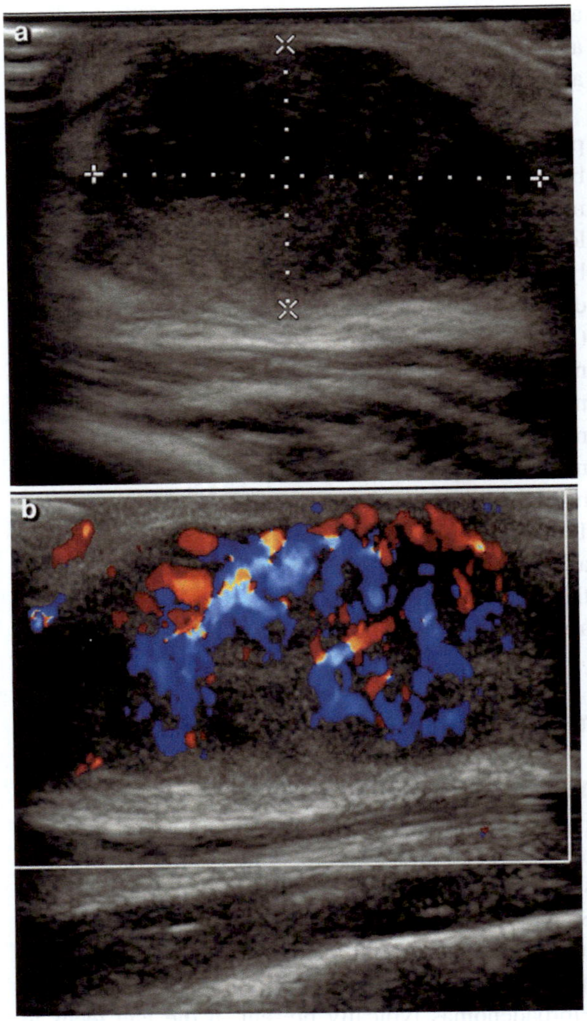

Fig. 17 Haemangioma. **a** US of a solid mass in a 6-month-old boy (between callipers) within the superficial soft tissues of the right breast. **b** Colour Doppler imaging shows high-flow internal vascular channels

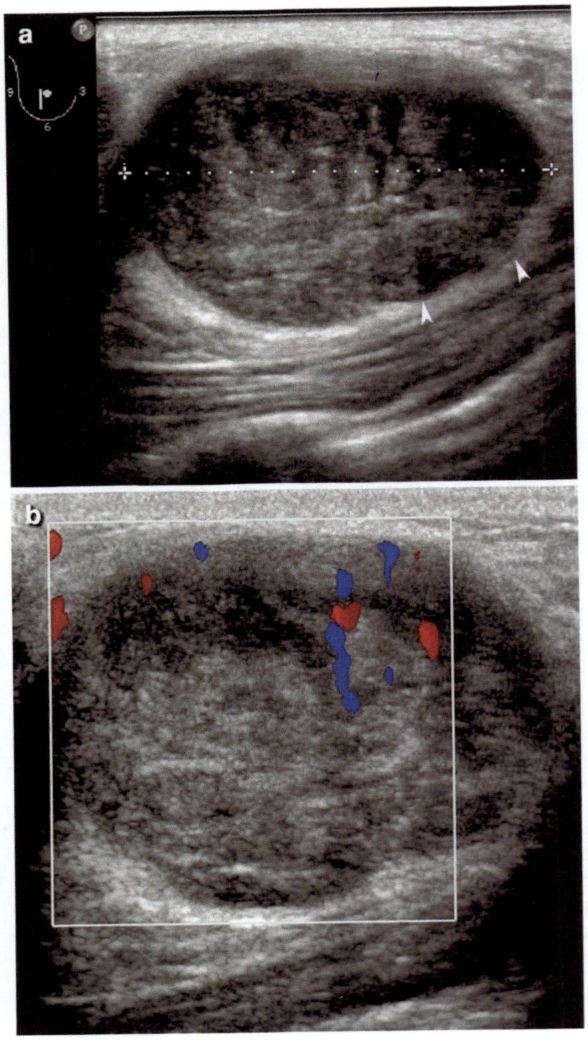

Fig. 18 Fibroadenoma. Longitudinal views of the right breast in a 15-year-old girl with a solitary painless breast mass. **a** A fairly uniform, well-defined, solid lesion containing low echoes is demonstrated with less than 3 macrolobulations (*arrows*) **b** Colour Doppler imaging shows minimal central vascularity

A juvenile variant, also known as a *giant fibroadenoma* (cellular fibroadenoma), refers to lesions in excess of 5 cm, which are characterised by rapid growth (Fig. 19). These occur in 5–10% of cases. The differential includes phyllodes tumour and benign virginal hypertrophy. Based on growth, these are usually enucleated. Atypical fibroadenomas are difficult to differentiate from phyllodes tumour, which is discussed below. Surgical excision is recommended in symptomatic fibroadenomas, giant fibroadenomas due to rapid growth and atypical fibroadenomas.

Despite the benign behaviour of fibroadenomas, they have been associated with an increased risk of invasive breast cancer. A large retrospective study of 1,835 patients with fibroadenoma diagnosed between 1950 and 1968 reported that the risk of invasive breast cancer was 2.15 (95th CI: 1.9,5.1) compared to controls. The risk was greatest in patients with benign proliferative disease in the parenchyma adjacent to the fibroadenoma (3.88, 95th CI: 2.1,7.3). Twenty per cent of patients who had a family history of breast cancer in addition to proliferative developed breast

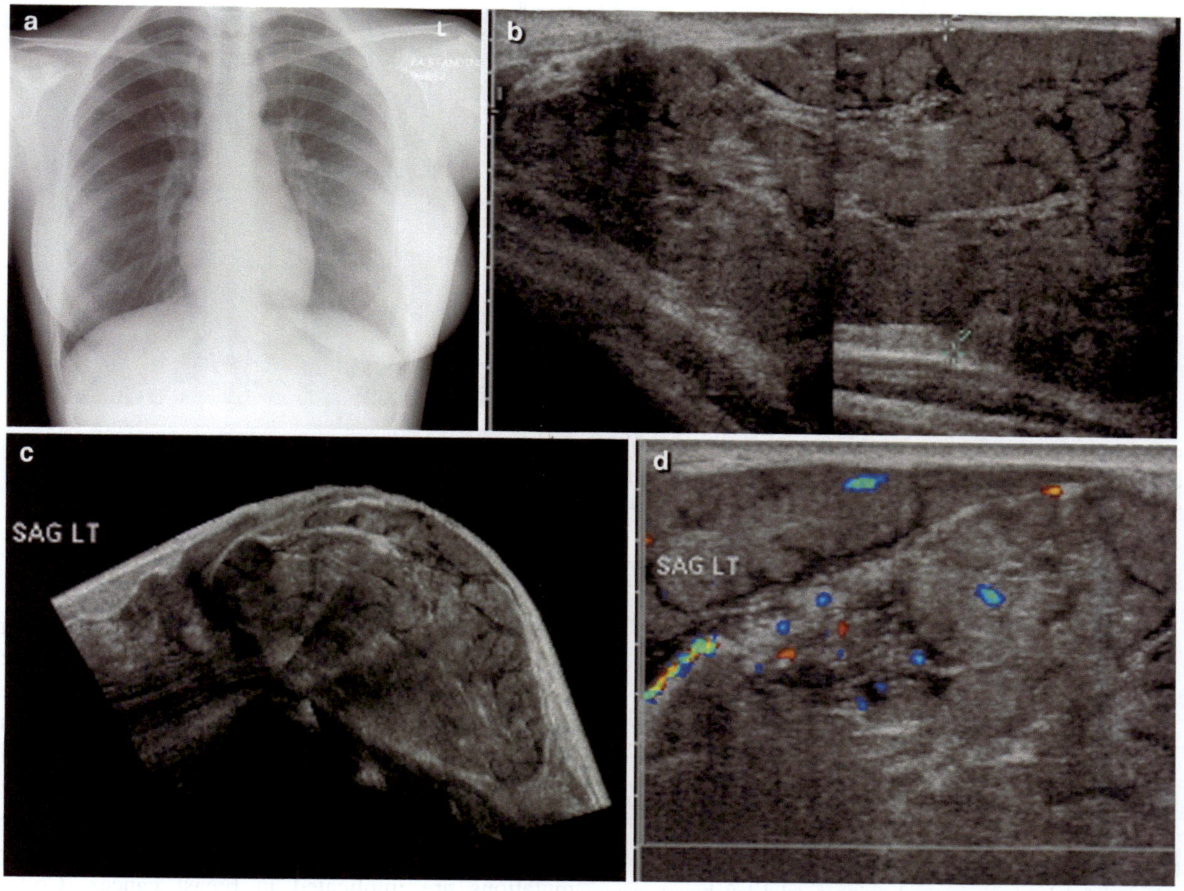

Fig. 19 Giant fibroadenoma. **a** Frontal chest radiograph in a 14-year-old girl with painful marked asymmetric enlargement of the left breast. **b** Composite longitudinal view of the left breast mass showing a solid heterogeneous lesion. **c** Panoramic longitudinal scan demonstrating the large solitary, encapsulated breast mass separate from the pectoralis major **d** Colour Doppler imaging reveals intralesional flow. The differential for this appearance is phyllodes tumour

cancer within the first 25 years of follow-up (Dupont et al. 1994).

15.2.2 Phyllodes Tumour

Phyllodes tumour is an extremely rare breast tumour that accounts for less than 1% of breast lesions. They are usually benign but can be malignant. The clinical findings and imaging features are similar to those of juvenile fibroadenoma and more often demonstrate a hypoechoic mass with a heterogeneous echotexture and peripheral cysts. Complete surgical excision is indicated with a 1-cm clear margin of normal tissue. Approximately 25% may recur if the borders are infiltrative or the surgical margins are positive and although rare 10% metastasise haematogenously, mainly to the lungs (Selamzade et al. 1999).

15.3 Malignant Masses

Malignant tumours of the breast in children are exceptionally rare. The most common presentations are secondary malignancies with breast metastases; primary malignancy is exceedingly rare. A cohort study of 237 patients with breast masses aged 10–20 years found that only one patient had a primary breast cancer and two patients had sarcomas that had metastasised to breast (Farrow and Ashikai 1969). Not withstanding this, a heightened awareness of breast cancer in the general population and the high prevalence of breast cancer in the adult population often serve to heighten the anxiety of adolescents presenting with a palpable breast abnormality or nipple discharge.

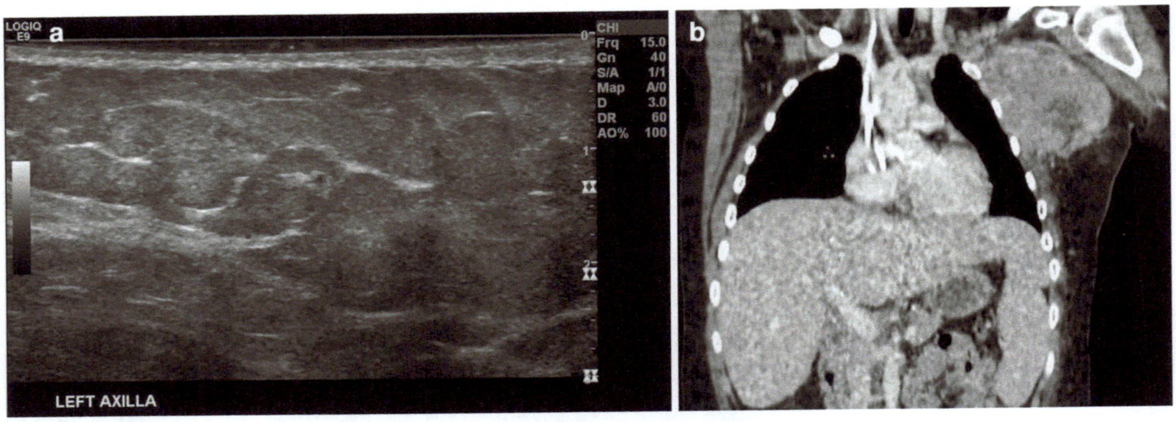

Fig. 20 Lymphoma. **a** High-resolution ultrasound of the left axilla and **b** Coronal reformatted CT image performed for staging in a child presenting with a large breast lump arising from the left axilla. The histopathological diagnosis was anaplastic large-cell lymphoma

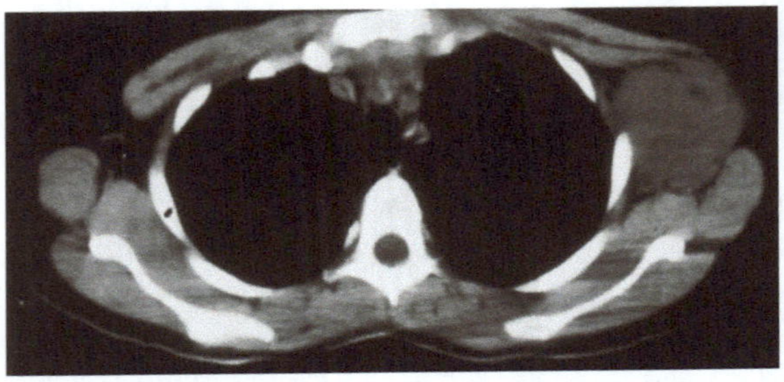

Fig. 21 Rhabdomyosarcoma: CT performed for staging in primary rhabdomyosarcoma showing a solid left breast mass arising from the axillary tail. Reproduced from Boothroyd and Carty (1994) with permission from Springer Publishers

15.3.1 Metastases

Metastatic deposits to the breast result from haematogenous or lymphatic spread. Primary tumours that metastasise to the juvenile breast include rhabdomyosarcoma (RMS), frequently of the alveolar histological subtype (Howarth et al. 1980), Hodgkin's lymphoma, non-Hodgkin's lymphoma (Fig. 20) and leukaemia (Chateil et al. 1998). Medulloblastoma, neuroblastoma, Langerhans cell histiocytosis, melanoma and renal carcinoma have been reported to metastasise to the breast (Chateil et al. 1998).

Metastatic alveolar RMS is usually seen in adolescents. The primary tumour may arise from the nasopharynx, body or extremities (Binokay et al. 2003). Bilateral involvement is seen as much as 30% of cases. Metastasis maybe solitary or multiple, unilateral or bilateral and appear as well- or ill-defined hypoechoic masses with variable echotexture.

15.3.2 Primary Breast Tumours

Primary Carcinoma

The overall risk of primary breast malignancy in children is very low (Ramirez and Ansfield 1968; Rogers et al. 1994). The most common primary malignancy in children and adolescents is a phyllodes tumour. Primary breast cancer in young females is extremely rare and usually due to a juvenile-secreting neoplasm (West et al. 1995) and the remainder are intraductal carcinomas. BRCA1 and BRCA2 gene mutations are implicated in breast cancer (Coffin 2002). The risk of developing breast cancer is 80% and ovarian cancer is 40–60% during their lifetime.

The diagnosis of breast cancer in children is challenging. Clinical and radiological investigations are non-specific and poor at differentiating between benign and malignant masses. US often demonstrates an irregular hypoechoic mass with heterogeneous echotexture. Malignant lesions appear taller-than-wide with variable acoustic shadowing (Venta et al. 1994). Even with image-guided biopsies yielding sufficient tissue for histological analysis, pathological confirmation can be problematic (Boothroyd and Carty 1994).

Sarcomas

Rhabdomyosarcoma is the most common paediatric soft tissue tumour. Rhabdomyosarcoma, fibrosarcoma, malignant fibrous histiocytoma and angiosarcoma may occur as primary breast tumours (Fig. 21). Alveolar rhabdomyosarcoma is the most common form; the tumour is locally invasive and spreads haematogenously. Prognosis is dependant upon local extent, histology, age at presentation and presence of metastatic disease.

Secondary Tumours

The latent period between exposure to radiotherapy and induction of a secondary treatment–related breast tumour is of the order of decades and usually not before 20 years. Chest wall radiation is typically instituted as part of multimodal therapy for Hodgkin's Lymphoma. Girls with Hodgkin's treated with chest radiotherapy have an 80-fold increased risk of breast cancer; ultimately, around 40% develop breast cancer in adulthood (Gold et al. 2003). Ten years after their chest wall radiation, they need to be referred to a breast family history clinic so that long-term surveillance can be undertaken.

16 Nipple Discharge

Nipple discharge can occur at any age. In the neonatal period, milky discharge reflects transient maternal hormonal influence. Non-lactational milky discharge in older children—galactorrhoea—has many causes. ROHN has classified the non-puerperal causes of lactation as: neurogenic, hypothalamic, pituitary, endocrine/hormonal, drug induced and idiopathic (Rohn 1984). A thorough history and physical examination is required to ascertain the likely underlying cause in order to target further imaging evaluation. Hormonal profiles should include serum prolactin, follicular stimulating hormone (FSH), luteinizing hormone (LH) and thyroid function studies. If hormonal profiles are abnormal, then an endocrinology opinion should be sought. Depending on the suspected underlying cause, cranial MRI or thyroid imaging may be appropriate.

Episodic serous to brown discharge can occur from the lactational areolar tubercles (Montgomery's tubercles). This is normally self-limiting. The tubercles may be palpable. The differential for bloody or serosanguinous discharge in children and adolescents includes mammary duct ectasia, intraductal papillomata, chronic cystic mastitis (De Silva and Brandt 2006b) and localised irritation or mechanical trauma (Loud and Micheli 2001). Mammary duct hyperplasia is rare in children or adolescents. Intraductal papilloma result from ductal cell proliferation, the malignant potential in adolescents, is low (Rosen 1985). Nipple discharge is also seen in interrupted puberty or with primary or secondary amenorrhoea (Fallat and Ignacio 2008).

Unilateral, intermittent or persistent nipple discharge merits further clinical evaluation. Gram staining of the discharge, hormonal profiles (prolactin, FSH, LH and thyrotropin) and breast US should be undertaken (Kelly et al. 2006). US will demonstrate a mass or ductal dilatation. If a single duct is involved, ductography has been advocated (Tabár et al. 1983) but its use in children and adolescents is rarely necessary. The technique employs sterile cannulation of an affected duct and hand injection of a small quantity of water-soluble contrast medium; standard mammograms are then obtained. Ductal filling defects are noted in intraductal papilloma and dilated cystic spaces in fibrocystic disease. Ductal injection with methylene blue aids perioperative localisation. Cytological evaluation of nipple discharge has low diagnostic sensitivity (Sakorafas 2001).

References

Binokay F, Soyupak SK, Inal M et al (2003) Primary and metastatic rhabdomyosarcoma in the breast: report of two pediatric cases. Eur J Radiol 48:282–284

Bock K, Duda VF, Hadji P et al (2005) Pathologic breast conditions in childhood and adolescence: evaluation by sonographic diagnosis. J Ultrasound Med 24:1347–1354

Boothroyd A, Carty H (1994) Breast masses in childhood and adolescence. A presentation of 17 cases and a review of the literature. Pediatr Radiol 24:81–84

Bower R, Bell MJ, Ternberg JL (1976) Management of breast lesions in children and adolescents. J Pediatr Surg 11:337–346

Brand IR, Sapherson DA, Brown TS (1993) Breast imaging in women under 35 with symptomatic breast disease. Br J Radiol 66:394–397

Bruni V, Dei M, Deligeoroglou E et al (1990) Breast development in adolescent girls. Adolesc Pediatr Gynecol 3:201–205

Cant PJ, Madden MV, Coleman MG et al (1995) Non-operative management of breast masses diagnosed as fibroadenoma. Br J Surg 82:792–794

Chateil JF, Arboucalot F, Pérel Y et al (1998) Breast metastases in adolescent girls: US findings. Pediatr Radiol 28:832–835

Chung EM, Cube R, Hall GJ et al (2009) From the archives of the AFIP: breast masses in children and adolescents: radiologic-pathologic correlation. Radiographics 29:907–931

Coffin CM (2002) The breast. In: Stocker JT, Dehner LP (eds) Pediatric pathology, 2nd edn. Lippincott Williams & Wilkins, Philadelphia, pp 993–1015

De Silva NK, Brandt ML (2006a) Disorders of the breast in children and adolescents, Part 1: disorders of growth and infections of the breast. J Pediatr Adolesc Gynecol 19(5):345–349

De Silva NK, Brandt ML (2006b) Disorders of the breast in children and adolescents, Part 2: breast masses. J Pediatr Adolesc Gynecol 19:415–418

Denoel C, Aguirre MF, Bianco G et al (2009) Idiopathic scoliosis and breast asymmetry. J Plast Reconstr Aesthet Surg 62:1303–1308

Dubois J, Garel L, Abela A et al (1997) Lymphangiomas in children: percutaneous sclerotherapy with an alcoholic solution of zein. Radiology 204:651–654

Dubois J, Patriquin HB, Garel L et al (1998) Soft-tissue hemangiomas in infants and children: diagnosis using Doppler sonography. Am J Roentgenol 171:247–252

Duflos C, Plu-Bureau G, Thibaud E et al (2004) Breast diseases in adolescents. In: Sultan C (ed) Paediatric and adolescent gynaecology, vol 7. Karger, Basel, pp 183–196

Dupont WD, Page DL, Parl FF et al (1994) Long-term risk of breast cancer in women with fibroadenoma. N Eng J Med 331:10–15

Elsheikh A, Keramopoulos A, Lazaris D et al (2000) Breast tumors during adolescence. Eur J Gynaecol Oncol 21:408–410

Fallat ME, Ignacio RC Jr (2008) Breast disorders in children and adolescents. J Pediatr Adolesc Gynecol 21:311–316

Farrow JH, Ashikai H (1969) Breast lesions in young girls. Surg Clin North Am 49:261–269

Feig SA (1984) Radiation risk from mammography: is it clinically significant? Am J Roentgenol 143:469–475

Ferguson CM, Powell RW (1989) Breast masses in young women. Arch Surg 124:1338–1341

Furnival CM, Irwin JRM, Gray GM (1983) Breast disease in young women. MJA 2:167–169

Garcia CJ, Espinoza A, Dinamarca V et al (2000) Breast US in children and adolescents. RadioGraphics 20:1605–1612

Gold DG, Neglia JP, Dusenbery KE (2003) Second neoplasms after megavoltage radiation for pediatric tumors. Cancer 97:2588–2596

Greydanus DE, Parks DS, Farrell EG (1989) Breast disorders in children and adolescents. Pediatr Clin North Am 36:601–638

Greydanus DE, Matytsina L, Gains M (2006) Breast disorders in children and adolescents. Prim Care Clin Office Pract 33:455–502

Haber HP, Wollmann HA, Ranke MB (1995) Pelvic ultrasonography: early differentiation between isolated premature thelarche and central precocious puberty. Eur J Pediatr 154:182–186

Hayes R, Michell M, Nunnerley HB (1991) Acute inflammation of the breast—the role of breast ultrasound in diagnosis and management. Clin Radiol 144:253–256

Hindle WH, Davis L, Wright D (1999) Clinical value of mammography for symptomatic women 35 years of age and younger. Am J Obstet Gynecol 180:1484–1490

Howarth CB, Caces JN, Pratt CB (1980) Breast metastases in children with rhabdomyosarcoma. Cancer 46:2520–2524

Huneeus A, Schilling A, Horvath E et al (2003) Retroareolar cysts in the adolescent. J Pediatr Adolesc Gynecol 16:45–49

Jackson VP (1990) The role of US in breast imaging. Radiology 1772:305–311

Kajava Y (1915) The proportions of supernumerary nipples in the Finnish population. Duodecim 31:143–170

Kelly VM, Arif K, Ralston S et al (2006) Bloody nipple discharge in an infant and a proposed diagnostic approach. Pediatrics 117:814–816

Kronemer KA, Rhee K, Siegel MK et al (2001) Gray scale sonography of breast masses in adolescent girls. J Ultrasound Med 20:491–496

Lee BB, Kim DI, Huh S et al (2001) New experiences with absolute ethanol sclerotherapy in the management of a complex form of congenital venous malformation. J Vasc Surg 334:764–772

Loud KJ, Micheli LJ (2001) Common athletic injuries in adolescent girls. Curr Opin Pediatr 13:317–322

Marshall WA, Tanner JM (1969) Variations in the pattern of pubertal changes in girls. Arch Dis Child 44:291–303

McKiernan JF, Hull D (1981) Prolactin, maternal oestrogens, and breast development in the newborn. Arch Dis Child 56:770–774

Miaux Y, Lemarchand-Venencie F, Cyna-Gorse F et al (1992) MR imaging of breast hemangioma in female infants. Pediatr Radiol 22:463–464

O'Donovan JC, Donaldson JS, Morello FP et al (1997) Symptomatic hemangiomas and venous malformations in infants, children, and young adults: treatment with percutaneous injection of sodium tetradecyl sulfate. Am J Roentgenol 1693:723–729

O'Hare PM, Frieden IJ (2000) Virginal breast hypertrophy. Pediatr Dermatol 17:277–281

Ogita S, Tsuto T, Tokiwa K, Takahashi T (1987) Intracystic injection of OK-432: a new sclerosing therapy for cystic hygroma in children. Br J Surg 748:690–691

Osborne MP, Boolbol SK (2009) Breast Anatomy and Development In: Harris JR, Lippman ME, Morrow M et al (eds) Diseases of the breast 4th edn. Lippincott Williams & Wilkins, Philadelphia, pp 1–12

Pacinda S, Ramzy I (1998) Fine-needle aspiration of breast masses: a review of its role in diagnosis and management in adolescent patients. J Adolesc Health 23:3–6

Ramirez G, Ansfield FJ (1968) Carcinoma of the Breast in Children. AMA Arch Surg 96:222–225

Ries LA, Eisner MP, Kosary CL, et al (eds) (2005) SEER cancer statistics review, 1975–2002. Bethesda, MD. National Cancer Institute, http://seer.cancer.gov/csr/1975_2002. Accessed 12 Oct 2010

Rogers DA, Lobe TE, Rao BN (1994) Breast malignancy in children. J Pediatr Surg 29:48–51

Rohn RD (1984) Galactorrhea in the adolescent. J Adolesc Health Care 5:37–42

Rosen PP (1985) Papillary duct hyperplasia of the breast in children and young adults. Cancer 56(7):1611–1617

Rudoy RC, Nelson JD (1975) Breast abscess during the neonatal period. Am J Dis Child 129:1031–1034

Sakorafas GH (2001) Nipple discharge: current diagnostic and therapeutic approaches. Cancer Treat Rev 27:275–282

Selamzade M, Gidener C, Koyuncuoglu M et al (1999) Borderline phyllodes tumour in an 11-year-old girl. Pediatr Surg Int 15:427–428

Shamberger RC (1996) Congenital chest wall deformities. Curr Probl Surg 33:469–542

Siegal A, Kaufman Z, Siegal G (1992) Breast masses in adolescent females. J Surg Oncol 51:169–173

Siegel MJ (2002) Chest. In: Siegel MJ (ed) Pediatric sonography, 3rd edn. Lippincott Williams & Williams, Philadelphia, pp 201–211

Stanhope R, Traggiai C (2004) Precocious puberty (complete, partial). Endocr Dev 7:57–65

Stavros AT, Thickman D, Rapp CL et al (1995) Solid breast nodules: use of sonography to distinguish between benign and malignant lesions. Radiology 196:123–134

Tabár L, Dean PB, Péntek Z (1983) Galactography: the diagnostic procedure of choice for nipple discharge. Radiology 149:31–38

Templeman C, Hertweck SP (2000) Breast disorders in the pediatric and adolescent patient. Obstet Gynecol Clin North Am 27:19–34

Vade A, Lafita VS, Ward KA et al (2008) Role of breast sonography in imaging of adolescents with palpable solid breast masses. Am J Roentgenol 191:659–663

Venta LA, Dudiak CM, Salomon CG (1994) Sonographic evaluation of the breast. Radiographics 14:29–50

Welch ST, Babcock DS, Ballard ET (2004) Sonography of pediatric male breast masses: gynecomastia and beyond. Pediatr Radiol 34:952–957

West KW, Rescorla FJ, Scherer LR et al (1995) Diagnosis and treatment of symptomatic breast masses in the pediatric population. J Pediatr Surg 130:182–187

Index

11β-Hydroxylase deficiency, 36
17,20 Desmolase deficiency, 36
17-Hydroxylase deficiency, 158
17β-Hydroxysteroid dehydrogenase type, 3, 130
17β-OH-dehydrogenase deficiency, 36
21-Hydroxylase deficiency—(see also Congenital adrenal hyperplasia-classic), 35, 39, 42, 140, 160
3β-Hydroxysteroid hydrogenase deficiency, 35–36
46,XX Disorders of sex development, 36, 39, 42–43
5α-Reductase deficiency, 35–36, 46–47
β-hCG level, 182, 199, 201–202, 206

A

Abdominopelvic cyst (see Cyst—abdominopelvic)
Acromegaly, 137, 156
Addison disease (see Adrenal insufficiency)
Adenomyosis, 205
Adenomyotic cyst, 205
Adnexa, 92
Adnexal
  masses, 185
  torsion (also see Ovarian Torsion), 185
  volume ratio, 175, 177, 190, 193
Adrenal
  adenoma, 140–141, 161
  androgen-secreting tumour, 132, 156
  cerebriform morphology, 40
  carcinoma, 140–141, 161–162
  insufficiency, 158, 159
  normal imaging appearances, 103, 106–107
  oestrogen-secreting tumour, 132–133
  rest tumour, 42, 160
Adrenarche, 117, 131
  exaggerated, 131–132
  premature, 115, 117, 130
Adrenocortical tumour, 116, 140, 161
Adrenocorticotropic Hormone deficiency, 140
Alphafetoprotein, 211
Amenorrhoea
  clinical assessment, 149
  endocrine investigations, 149
  primary, 148, 151
  secondary, 148–149
American Society of Reproductive Medicine Classification, 66–67
Anaesthesia, 2–3
Androgen Excess Society diagnostic criteria, 156
Androgen insensitivity syndrome
  complete, 5, 44, 164–166
  diagnostic criteria, 165
  imaging, 44–45, 165
  mild, 164
  partial, 44–45, 164–165
Androgen receptor, 44
  mutation, 44, 164
Anorexia nervosa, 148, 150
Anosmia, 125
Anovulation, 147
Anti-Müllerian hormone, 22, 33–34, 127, 130, 160
Assessment of skeletal maturity (see Bone age)
Autoimmune oophoritis, 148, 158, 160

B

Balanced X chromosome translocations, 158
Bartholins glands, 30
Beckwith-Wiedemann syndrome, 141, 161, 218
Blepharophimosis-ptosis-epicanthus inversus syndrome, 158
Blood dyscrasia, 147
Body mass index, 16, 118, 134
Bone age
  automated analysis, 108
  Fels method, 105, 118
  Greulich and Pyle, 105, 118
  Tanner-Whitehouse methodologies, 105
Bone mineral
  content, 108
  density, 109
Breast
  abscess, 233–234
  amastia, 233
  aplasia, 232
  asymmetry, 231–232
  athelia, 232
  clinical evaluation, 230
  cyst, 234–235

G. Mann et al. (eds.), *Imaging of Gynecological Disorders in Infants and Children*, Medical Radiology. Diagnostic Imaging, DOI: 10.1007/978-3-540-85602-3, © Springer-Verlag Berlin Heidelberg 2012

B (*cont.*)
development, 117, 132, 149, 226–227
embryology, 226
fibroadenoma, 239–240
fibrocystic disease, 236
galactocele, 236
giant fibroadenoma, 240
haemangioma, 238
haematoma, 237
hypomastia, 233
hypoplasia, 231–232
lobule, 228
lymphangioma, 237
lactiferous ducts, 226
lymphatic drainage, 228
lymphoma, 242
macromastia, 233
malignant masses, 241–242
mamma aberrata, 230
mammary duct ectasia, 236
mammary ridge, 226
mammography, 228
management of solid mass, 238
metastases, 241
milk lines, 226
nipple discharge, 243
phyllodes tumour, 240
polymastia, 230
polythelia, 230
postnatal development, 226
primary carcinoma, 242
primary mammary bud, 226
pseudomamma, 230
retroareolar cyst, 235
phabdomyosarcoma, 242
secondary mammary bud, 226
secondary tumours, 243
supernumerary tissue, 230
Tanner staging, 227
ultrasound, 228
vascular malformation, 237
vascular supply, 228
virginal hypertrophy, 233
Bulimia nervosa, 148

C
Canal of Nuck, 24, 30
cyst, 24, 61
hydrocele, 61
Carcinoma
adrenal, 140–141, 161–162
breast primary, 242
ovarian, 210
Carney complex, 141
Cell
granulosa, 34
Leydig, 33–34, 116, 138
Sertoli, 33, 129
theca, 34
Cervical
atresia, 56
stenosis, 147, 149
Cervicovaginal atresia, 68
Cervix uterus
anatomy, 84, 86
MRI appearances, 88–89
ultrasound appearances, 86
Chemotherapy, 119, 158
Choriocarcinoma, 201–202, 211
Chromosomal sex, 22, 32
Classification
American Society of Reproductive Medicine, 66–67
clinico-embryological, 67
PVE, 41
Prader, 41
Clear cell carcinoma, 221
Clinico-embryological Classification, 67
Cliteromegally, 61–62
Clitoris, 28–29
Cloaca, 27, 35
Cloacal
malformation, 7, 51–52, 56–59, 70
membrane, 27–28, 35
Colour Doppler, 6–7
Complete androgen insensitivity syndrome (see androgen insensitivity syndrome)
Complete hydatiform mole, 174, 201
Computed Tomography
bowel preparation, 15
contrast medium, 14
indications, 13
scanning parameters, 13
Congenital adrenal hyperplasia
classic, 35, 39, 116, 130, 132–133, 139–140, 161
lipoid, 160
non-classic, 39, 130–133, 139
virilising, 148
Congenital androgen insensitivity syndrome (see Androgen insensitivity syndrome)
Congenital disorders of glycosylation, 158
Constitutional delay in growth and puberty, 148
Corpus albicans, 97
Corpus luteum, 97, 100–101
Corpus luteum cyst, 179–184
Cortical cord (see secondary sex cord)
Craniopharyngioma, 116, 119, 135
Cryptomenorrhoea, 147, 185
Criteria
Androgen Excess Society diagnostic, 156
Rotterdam consensus, 156
Cryptomenorrhoea, 147, 185
Cushing syndrome, 118, 130, 137, 140, 148, 156, 160
Cyst
abdominopelvic, 52
Bartholin duct, 61
duplication, 52–53
Gartner duct, 61–62
hymenal, 61
Kobelt, 195
mesonephric, 61, 195
mesothelial, 195

Müllerian, 61
neonatal ovarian (see Ovarian cyst—neonatal)
paramesonephric, 195
paratubal, 195
paraurethral, 61
paraurethral, 182
peritoneal inclusion, 195
Skene duct, 61
urothelial, 61
vaginal wall inclusion, 61
Wolffian, 195
Cystography, 13

D

Daughter cyst sign, 52–53
Defects in androgen biosynthesis (also see Androgen insensitivity syndrome), 36, 43, 119, 127
Defects in testis determination, 42, 130
Dehydroepiandrosterone, 83
Dehydroepiandrosterone sulphate, 83
DeMorsier syndrome (see Septo-optic dysplasia)
Denys-Drash syndrome, 39–40
Dermoid cyst (also see Ovarian teratoma), 16, 182, 188–189
Development
fallopian tubes, 34
ovaries (also see gonadal differentiation), 3, 40, 46
cervix, 26, 35
external genitalia, 28–29, 38
fallopian tubes, 26
uterus, 26, 35
vagina, 26, 28, 38
Differentiation
external genitalia, 22
gonadal, 3, 22–24, 40, 46
Müllerian duct differentiation, 22–26
sexual, 23
DiGeorge syndrome, 158
Disorders of sex development
aetiology, 35
classification, 35
clinical assessment and management of delayed presentations, 37
initial clinical assessment and management, 35
long term clinical management, 48–49
nomenclature, 32
radiological assessment, 35
Dominant (Graafian) follicle, 97, 103, 155
Double wall sign, 52–53, 63
Dual-energy X-ray absorptiometry, 109
Ductal differentiation, 22
Duplication cyst (see Cyst—duplication)
Dysfunctional uterine bleeding, 147
Dysgerminoma, 165, 211, 214
Dysmenorrhoea, 146–147, 176

E

Eating disorders, 148
Ectopic pregnancy (see Pregnancy—ectopic gestation)
Empty sella syndrome, 148, 152
Endocrinology of female reproductive tract
childhood, 83
during puberty, 83
infancy, 82
onset of puberty, 83
Endodermal sinus tumour, 168, 210–211
Endometrial polyp, 147
Endometrioma, 182–184, 187, 196, 202–204
Endometriosis
aetiology, 202
imaging, 202–204
staging, 203
Endometritis, 147, 175, 198
Endometrium (also see menstrual cycle), 3, 13, 86, 97–99, 102, 104
Epitheliod site trophoblastic tumour, 174, 201
Epoophoron, 26, 29–30
External genitalia differentiation, 22

F

Fallopian tubes
anatomy, 92, 96
isolated torsion, 193
imaging, 92
Fibroid uterus (see Uterine—leiomyoma)
Fitzhugh-Curtis syndrome, 198
Follicle stimulating hormone, 82, 117, 123
Follicle stimulating hormone deficiency, 117, 129, 132
Foreign body (see Vaginal—foreign body)
Fragile X Mental Retardation-1 gene, 160
Fragile X permutations, 158
Fundocervical ratio, 6, 97

G

Galactorrhoea, 152, 243
Galactosaemia, 158
Gartner duct (see Cyst—Gartner duct)
Gartner's pseudocyst, 68
Genital outflow tract stenosis, 56
Genital prolapsed, 61
Genital Renal Ear and Skeletal syndrome, 76
Genital ridge
agenesis, 68
hypoplasia, 68
Genital tubercle, 35, 41–42
Genitography
contraindications, 13
indications, 11
technique, 12
Genotype
Germ cell tumour, 54, 152, 210–214
Germinoma, 135–136
Gestational trophoblastic neoplasia, 201
Gonad
bipotential (see also Indifferent gonad), 33
intraabdominal, 45
labial, 37, 63, 164–165
streak, 38, 43, 129–130, 158–160
Gonadal

G (*cont.*)
agenesis, 148
differentiation, 24
dysgenesis, 119, 127, 129–130, 148, 158
complete, 35–36, 46–47
partial, 33, 43
ridge, 22–23
sexual differentiation, 22–24
Gonadoblastoma, 39, 127, 152, 165, 211
Gonadotoxic drugs, 148
Gonadotropin, 82–84, 96
Gonadotropin
receptor gene mutations, 158
releasing hormone, 83, 117
releasing hormone-releasing neurones, 116, 123
Gorlin Syndrome, 218
Granulosa cell, 34
Granulosa-theca cell tumour, 214
Growth hormone
deficiency, 120–121, 125–126
excess, 137
Growth spurt, 117, 125
Gubernaculum, 24
Gynaecological tract obstruction, 51–52, 56–58, 78, 163, 185–186

H
Haemangioma, 169
Haematocolpos, 78, 163, 186
Haematometrocolpos, 163, 186
Haematosalpinx, 184, 194, 196, 201
Haemoperitoneum, 182–184, 195, 201, 206
Haemorrhagic ovarian cyst (see Ovarian cyst—Haemorrhagic)
Haemosiderosis, 148
Height-target, 117, 131
Herlyn–Werner–Wunderlich syndrome, 76, 79
Hermaphrodite (also see ovotesticular disease), 33
Holoprosencephaly, 119–121, 135
Human Papilloma Virus, 221
Hydatid, 26
Hydatid cyst of Morgani, 195
Hydatiform mole, 174, 201
Hydranencephaly facial cleft syndrome, 121
Hydrocolpos, 51–52, 56–58, 60
Hydrometrocolpos, 56, 58
Hydrosalpinx, 195
Hymen
anatomy, 27
atresia, 68
imperforate, 56, 61, 149, 163–164, 185
septate, 68
Hyoscine-N-butylbromide, 9
Hyperandrogenaemia, 156
Hyperandrogenism, 156
Hypercalcaemia, 211
Hypergonadotropic hypogonadism, 119, 127, 149, 157
Hypermenorrhoea, 147
Hyperparathyroidism, 137
Hyperprolactinaemia, 137, 148–149, 155
Hyperthyroidism, 148, 152
Hypogonadotropic hypogonadism, 119, 121, 125, 151
Hypogonadotropic hypogonadism—idiopathic, 151–152
Hypomenorrhoea, 147
Hypooestrogenism, 150
Hypoparathyroidism, 158–159
Hypophosphatemic rickets, 138
Hypopituitarism
congenital, 47
idiopathic, 119
Hyposmia, 125
Hypothalamic
glioma, 119, 135
hamartoma, 116, 133–135, 151
infiltration, 148
irradiation, 148
tumour, 148, 150–151
Hypothalamic-pituitary-gonadal axis, 102, 117, 130, 149
Hypothyroidism, 117–118, 120, 129–130, 139, 147, 152, 155, 159

I
Idiopathic Hypogonadotropic Hypogonadism (see Hypogonadotropic Hypogonadism—Idiopathic)
Imperforate hymen, 16, 56, 61, 149, 162
Implantation, 97
Indifferent gonad, 22–23, 26, 33
Infundibulopelvic ligament, 24–25, 93–94
Inguinal hernia, 45, 51, 53, 61–62, 164
Inhibin, 97, 138
Interlabial mass, 56, 60–61
Intermenstrual bleeding, 147
Intersex (also see Disorders of sex development), 32–37
Isolated premature
adrenarche, 115, 117, 130
menarche, 117, 131
thelarche, 117, 130–131, 231

J
Junctional zone (also see Uterus-junctional zone), 88, 102
Juvenile granulosa cell tumour, 116, 138–139

K
Kallman syndrome, 119, 121–125, 148

L
Labia
majora, 28–29, 35, 40
minor, 28–29, 35
Labial
gonad, 37, 63, 164–165
hypertrophy, 61
Labioscrotal folds, 28, 35
Langerhans cell histiocytosis, 116, 119, 126–127, 148
Leptin, 83
Leucorrhoea, 167
Leydig cell, 33–34, 116, 138
Leydig cell hypoplasia, 36

Li-Fraumeni syndrome, 141, 161, 218
Ligament
broad, 96
cardinal, 87
infundibulopelvic, 93–94
ovarian, 94
round, 94
sacrospinal, 94
uterosacral, 94
Longitudinal septum (see Septum—longitudinal)
Luteinising hormone, 82, 117, 119, 123, 127
deficiency (see also Leydig cell hypoplasia), 36, 82, 119–120
receptor defect, 119, 127
Lymphoma, 210
Lynch familial neoplasia, 161

M
Maffucci's syndrome, 138
Magnetic Resonance Angiography, 11
Magnetic Resonance Imaging
coil selection, 9
contraindications, 8
Diffusion Weighted Imaging, 11
fetal, 18
field strength, 8
indications, 8
parallel imaging, 9
patient preparation, 8
scanning planes, 10
T1-weighted imaging, 11
T2-weighted imaging, 10
Magnetic Resonance Urography, 11
Mammography, 228
Masculinisation—XX female, 33
Massive ovarian oedema, 193, 218
Mature cystic teratoma (also see ovarian teratoma), 179, 188
Mayer-Rokitansky–Küster–Hauser syndrome, 68, 75, 162
McCune-Albright syndrome, 116, 130, 135–137
Meconium calcifications, 16
Menarche, 83–85, 96, 117, 129, 146–148
Menometrorrhagia, 147
Menorrhagia (see Hypermenorrhoea)
Menstrual cycle
endocrinology, 97
follicular phase, 97
luteal phase, 97
MR imaging of endometrium, 101, 104
ovulation, 97
US imaging of endometrium
Menstruation, 97
Proliferative (follicular) phase, 98
Secretory (luteal) phase, 98
Menstrual disorders—classification, 146–147
Mermaid syndrome, 58
Mesonephric
cyst (see Cyst—mesonephric)
duct, 23, 25–26
Mesonephros, 22, 25
Mesosalpinx, 92
Mesothelioma, 205, 210
Mesovarium, 24–25
Metanephros, 25
Metrorrhagia, 147
Midline brain abnormalities, 119
Mittelschmerz, 174–175, 177
Mosaicism, 36–37, 43
Mucocolpos, 163
Mucocutaneous candidiasis, 158–159
Müller's tubercle, 26–27, 35
Mullerian duct (see also Paramesonephric duct), 33–34, 43, 66–67
agenesis, 66–67, 162
disorder of lateral fusion, 73–74, 162
disorder of vertical fusion, 68, 162
hypoplasia, 162
organogenesis, 26
Multicystic dysplastic kidney, 77, 164
Multifollicular morphology, 100, 151
Multiple Endocrine Neoplasia type 1, 137, 141, 161
MURCS association, 75, 162
Mutation
STK11 (Serine/threonine kinase 11) gene, 116, 138
CYP21A2 gene, 160
DAX-1 (dosage-sensitive sex reversal-adrenal hypoplasia, 36
p53 gene, 141
SF1 (Steroidogenic factor 1), 36, 43
SOX-9 (SRY box 9), 34
SRD5A2 gene, 46
SRY (sex-determining region of the Y chromosome), 36, 116, 129
WT-1 (Wilm's Tumour-1), 36, 43
CHD7 (Chromodomain helicase-DNA-binding protein 7 gene), 116, 123
FGF8 (Fibroblast Growth Factor 8) gene, 116, 123
FGFR1 (Basic fibroblast growth factor receptor) gene, 116, 123
HESX1 (HESX homeobox 1) gene, 116, 120–121
KAL1 (Anosmin-1) gene, 116, 123
LHX3 (LIM homeobox 3 LHX3) gene, 116, 120
LHX4 (LIM homeobox 4 LHX4) gene, 16, 120
POU1F1 (POU class 1 homeobox 1) gene, 116, 120
PROK2 (Prokineticin-2) gene, 116, 123
PROKR2 (Prokineticin-2 receptor) gene, 116, 123
PROP1 (PROP paired-like homeobox 1) gene, 116, 120
SOX2 (SRY [sex determining region Y]-box 2) gene, 116, 120
SOX3 (SRY [sex determining region Y]-box 3) gene, 116, 120
TBX19 (T-box 19) gene, 116, 120
Myometrium, 86, 88, 101–102

N
Nabothian cyst, 91
Neonatal ovarian cyst (see Ovarian cyst—neonatal)
Neuroblastoma, 210
Neurofibromatosis type 1, 116, 118, 134–135, 218
Nonclassical congenital adrenal hyperplasia, 148
Noonan syndrome, 118

O

Obstruction of the gynaecological tract, 51–52, 56–58, 78, 163, 185–186
Olfactory
  bulbs, 124–125
  gyri, 124
  placode, 123
  sulci, 124, 125
Oligomenorrhoea, 146–147, 152, 155
Oligoovulation, 147
Ollier's syndrome, 138
Oopherectomy, 119, 148
Optic
  nerve hypoplasia, 121
  pathway glioma, 116, 134, 135
Oral contraceptives, 147
Ovarian
  androgen-secreting tumour, 132, 156
  artery, 88
  autonomous cyst (see Ovarian – functioning cyst)
  carcinoma, 210
  dominant follicle, 97, 103, 155
  dysgenesis, 129
  functional tumours, 138, 140
  germ cell tumour (see Germ cell tumour)
  irradiation, 148, 160
  ligament, 24–25
  premature failure, 129, 147–148
  primary insufficiency, 127, 158–160
  oestrogen-secreting tumour, 130, 139
  secondary tumours, 218
  teratoma
    immature, 210–211
    mature cystic, 6, 217
  thecoma, 215
  torsion, 119, 148, 190
Ovarian cyst
  adolescent, 179
  benign masses, 179
  childhood, 177–178
  complex, 50, 53–55
  definition, 177
  dermoid, 16, 182, 188–189
  fetal, 18
  follicular, 182
  functioning, 116, 130, 133, 136–137, 147
  giant, 54
  haemorrhagic, 180–181, 184
  indications for surgical resection, 182
  luteal, 177
  neonatal, 52, 54
  theca lutein, 179
  epithelial, 210
Ovary
  anatomy, 94
  cortex, 22, 33, 105
  descent, 24, 34
  ectopic, 24, 36
  follicle, 95–96
  inguinal, 24, 33, 164–165
  medulla, 33, 94, 105
  multifollicular, 100
  neonatal, 3–5, 36, 38
  streak, 129, 148
  stroma, 84, 94, 101
  supernumerary, 25
  ultrasound appearances at puberty, 9, 100
  ultrasound appearances in prepubertal child, 94, 98
  ultrasound appearances in the neonate, 94, 98
  volume normative data, 99
  zonal anatomy on MR, 102, 105
Overvirilisation—XX female, 33
Ovotesticular disorder of sexual differentiation, 36, 47–48
Ovotestis, 47–48
Ovulation (see Menstrual cycle—ovulation)

P

Pallister-Hall Syndrome, 135
Paramesonephric
  differentiation, 26
  duct, 23–26
Parametrium, 93
Paraneoplastic syndrome, 211
Paraphooron, 26, 29–30
Paraurethral
  cyst, 61
  glands, 28–29
Partial androgen insensitivity syndrome (see Androgen insensitivity syndrome—partial)
Partial hydatiform mole, 174, 201
Pectus excavatum, 232
Pelvic
  abscess, 16–17
  free fluid, 173, 181, 184, 192, 205–206
  inflammatory disease, 198
  irradiation, 158
  pain
    acute, 174–176
    causes, 174–175
    chronic, 174–176
    cyclical, 176
  radiotherapy, 117, 119
PELVIS syndrome, 169
Perihepatitis, 198
Perimetrium, 86
Periovulation, 91, 103
Peritoneal inclusion cyst, 195
Peutz-Jeghers syndrome, 116, 138
Pituitary
  abscess, 148
  adenoma, 118, 136, 140–141, 148, 151
  agenesis, 119–120
  apoplexy, 153
  ectopic, 47
  hypophysitis, 148
  infiltration, 148
  irradiation, 148
  macroprolactinoma, 148
  normal MR appearances, 103, 107–108
  resection, 148
  stalk interruption syndrome, 119

transcription factor mutations, 120–121
tumours, 151
Placental
aromatase deficiency, 36
site trophoblastic tumour, 174, 201
Poland syndrome, 232
Polycystic ovarian morphology, 155
Polycystic ovarian syndrome, 141, 147–148, 155–157
Polyglandular failure
Type I, 158–159
Type II, 158–159
Polymenorrhoea, 147
Polyostotic fibrous dyplasia, 135, 137–138
Portio supravaginalis cervicalis, 86, 93
Portio vaginalis cervicalis, 86
Postcoital bleeding, 147
Posterior pituitary-ectopic, 47
Post-traumatic hypopituitarism, 126, 153
Pouch of Douglas (see Rectouterine Pouch)
Prader Classification, 41
Precocious puberty (see Puberty—precocious)
Pregnancy
ectopic gestation, 200
intrauterine gestation, 199
molar, 200
Premature
adrenarche, 115, 117, 130
menarche, 117, 131
thelarche, 117, 130–131, 231
ovarian failure (see Ovarian—premature failure)
thelarche, 227, 231
Primary Ovarian Insufficiency, 127, 158, 160
Primary sex cord, 22–23
Primitive germ cell (see Primordial germ cell)
Primordial germ cell, 22–23
Progesterone, 97, 100
Prolactin, 83–84
Prolactin deficiency, 120, 136
Prolactinoma, 147, 149, 152, 156
Prolapsed
ectopic cecouteroecele, 61
ectopic uteroecele, 61
urethra, 61
Pronephros, 25
Pseudohermaphrodite
female, 33
male, 33
Pseudohypoparathyroidism Type Ia, 158
Psychogenic stress, 147
Pubertal development
biochemical evaluation, 118, 129–130
clinical assessment of abnormal puberty, 117
radiological assessment of pubertal stage, 115, 118, 129–131
Puberty
delayed, 83, 103, 108, 119
endocrine changes, 83
gonadotropin dependent precocious (see Puberty—true precocious)
gonadotropin independent precocious (see Puberty—pseudo-precocious)
isosexual, 138
non-isosexual development, 35, 47
normal development, 117
physical changes, 84
precocious, 61, 103, 106, 108, 116–118, 131–134, 138, 215
pseudo-precocious, 117, 131, 133, 138, 215
true precocious, 117, 130, 134
PVE classification, 41

Q
Quantitative
Computed Tomography, 110
Quantitative Ultrasound, 111

R
Radiographs, 15
Rathke's cleft cyst, 153, 155
Rectal duplication, 61
Rectouterine Pouch
anatomy, 91
free fluid, 91, 96
imaging, 88, 91
Renal agenesis, 68, 77, 165
Rete ovarii, 22
Rhabdomyosarcoma
genitourinary, 60, 61, 168, 218, 219, 220, 221
uterus and cervix, 210
vagina, 60, 61, 168, 210
Rotterdam consensus criteria, 156

S
SACRAL syndrome, 169
Sarcoidosis, 148
Sarcoma botryoides, 61
Schizencephaly, 121
Secondary sex cord, 22–23
Sedation, 2–3
Septo-optic dysplasia, 16, 119, 121, 135
Septum
longitudinal, 149
transverse, 56, 149
Sertoli cell, 33, 129
Sertoli–Leydig cell tumour, 116, 138, 212, 214–215
Sex
cord
primary, 22–23
secondary, 22–23
determination, 34
differentiation
female, 33
male, 33
reversal (see also Swyer syndrome), 33, 43
Sexually transmitted diseases, 147
Sheehan's syndrome, 148
Sign
beads-on-a-string, 196
daughter cyst, 52–53
dermoid mesh, 189

S (*cont.*)
dermoid plug, 189
double wall, 52–53, 63
flapping sail, 174, 180, 182, 194–196
shading, 202, 205
split, 196
string of beads, 196
string of pearls, 157
tip of the iceburg, 189
waist, 196
whirlpool, 182, 193
Sinovaginal
bulb, 26
node, 26–27
Sirenomelia, 58
Skeletal maturity score, 105
Skene
duct cyst (see Cyst—Skene duct)
glands, 28–29
Spasmolytic agents, 8
Squamous cell carcinoma, 217, 221
SRY
gene, 33
protein, 22, 26, 35
StAR protein
mutatation, 160
protein deficiency, 36
Stratum
basalis, 99
functionalis, 99
Streak
gonad (see Gonad—streak)
ovary (see Ovary—streak)
Structural anomalies of reproductive system
classification systems, 41, 66–68
MRI protocol, 69
Suspensory ligaments, 93
Swyer syndrome, 129, 158
Symphyseal diastasis, 15

T
Tanner staging—Breast, 227
Teratomas (see Ovarian teratoma)
Thalassaemia, 158
Theca cell, 34
Thecoma, 215
Thelarche (also see Breast—development), 84, 118, 131, 227
Thelarche variant, 115, 117, 131
Thyroid dysfunction, 148, 155
Thyroid stimulating hormone deficiency, 116
Transabdominal ultrasound (see Ultrasound—transabdominal)
Transperineal ultrasound (see Ultrasound—transperineal)
Transrectal ultrasound (see Ultrasound—transrectal)
Transvaginal ultrasound (see Ultrasound—transvaginal)
Transverse septum, 56, 149
Traumatic brain injury, 148
Trisomy X, 158
Trophoblast, 97
True Hermaphrodite (also see ovotesticular disease), 33
Tuberculosis, 148
Tubo-ovarian abscess, 174–175, 180, 182, 190, 193, 196–198
Tumour
adrenal androgen-secreting, 132, 156
adrenal oestrogen-secreting, 132–133
adrenal rest, 42, 160
adrenocortical tumour, 160, 162
germ cell, 54, 152, 210–214
granulosa-theca cell, 214
hypothalamic, 148, 150–151
ovarian functional, 138, 140
ovarian oestrogen-secreting, 130, 139
ovarian secondary, 218
pituitary, 151
placental site trophoblastic, 174, 201
Sertoli-Leydig cell, 116, 138, 212, 214–215
virilising, 160, 162
Turner mosaic
45,XO/46XX, 130
45,XO/46XY, 129
Turner syndrome
45,XO, 119, 127–130
45,X, 158
45,X and 46,XY mosaicism, 158

U
Ultrasound
3D, 67, 69
antenatal, 17
hysterosonography, 69
indications, 3, 8
patient preparation, 4
probe selection, 4
scanning planes, 5, 7
transabdominal, 3
transperineal, 6, 16
transrectal, 8
transvaginal, 7–8, 69
Undermasculinisation—XY male, 33
Undervirilisation—XY male, 33
Undifferentiated gonad (see indifferent gonad)
Urethral
folds, 28, 35
groove, 28, 35, 42
polyp, 61
Urogenital
membrane, 27–28
ridge (see gonadal ridge)
Urogenital sinus, 12, 27–28, 35, 37, 40–41, 56–58, 63
Urogenital sinus anomalies, 68, 71
Urorectal septum, 27–28, 35
Urothelial cyst (see Cyst—urothelial)
Uterine
artery, 88
artery Doppler, 95
dysfunctional bleeding, 147
Uterus
agenesis, 65–66, 148
anatomy, 86
anteflexion, 87
anteversion, 87

arcuate, 73
bicornuate, 72–73
corpus, 86, 88, 97, 100–101
DES-exposed, 66, 74
didelphys, 4, 9, 73–74, 76–77, 163–164, 185, 187, 189
fibroid, 204–205
fundal-cervical ratio, 6
fundus, 88, 90, 95
hypoplastic, 66, 68
hypoplasia, 66, 147
isthmus, 86
junctional zone, 205
leiomyoma, 204–205
length, 94, 97
lipoleiomyoma, 204
neonatal, 3–5, 167
retroversion, 87
septate, 72–73
shape, 97
ultrasound appearances at puberty, 86
ultrasound appearances in infancy, 86, 92
ultrasound appearances in infancy prepubertal child, 86, 93
unicornuate, 68, 74
volume, 6, 11
zonal anatomy on MR (also see Menstrual cycle—MR imaging of endometrium), 104
Utero-ovarian ligament (see ovarian ligament), 34
Uterosacral ligament, 24–25

V

VACTERL association, 58
Vagina
anatomy, 84–85
atresia (agenesis), 56, 68, 149, 185
duplication, 68, 78
hypoplasia, 78, 185
longitudinal septum, 186
MRI appearances, 85–86
septa, 185–186
stenosis, 68, 149, 185
transverse septum, 67, 78, 185
ultrasound appearances, 84–85
Vaginal
bleeding, 166–167
discharge, 61–63, 166
foreign body, 13, 149, 167–168
rhabdomyosarcoma, 7, 60–61, 168, 210, 218, 220–221
Vaginography, 13
Van Wyk-Grumbach syndrome, 116, 139
VCUAM Classification, 67–68
Vestibular glands, 29–30
Vestigial remnants of the genitourinary system, 29–30
Virilisation, 130, 138, 140, 215
Virilising tumour (see also Adrenocortical tumour), 160, 162

W

Wegener's granulomatosis, 148
Weight-loss, 148–149
William's syndrome, 118
Wilm's tumour screening, 39
WNT4 deficiency, 75
Wolffian duct (see also Mesonephric duct), 33–34, 40
Wolffian vestiges, 30

X

X-chromosome, 22, 33
XX gonadal dysgenesis, 119, 127, 129

Y

Y-chromosome, 22, 33

MIX
Papier aus verantwortungsvollen Quellen
Paper from responsible sources
FSC® C105338

If you have any concerns about our products,
you can contact us on
ProductSafety@springernature.com

In case Publisher is established outside the EU,
the EU authorized representative is:
Springer Nature Customer Service Center GmbH
Europaplatz 3, 69115 Heidelberg, Germany

Printed by Libri Plureos GmbH
in Hamburg, Germany